NEW DEVELOPMENTS IN MEDICAL RESEARCH

ADVANCES IN HYPERTENSION RESEARCH

NEW DEVELOPMENTS IN MEDICAL RESEARCH

Additional books in this series can be found on Nova's website under the Series tab.

Additional e-books in this series can be found on Nova's website under the e-book tab.

NEW DEVELOPMENTS IN MEDICAL RESEARCH

ADVANCES IN HYPERTENSION RESEARCH

RAMÓN RODRIGO
EDITOR

New York

For permission to use material from this book please contact us:
Telephone 631-231-7269; Fax 631-231-8175
Web Site: http://www.novapublishers.com

Library of Congress Cataloging-in-Publication Data

ISBN: 978-1-62948-857-8

Library of Congress Control Number: 2013956178

Published by Nova Science Publishers, Inc. † New York

Contents

Preface

High blood pressure, termed hypertension, is a disease afflicting almost 1 billion people worldwide and given the current epidemiological trends, it is expected to keep increasing. It is a leading cause of morbidity and mortality. It is noteworthy that one-third of patients in this condition are not aware they have the condition, as this disease is usually asymptomatic for many years, even decades, until it finally damages certain critical organs and the only reliable way to detect its occurrence is to regularly check blood pressure. Therefore, this disease is sometimes called the "silent killer" due to the deleterious damaging effects derived from hypertension, such as stroke, myocardial infarction, renal dysfunction, visual problems, among others. The complications of hypertension are often referred to as end-organ damage because damage to these organs is the end result of chronic (long duration) high blood pressure. If hypertension is not treated, there will be organ damage to kidneys, heart, and brain which is generally not reversible. Death in hypertensive patients most often occurs from heart failure, chronic renal failure, and stroke.

It is of interest to mention that about 95% of cases do not have an identifiable cause for hypertension, thus giving rise to the condition known as "primary" or "essential" hypertension, while those cases with a known direct cause, such as kidney disease, endocrine causes, among others, are termed "secondary hypertension. Although is it known that in primary hypertension the process of sodium excretion is impaired, probably due to multigenic and environmental factors, its cause is unknown and its pathophysiology is yet to be completely elucidated. On the other hand, while the causes of secondary hypertension are known, the molecular mechanisms leading to hypertension in these conditions are incomplete or have yet to reach consensus in the scientific community.

The present book is intended for health science researchers and professors, as well as those in the biomedical areas. It is also intended for physicians, especially those in disciplines such as cardiology, nephrology and gynecology. Graduate and undergraduate students of biomedical and health science professions with an interest in hypertension will also be provided with a valuable resource to keep up with the latest trends in hypertension research. Readers will find in this book an organized approach to hypertension research with an emphasis in providing a mechanistic and molecular rationale to its diagnosis and treatment.

Prevention of hypertension can be best achieved though lifestyle adjustment, in which proper diet and exercise are key components. In brief, it is important to maintain a healthy weight, reduce salt intake, reduce alcohol intake and reduce stress. It is important to screen, diagnose, treat and control hypertension in its earliest stages. This aim can be accomplished by increasing public awareness and increasing the frequency of screenings for the condition.

Multiple guidelines for an effective management of hypertension have been published. These guidelines need to be updated both to respond to some specific concerns and to address a number of issues for which considerable new evidence has been obtained from epidemiological surveys and therapeutic trials. Considerable effort is being devoted to the improvement of our knowledge on hypertension. In order to contribute to the updated relevant mechanisms accounting for hypertension, as well as to give some clues for new therapeutic strategies, this book is structured around six chapters, following a brief preface

Chapter 1. Oxidative Stress and Hypertension

It is well known that reactive oxygen and reactive nitrogen species play a key role in the modulation of vasomotor system. Moreover, these species are mediators of vasoconstriction (superoxide anion) and vasodilation (nitric oxide) effects. The occurrence of oxidative stress leads to decreased bioavailability of nitric oxide, decreased synthesis of prostacyclin and directly increased vasoconstriction.

One of the major contributors to endothelial dysfunction is a decrease in nitric oxide (NO) bioavailability, impaired NO signaling, and an increase in the amount of reactive oxygen species (ROS). In the endothelium NO is produced by endothelial nitric oxide synthase (eNOS), for which l-arginine is a substrate. Arginase, an enzyme critical in the urea cycle also metabolizes l-arginine, thereby directly competing with eNOS for their common substrate and constraining its bioavailability for eNOS, thereby compromising NO production. Arginase expression and activity is upregulated in many cardiovascular diseases including ischemia reperfusion injury, hypertension, atherosclerosis, and diabetes mellitus.

Chapter 2. Endothelial Dysfunction and Hypertension

Endothelial dysfunction and resulting vascular pathology have been identified as an early hallmark of multiple diseases, including hypertension. Oxidative stress is believed to be a central mechanism in its generation. There are several methods for the assessment of endothelial dysfunction, with advantages and disadvantages specific of each method. Early diagnosis and treatment of endothelial dysfunction would be especially beneficial because it may precede the development of hypertension and atherosclerosis, and through a timely treatment prevent their development. The nature of these therapies is diverse and goes from lifestyle changes to molecules acting as transcription enhancers.

Chapter 3. Hypertension in Preeclampsia

Preeclampsia (PE) is a multisystem syndrome of pregnancy characterized by hypertension and proteinuria. Its origin is widely accepted to be the placenta. Placental hemodynamics are believed to be crucial to the development of this pathology and, interestingly, depend mainly on local factors, because of their lack of autonomic innervation. In this chapter PE is considered to be a condition determined by an exacerbated systemic inflammatory response that is associated with endothelial dysfunction.

This chapter takes into consideration the role of endothelin, thromboxane, superoxide, angiogenic imbalance and decreased formation of vasodilators such as nitric oxide, prostacyclin and endothelial derived hyperpolarizing factor as mediators involved in the pathogenesis of preeclampsia for an updated mechanistic approach centered around oxidative stress, while proposing potential therapies for PE.

Chapter 4. Hypertension in Renovascular Disease

Renovascular hypertension is among the most common causes of secondary hypertension worldwide. It is characterized by a stenosis of the renal arteries, generally secondary to a atherosclerotic peripheral vascular disease. The renal artery stenosis determines a complex series of pathophysiological responses that determine hypertension and progressive kidney damage. This chapter deals with several pathophysiological mechanisms in this disease, including the Renin-Angiotensin-Aldosterone System, stimulation of the sympathetic nervous system, endothelial dysfunction, oxidative stress and increased proinflammatory cytokine release. Current consensus on treating renovascular disease is analyzed under a critical lense while providing perspectives for the advancement of new therapies with basis on the pathophysiological mechanisms explained in this chapter.

Chapter 5. Hypertension in Metabolic Syndrome

Metabolic syndrome (MS) is a highly prevalent pathological condition which can be defined as a cluster of metabolic disorders that are associated with an increased risk of type 2 diabetes (T2D) and cardiovascular disease (CVD). Among the disorders present in the metabolic syndrome is hypertension, which is by itself an important cardiovascular risk factor. In the pathophysiology of hypertension in metabolic syndrome, which is a proinflammatory state and a systemic oxidative stress condition, there are three mainly mechanisms involved: sympathetic hyperactivation, increased renin-angiotensin-aldosterone activity and endothelial dysfunction. Recent developments show a new cellular type involved in the pathogenesis of this disease, the perivascular adipose tissue. The adipose tissue releases a large amount of mediators that contributes to hypertension in metabolic syndrome. This chapter analyses the current patophysiological consensus on hypertension in metabolic syndrome, based on clinical and animal models. Although the most accepted therapy of hypertension in metabolic syndrome is the same used in essential hypertension, this chapter also analyses new studies reviewing the beneficial effects of antioxidant therapy in metabolic syndrome.

Chapter 6. Hypertension in Chronic Kidney Disease

Chronic kidney disease is an increasingly important public health issue owing to its high morbi-mortality and steadily increasing prevalence. The treatment of hypertension in the context of CKD is being considered a fundamental therapeutic target to researchers around the world, because the cause-effect relationship of CKD and hypertension is cyclic. For this reasons many clinical guidelines emphasize the importance of decreasing blood pressure to slow progression of renal disease and reduce cardiovascular morbidity and mortality In order to accomplish such an objective, however, a better understanding of the pathophysiology and the mechanisms of hypertension in context of CKD is needed. To this end, this chapter analyses the role of sodium homeostasis, the symphathetic nervous system, the Renin-Angiotensin-Aldosterone System, Oxidative stress, Urotensin II and Uric acid, then evaluates therapies oriented to neutralizing the aforementioned factors.

In: Advances in Hypertension Research
Editor: Ramón Rodrigo

ISBN: 978-1-62948-857-8

Chapter 1

Oxidative Stress and Hypertension*

Ramón Rodrigo† and Matías Libuy
[1]Molecular and Clinical Pharmacology Program, Institute of Biomedical Sciences, Faculty of Medicine, University of Chile, Chile

Abstract

Hypertension is considered to be the most important risk factor in the development of cardiovascular disease. It occurs as an imbalance of vasodilating forces over vasoconstricting ones with predominance of the latter. Although low levels of reactive oxygen species could exert an important role in the homeostasis of the vascular wall, their excess may be harmful. Thus, ROS may act not solely as mediators of vasoconstriction, but also contributing to impair endothelium-dependent vasodilation in part by decreasing nitric oxide bioavailability, a pathophysiological condition leading to hypertension. The development of oxidative stress in the vascular wall is found in clinical settings such as essential hypertension or preeclampsia, among others. These data strongly suggest the involvement of oxidative stress as one of the factors able to modulate blood pressure. On the other hand, antioxidant vitamins are able to reduce BP in hypertensives without an established damage of the vascular wall, pointing to a potential therapeutic role of antioxidants in these patients. The aim of this chapter was to present an update of the studies related to the novel contribution of oxidative stress in the pathophysiology of hypertension and the suitability of antioxidants as antihypertensive agents.

Keywords: Oxidative stress; essential hypertension, antioxidants

* Supported by FONDECYT, grant 1120594.
† Corresponding author: Dr. Ramón Rodrigo. Molecular and Clinical Pharmacology Program; Institute of Biomedical Sciences; Faculty of Medicine, University of Chile; Independencia 1027, C.P 8380453, Santiago 7, Chile. Telephone: 56-2-29786126 Fax: 56-2-29786126; 2E-mail: rrodrigo@med.uchile.cl.

Abbreviations

ACE	angiotensin I-converting-enzyme
ACEI	angiotensin I-converting-enzyme inhibitors
ADMA	asymmetric dimethyl arginine
Ang-II	angiotensin II
AT_1	angiotensin II type 1 receptor
AT1-AA	autoantibodies to angiotensin II type 1 receptor
BP	blood pressure
CAT	catalase
DASH	dietary approaches to stop hypertension
EDHF	endothelium-derived hyperpolarizing factor
eNOS	endothelial nitric oxide synthase
ERα	estrogen receptor α
ET-1	endothelin-1
hsCRP	high sensitivity C-reactive protein
HSP60	heat shock protein 60
IL-6	interleukin-6
MCSF	macrophage colony stimulating factor
MCP-1	monocyte chemoattractant protein-1
MDA	malondialdehyde
MEGJs	myoendothelial gap junctions
MHC	major histocompatibility complex
NAC	N-acetyl-L-cysteine
NADPH oxidase	reduced nicotinamide adenine dinucleotide phosphate- oxidase
NO	nitric oxide
NPG	normal pregnancy
PAI-1	plasminogen activator inhibitor-1
PE	preeclampsia
PPP	primary prevention project
p38 MAPK	p38 mitogen-activated protein kinase
p67	phox-67 NADPH oxidase subunit
ROS	reactive oxygen species
sFlt1	soluble fms-like tyrosine kinase 1 factor
SIRT-1	sirtuin-1
SOD	superoxide dismutase
TLRs	toll-like receptors
U-II	urotensin II
VSMC	vascular smooth muscle cells

1. Introduction

Accumulating evidence indicates that oxidative stress is one of the fundamental mechanisms responsible for the development of hypertension [1]. Indeed, reactive oxygen species (ROS) could play an important role in the homeostasis of the vascular wall, thereby leading to the development of elevation of BP [2-4]. ROS are important molecules regulating numerous physiological processes. However, their excessive production is harmful as these species also participate in pathological processes occurring in the vascular wall, such as atherosclerosis, vascular inflammation and endothelial dysfunction. The vasculature is a rich source of ROS, which under pathological conditions play an important role in vascular injury, as well as in hypertensive end-organ damage. Vascular ROS are produced in endothelial, adventitial, and vascular smooth muscular cells (VSMC) when stimulated by hormones such as angiotensin II (Ang-II) [5], endothelin-1 (ET-1) [6] and urotensin II (U-II) [7], among others. In addition, increased ROS production may be generated by mechanical forces, such as both unidirectional laminar and oscillatory shear stress occurring during elevation of BP [8]. The overproduction of ROS enough to overwhelm the antioxidant defense system, i.e., oxidative stress, results in an imbalance between vasoconstriction and vasodilatation forces, in favor of the first [9]. The pathological effects of ROS in the vascular wall result simultaneously from their direct actions modifying vascular cell functions and from their ability to scavenge and remove several beneficial vasoprotective compounds such as nitric oxide (NO) [10]. The mechanisms whereby oxidative stress mediates hypertension and cardiovascular disease are not clear. Cumulated data from animal studies point to a causative role for oxidative stress in the pathogenesis of hypertension [11]. However there is still no solid evidence that oxidative stress causes hypertension in humans, although reduced nicotinamide adenine dinucleotide phosphate-oxidase (NADPH oxidase) has been identified as one of the main ROS sources [12]. Recent studies about oxidative stress related to biomarkers are just emerging and could warrant the development of new mechanistic and therapeutic approaches in some human models. The aim of this chapter was to present an update of experimental and clinical studies related with the role of oxidative stress in the mechanism of hypertension, as well as the therapeutic opportunities based on the antioxidant system reinforcement.

2. Pathophysiology

The contribution of oxidative stress to the pathogenesis of hypertension is supported by a great body of evidences. There are a number of sources of ROS, including neutrophil-like membrane-associated NADPH oxidase, xanthine oxidase, myeloperoxidase, uncoupled endothelial nitric oxide synthase (eNOS) and spillover from mitochondrial respiratory chain [13], as it is shown in Figure 1.1. In addition, the occurrence of this disturbance may be caused by decreased antioxidant enzyme activity (superoxide dismutase [SOD], catalase [CAT]) and reduced levels of ROS scavengers (e.g., vitamin E, glutathione), all acting as contributing factors to the development of oxidative stress. These findings are based, in general, on increased levels of plasma thiobarbituric acid-reactive substances and 8-isoprostanes, biomarkers of lipid peroxidation and oxidative stress [14, 15]. Indeed, ROS of vascular origin contribute importantly to peripheral vascular resistance and arterial pressure under pathophysiological conditions such as hypertension [11]. In addition, polymorphonuclear leukocytes and platelets, rich superoxide sources, also participate in vascular oxidative stress and inflammation in hypertensive patients [16, 17]. In this setting, the elevation of BP has been associated with ROS abundance and frequently also with an impairment of endogenous antioxidant mechanisms. Uric acid, synthesized together with superoxide, stimulates proliferation, Ang II production, and oxidative stress in VSMC [18]. Accordingly, increased biomarkers of oxidative stress are found in human hypertensive subjects, as well as in various animal models of hypertension [14, 19-21], but further studies are still lacking.

2.1. Vascular Oxidative Stress

Oxidative stress constitutes a unifying mechanism of injury of many types of disease processes. The ROS family comprises many molecules that have divergent effects on cellular function, such as regulation of cell growth and differentiation, modulation of extracellular matrix production and breakdown, inactivation of NO, and stimulation of many kinases and proinflammatory genes [22-24]. Importantly, many of these actions are associated with pathological changes observed in cardiovascular disease. ROS are produced by all vascular cell types, including endothelial, smooth muscle, and adventitial cells, and can be formed by numerous enzymes. Enzymatic sources of ROS that are important in vascular disease and hypertension are xanthine oxidase, uncoupled NOS, and NADPH oxidase. In pathological conditions, ROS production in vascular tissues, particularly superoxide anions, has been implicated as playing an important role in vascular events such as inflammation, endothelial dysfunction, cell proliferation, migration and activation, extracellular matrix deposition, fibrosis, angiogenesis, all important processes contributing to cardiovascular remodeling in hypertension, atherosclerosis, diabetes, cardiac failure, myocardial ischemia-reperfusion injury, vascular remodeling after angioplasty and ischemic stroke [25-27]. These effects are mediated through redox-sensitive regulation of multiple signaling molecules and second messengers [28-30]. The elevation of BP has been associated with ROS abundance and frequently also with an impairment of endogenous antioxidant mechanisms [11]. Superoxide, the first ROS formed by one electron reduction of molecular oxygen, and superoxide-derived ROS have multiple pathophysiological actions in the artery wall, including an impairment of endothelium-dependent vasodilation. In agreement with this view, in human hypertension, biomarkers of systemic oxidative stress are elevated [14].

Mouse models with genetic deficiency in ROS-generating enzymes have lower BP compared with wild-type counterparts, and Ang-II infusion fails to induce hypertension in these mice [31, 32]. In addition, in cultured VSMC and isolated arteries from hypertensive rats and humans, ROS production is enhanced, redox-dependent signaling is amplified, and antioxidant bioactivity is reduced [5]. It should be mentioned that in patients with never-treated mild-to-moderate hypertension, lipid peroxidation and oxidative stress were not found increased [33], suggesting that ROS may not be critical in the early stages of human hypertension, but could be more important in severe hypertension. In addition, classical antihypertensive agents such as β-adrenergic blockers, angiotensin I converting enzyme inhibitors (ACEI), angiotensin II type 1 receptor (AT_1) antagonists, and Ca^{2+} channel blockers may be mediated, in part, by decreasing vascular oxidative stress [6]. It is of interest to note that increased ROS production in vascular tissues has also effects other than elevation of BP. Particularly superoxide anions, has been implicated as playing an important role in vascular events such as vascular remodeling after angioplasty, atherosclerosis, myocardial infarction, and ischemic stroke [27]. Thus, therapeutic strategies should aim to restore the bioavailability of NO, either scavenging ROS or through down-regulation of their generation and/or up-regulation of eNOS activity and antioxidant enzymes.

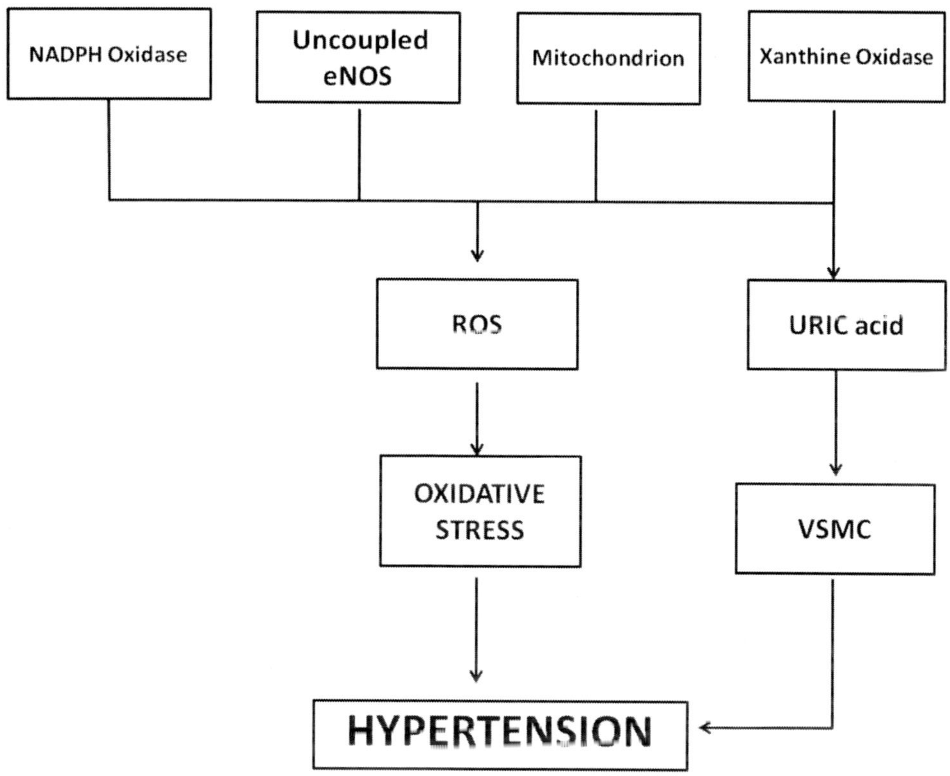

Figure 1.1. Pathophysiological pathways of oxidative stress in hypertension.
NO, nitric oxide; eNOS, endothelial nitric oxide synthase; ROS, reactive oxygen species; VSMC, vascular smooth muscle cells.

2.2. Inflammation

Inflammatory mechanisms are important participants in the pathophysiology of hypertension and cardiovascular disease. Markers of inflammation have been shown to be up-regulated in different forms of cardiovascular disease, and to correlate with vascular risk. Atherosclerosis is characterized by chronic inflammation of the vascular wall. The I-kappaB (I-NF-kappaB)/nuclear factor-kappaB (NF-kappaB) system is considered a major intracellular inflammatory pathway, mediating most of the vascular inflammatory responses [34]. The role of inflammation in atherosclerosis has been well established, leading to the concept that atherosclerosis in an inflammatory disease [35, 36]. Endothelial dysfunction leads to an increase of the expression of adhesion molecules in endothelial cells, such as VCAM-1, especially in regions with unusual shear stress (low average shear stress but high oscillatory shear stress). This leads to adherence of monocytes and T-lymphocytes. After adhesion, leukocytes migrate into the underlying intima in response to chemoattractant stimuli, including chemokines such as monocyte chemoattractant protein-1 (MCP-1). This inflammatory process stimulates migration and proliferation of VSMC that become intermixed with the area of inflammation to form an intermediate lesion. If inflammation continues, an increased number of monocytes and lymphocytes accumulate in the arterial wall, due to emigration from the blood and multiplication in the lesion, perpetuating the inflammation process [35]. Recent evidence suggests a potential link between vascular inflammation and hypertension. Cross sectional studies in hypertensive individuals have shown increased plasma and vascular tissue levels of CRP, cytokines such as TNF-α and interleukin-6 (IL-6), such as MCP-1 and plasminogen activator inhibitor-1 (PAI-1), and adhesion molecules such as P-selectin and sICAM-1 [37].

2.2.1. Monocytes – Macrophages – Foam Cells

After adhesion to the endothelium and migration to the subendothelial space, monocytes mature into macrophages under the influence of macrophage colony stimulating factor (MCSF), which is over-expressed in the inflamed intima [38]. Macrophage differentiation is a necessary step for atherosclerosis and is associated with up-regulation of pattern recognition receptors for innate immunity, including scavenger receptors and toll-like receptors (TLRs) [38]. Macrophages internalize oxLDL via scavenger receptors. The accumulation of cholesteryl esters in the cytoplasm leads to the formation of foam cells. Toll-like receptors bind certain ligands and initiate a signal cascade leading to macrophage activation [36]. Besides ligands such as bacterial toxins, TLRs can be activated by oxLDL and heat shock protein 60 (HSP60), which is highly expressed in atherosclerotic lesions of increasing severity [39]. Macrophage activation in atheroma leads to release of vasoactive molecules, ROS and metalloproteinases that may degrade matrix components. The loss of matrix components may subsequently lead to destabilization of plaques involving increased risk for plaque rupture and thrombosis.

2.2.2. T-Cells

T-cells are present in atherosclerotic lesions, with a majority of CD4+ T-cells over CD8+ T-cells. Major histocompatibility complex (MHC) class II–expressing macrophages and dendritic cells can be detected close to these T cells. This implies a possible immune activation of T-cells in atherosclerotic lesions through processing and presentation of antigens by macrophages. Also, the atherosclerotic lesion contains cytokines that promote a T-helper 1 response, inducing activated T cells to differentiate into T-helper 1 effector cells. T-cell activation results in the secretion of cytokines, including interferon-γ and TNF-α and β that amplify the inflammatory response [35].

2.3. Endothelial Dysfunction

Dysfunction of the endothelium has been implicated in the pathophysiology of different forms of cardiovascular disease, including hypertension, coronary artery disease, chronic heart failure, peripheral artery disease, diabetes, and chronic renal failure [40]. Endothelial dysfunction may be defined as impairment characterized by a shift of the actions of the endothelium toward reduced vasodilation, a proinflammatory state, and prothrombotic setting. The pathophysiology of endothelial dysfunction is complex and involves multiple mechanisms. It is characterized by unbalanced concentrations of vasodilating and vasoconstricting factors, the most important being represented by NO and Ang-II, respectively [41]. Nitric oxide is recognized as one of the major mediators of the maintenance of vascular homeostasis, and a decrease in NO bioavailability is associated with endothelial dysfunction [42]. In this context, the causes of reduced vasodilatory responses in endothelial dysfunction include reduced NO generation, oxidative excess and reduced production of endothelium-derived hyperpolarizing factor (EDHF). Reduced NO bioavailability could be due to either reduced formation or accelerated degradation of this vasodilator. The mechanism, by which oxidative stress mediates endothelial cell function, and ultimately vascular reactivity, is not fully understood. Although these mechanisms may be multifactorial, there is a growing body of evidence that increased production of ROS may contribute considerably as a causative factor in endothelial dysfunction by reducing NO bioavailability and uncoupling eNOS [43]. The endothelium, the media and also the adventitia produce large amounts of ROS, which will attenuate endothelial mediated dilation, although the mechanisms underlying endothelial dysfunction are located in addition to the endothelium in the smooth muscle cell layer [44]. Superoxide combines with NO, which is synthesized by eNOS, to form peroxynitrite. The consequence is an overall increase in ROS and reduced ability of endothelium-dependent vasodilation. Under settings associated with oxidative stress the vasculature per se produces large amounts of superoxide via elevated expression of NADPH oxidase [41].

3. Clinical Settings

3.1. Essential Hypertension

Essential hypertension is characterized by increased peripheral vascular resistance to blood flow, due in large part to vascular remodeling. Clinical studies have demonstrated that essential hypertensive patients produce excessive amount of ROS [45, 46], and have abnormal levels of antioxidant status [47], thereby contributing to the accumulating evidence that increased vascular oxidative stress could be involved in the pathogenesis of essential hypertension [3, 48]. Also vascular changes in hypertension are associated with mechanical and humoral factors that modulate signaling events, resulting in abnormal function, media growth, extracellular matrix deposition and inflammation. Inflammatory processes are important participants in the pathophysiology of hypertension and cardiovascular disease [49]. Recent evidence suggests that inflammation is present in the vasculature in animal models of hypertension. Inflammatory markers, such as C-reactive protein, are associated with vascular lesions in humans, and are predictive of cardiovascular outcome. In a recent study, chronic low grade low-grade inflammation has been identified as an integral part in the pathogenesis of vascular disease. Indeed, several clinical studies have demonstrated increased numbers of well recognized pro-inflammatory markers, such as high sensitivity C-reactive protein (hsCRP), in patients with hypertension, even after adjustment for potential confounding factors. Furthermore, elevated hsCRP levels have also been shown to be predictive for the development of hypertension in prehypertensive and normotensive patients. Oxidative stress also appears to be a key feature in the reduced availability of NO and is aggravated by increased circulating Ang II. Importantly, there is some evidence that drugs commonly used in the management of hypertension, such as statins, angiotensin converting enzyme inhibitors and Ang II receptor blockers have anti-inflammatory properties that can positively influence outcomes in patients with hypertension. The inflammatory state in hypertension may pose a new therapeutic target for future drug design [50].

3.2. Preeclampsia

Preeclampsia (PE) is a multisystem disorder that remains a major cause of maternal and foetal morbidity and death. To date, no treatment has been found that prevents the development of the disease. Endothelial dysfunction is considered to underlie its clinical manifestations, such as maternal hypertension, proteinuria, and edema; however, the precise biochemical pathways involved remain unclear. A current hypothesis invokes the occurrence of oxidative stress as pathogenically important, as suggested by the fact that in PE, the placental and circulating levels of lipid peroxidation products [F2-isoprostanes and malondialdehyde (MDA) are increased] and endothelial cells are activated. A potential mechanism for endothelial dysfunction may occur via NF-kappaB activation by oxidative stress. Alternatively, the idea that the antiangiogenic placental soluble fms-like tyrosine kinase 1 factor (sFlt1) is involved in the pathogenesis of this disease is just emerging; however, other pathophysiological events seem to precede its increased production [51].

3.2.1. Endothelium-Derived Hyperpolarizing Factor

Hypothetically, endothelial dysfunction in small arteries might be the most severe, and because uterine circulation is of unique importance during pregnancy, the abnormalities in the myometrial arteries might further aggravate the disease process. The results of *ex vivo* studies are controversial; however, with reported findings ranging from almost total abolishment [52, 53] to reduction [54, 55] to preservation [54, 56] of endothelium-dependent responses. Several endothelium-derived vasodilator substances—nitric oxide (NO), prostacyclin (PGI2), and EDHF—are involved in endothelium dependent relaxation at the level of resistance vasculature. Considering the many ways by which availability and/or synthesis of NO could be reduced in PE, the hypothesis regarding up-regulation of ''backup'' endothelial pathways like EDHF seems to be reasonable. However, data about the compromised pathways in endothelium-dependent dilation at the level of small arteries in PE are also rather conflicting, indicating the possible involvement of NO [57-59], PGI2 [60, 61], and particularly, EDHF [56, 62], the contribution of which is increasingly appreciated for small artery maintenance [63, 64].

In this line, EDHF-type responses may be mediated simultaneously by several factors or pathways, depending on the type of vasculature, the species, and the physiological environment [65]. Recent evidence suggests that myoendothelial gap junctions (MEGJs), either alone or in combination with H_2O_2 and/or cytochrome P450 2C9 (CYP2C9) products of arachidonic acid, are involved with EDHF-mediated responses in small subcutaneous arteries in PE [62], whereas MEGJs alone conferred the EDHF pathway in women with a normal pregnancy (NPG) [65]. According to this, Luksha et al., demonstrated that in PE, myometrial arteries have a significantly reduced response to the endothelium-dependent agonist BK and that EDHF-type, rather than NO-mediated, responses are impaired in myometrial and subcutaneous [62] arteries isolated from women with PE. The contribution of MEGJs as a common pathway of EDHF-type responses in arteries from women with NPG became reduced in subcutaneous arteries [62] and even more severely impaired in myometrial arteries from women with PE. However, the attenuated role of MEGJs in PE is partly compensated through contribution of H_2O_2.

3.2.2. Response to Agonistic Autoantibodies to the Angiotensin II Type I Receptor

Recent studies have suggested that the production of agonistic autoantibodies to the angiotensin II type I receptor (AT1-AA) may be an important link between placental ischemia and the development of hypertension in preeclamptic women [66-72]. Several studies have demonstrated that chronic infusion of purified rat AT1-AA, at rates to mimic the increase observed in placental ischemic pregnant rats, significantly increased BP [73, 74]. These increases in arterial pressure were associated with significant increases in local ET-1, circulating sFlt-1 and soluble endoglin, and placental secretion of sFlt-1. These factors were normalized by administration of AT1 receptor antagonist, illustrating the importance of AT1-AA activation of the AT1 receptor in stimulating the BP increase and soluble factors in response to placental ischemia in pregnant rats. In this line, Recently, Irani et al., [75] demonstrated that injection of human AT1-AA stimulated PE features including elevated tumor necrosis factor-α in pregnant but not virgin mice. Furthermore, coinjection of AT1-AA with a TNF-α neutralizing antibody decreased the bioavailability of the circulating cytokine and attenuated much of the PE like features associated with AT1-AA induced hypertension in pregnant mice. The authors concluded that AT1-AA is a novel stimulus for the elevation in circulating TNF-α during PE. TNF-α activation could lend to the excess ROS, sFlt-1, or interleukin-6 in this rat model of AT1-AA induced hypertension as well, however, these factors were not examined in this investigation, but could be the subject of future studies. Parrish et al., [74] demonstrated that AT1-AA's contribute to placental oxidative stress; one mechanism whereby the AT1-AA mediates hypertension during pregnancy. However, it is unclear how early in gestation the onset of AT1-AA production occurs. A better understanding of the pathophysiology of AT1-AA production in PE may lead to novel therapeutic targets for the treatment of the disease and /or a marker for predicting patient risk of developing PE.

3.2.3. Asymmetric Dimethyl Arginine

The generation of NO by eNOS could be down-regulated in PE by hypoxia and by increased levels of asymmetric dimethyl arginine (ADMA), as well as by a diminished enzyme expression. An elevated ADMA concentration has been attributed to hypertension [76], hyperlipidemia [77], and hyperhomocysteinemia [78, 79], all alterations likely to be found in PE. Accordingly, ADMA has been reported to be elevated in the plasma of women with PE [80], which could directly interfere with NO and induce endothelial dysfunction, due to its ability to behave as an endogenous competitive inhibitor of eNOS. Elevated circulating ADMA concentrations, in combination with low plasma arginine levels, have been suggested to be of pathophysiological importance in pregnancies complicated with PE [81]. In addition, ADMA causes an uncoupling, where the activity of the enzyme for NO production is decreased in association with an increase in eNOS-dependent superoxide anions formation [82]. Women at risk of PE, having a high resistance in the placental circulation, a foetus with a low weight for gestational age, or both, show elevated concentrations of ADMA, which is a potential contributory factor for the development of PE and is associated with endothelial dysfunction [83]. ACEI and AT_1 blockers can diminish ADMA generation, otherwise stimulated by angiotensin II [84], but the latter mechanism is not well understood. Recently, the association of increased plasma levels of ADMA and PE has been called into question by a study reporting no significant differences between preeclamptic and normal pregnant women [85]. The authors also showed lack of ethnicity-related differences in ADMA concentration in White, African, indigenous, and multiethnic pregnant women, thus suggesting that PE in low- and high-risk populations may have distinct underlying causes.

4. Experimental Models

Reactive oxygen species have an important pathogenic role in organ damage as shown in Table 1.1. NADPH oxidase has been shown to be important in the development of salt-sensitive hypertension [86, 87]. A recent study suggests that the expression of p67 (phox), a subunit of NADPH oxidase, was increased in response to a high-salt diet in the outer renal medulla of the Dahl salt-sensitive rat, an animal model for human salt-sensitive hypertension. The higher expression of p67, but not the other subunits, was associated with higher NADPH oxidase activity and salt sensitivity in SS rats compared with a salt-resistant strain. Genetic mutations of the SS allele of p67 were found in the promoter region and contributed to higher promoter activity than that of the salt-resistant strain [86]. Inhibition of AT_1 receptors may elicit beneficial effects on HF-induced hypertension and vascular injury in subjects that have genetically enhanced sodium-sensitive BP [88]. Recently, it was demonstrated a strong association between BP and some oxidative stress–related parameters [89]; thus, systolic and diastolic BPs of hypertensives were negatively correlated with plasma antioxidant capacity and positively correlated with both plasma and urine 8-isoprostane, a recognized biomarker of oxidative stress in vivo. In the context of oxidative stress in the vasculature it is particularly important to note that increased superoxide reacts extremely rapidly with NO to form peroxynitrite, thereby elevating vascular resistance and promoting vasoconstriction [90]. Formation of peroxynitrite is a pathophysiological process, because NO is an essential endogenous vasodilator. Thus, therapeutic strategies should aim to restore bioavailability of NO, scavenging ROS by antioxidant agents.

4.1. Role of Oxidative Stress in the Kidney

Evidence suggests a key role for ROS in the pathophysiological processes of several renal diseases; these diseases are considered causes and consequences of hypertension. One of the underlying mechanisms of ROS-mediated tubulointerstitial injury is the exposure of tubular cells to LDL, which may result in tubulointerstitial damage due to NADPH oxidase-mediated ROS production [91]. Ang-II has a pivotal role not only in the progression of tubulointerstitial injury but also in obstructive nephropathy [92, 93]. It activates NADPH oxidase and, subsequently, generates superoxide that leads to hypertrophy of the renal tubular cells [94]. There is evidence suggesting that a high-fat diet induces renal inflammation and elevation of BP via ROS in spontaneously hypertensive rats [95]. Additionally, metabolic syndrome is a risk factor for chronic kidney disease that is at least in part independent of diabetes and hypertension and probably mediated by ROS. Moreover, the onset and maintenance of renal damage may worsen metabolic syndrome features, such as hypertension, leading to potential vicious cycles [28].

4.2. Role of Oxidative Stress in the Central Nervous System

In addition to the kidney and the vasculature itself, the sympathetic nervous system, which is regulated in the central nervous system, is involved in the pathogenesis of hypertension [96]. Recent studies strongly suggest that central sympathetic outflow is increased in hypertension [97].There is also evidence that increased ROS generation in the brainstem contributes to the neural mechanisms of hypertension in hypertensive rats [98]. The rostral ventrolateral medulla is the major vasomotor center and is essential for the maintenance of basal vasomotor tone [99, 100]. Some findings strongly indicate that ROS in the rostral ventrolateral medulla is increased in stroke-prone spontaneously hypertensive rats and thereby contributes to the neural mechanisms of hypertension through activation of the sympathetic nervous system. The paraventricular nucleus of the hypothalamus is most likely also involved in the ROS-mediated neural mechanism of hypertension [101, 102]. There is evidence that other regions of the brain are likewise involved in ROS mediated hypertension. These investigations suggest that increased intracellular superoxide production in the subfornical organ is critical to the development of Ang-II-induced hypertension [103].

5. Therapy

Oxidative stress can play a pivotal role in the elevation of BP. Therefore, if oxidative stress is indeed a cause of hypertension, it should be expected that antioxidants have beneficial effect on hypertension control; i.e together with inducing a reduction of oxidative damage, antioxidant should result in a reduction in BP. Thus, oxidative stress could be considered a therapeutic target in the management of hypertension. The deleterious ROS effects would be, to a large extent, prevented by various antioxidant systems. Theoretically, agents that reduce oxidant formation should be more efficacious than nonspecific antioxidant scavengers in ameliorating oxidative stress. Therefore, it seems reasonable to suggest a beneficial effect in hypertension exerted by several antioxidants, such as ascorbic acid (vitamin C), α-tocopherol (vitamin E), glutathione, BH_4, and N-acetylcysteine, among others. These compounds, acting at different levels of ROS and RNS cycles, have shown to improve endothelial function and NO bioaction in cultured cells, and in animal and human clinical studies of vascular reactivity. In support of this view, epidemiological studies suggest that individuals with higher antioxidant intake have reduced cardiovascular risk. Based on experimental evidence of the importance of oxidative stress in vascular damage, there has been great interest in developing strategies that target ROS in the treatment of hypertension and other cardiovascular diseases. Therapeutic approaches that have been considered include mechanisms to increase antioxidant bioavailability or to reduce ROS generation by decreasing activity of superoxide-generating enzymes. Gene therapy targeting oxidant systems are also being developed, but their use in clinical hypertension remains unclear. This chapter presents the available evidence for the potential role of antioxidants in the prevention and treatment of hypertension associated with oxidative stress, as supported by experimental investigations, observational findings, clinical trials, and epidemiological data pointing to an antihypertensive effect of these compounds. The main antioxidants of human use will be presented below.

Table 1.1. Oxidative stress pathophysiologial approaches in animal models of hypertension

Pathophysiological Pathway	Model	Reference
Deficient in ROS-generating enzymes	Rat	Landmesser et al., 2002; Landmesser et al., 2003.
Increased renal expression of the NADPH oxidase p47phox and endothelial NO synthase	Dhal Rat	Tojo et al., 2003
Increased expression of NADPH oxidase subunit p67(phox) in the renal medulla	Dhal rat	Feng et al., 2012
Vascular oxidative stress and endothelial dysfunction in Dahl salt-sensitive rats.	Dhal rat	Kosaka et al.,2013
ROS in the rostral ventrolateral medulla is increased and thereby contributes to the neural mechanisms of hypertension through activation of the sympathetic nervous system	SHR-stroke prone	Hirooka et al., 2010
The paraventricular nucleus of the hypothalamus is most likely also involved in the ROS-mediated neural mechanism of hypertension.	2K1C rat	Campos et al., 2010
Exposure of tubular cells to LDL, which may result in tubulointerstitial damage due to NADPH oxidase-mediated ROS production	Human	Piccoli et al., 2009

5.1. Vitamin C

Vitamin C (ascorbic acid) is a potent water-soluble antioxidant in humans. It is a six-carbon lactone synthesized from glucose in the most mammalian species, mainly in liver, but not in humans. Vitamin C is an electron donor and therefore a reducing agent. When ascorbate acts as an antioxidant or enzyme cofactor, it becomes oxidized to dehydroascorbic acid. The latter can be used by cells to regenerate ascorbate, and directly or indirectly, it can change the redox state of many other molecules. Vitamin C performs against oxidation of lipids, proteins and DNA, subsequently protecting their structure and biological function. In addition, on the vascular wall vitamin C behaves as enzyme modulator exerting up-regulation on eNOS and down-regulation of NADPH oxidase [104]. It was demonstrated that vitamin C inhibits the effects of ET-1 of impairing endothelium-dependent and endothelium-independent vasodilation and the stimulation of IL-6 release in humans in vivo. This suggests that the mechanism by which ET-1 impairs vascular function and stimulates release of IL-6 involves increased oxidative stress [105]. Most studies have demonstrated an inverse relationship between plasma ascorbate levels and BP in both normotensive and hypertensive populations [14, 106]. In a recent study, a decreasing trend was observed with vitamin C levels and risk of hypertension in women but not in men [107]. Vitamin C supplementation is associated with reduced BP in hypertensive patients, with systolic BP falling by 3.6–17.8 mmHg for each 50 μmol/l increase in plasma ascorbate [14, 108, 109]. Nevertheless, there are several small and short-term clinical trials in which the effect of vitamin C supplements on BP have yielded inconsistent findings [108, 110-112]. The lack of antihypertensive efficacy observed in studies using supplementation with vitamin C alone could be due to the pharmacokinetics of vitamin C and/or the decreased bioavailability of NO under conditions of oxidative stress. It is of interest to take into account that the antihypertensive effect of vitamin C is expected to occur at 10 mmol/L, a plasma concentration required to compete efficiently with the reaction of NO with superoxide, due to their high reaction rate constant that is even higher than that for the reaction between SOD and superoxide [113]. However, it should be remarked that this concentration is unobtainable in humans following oral administration. Indeed, the lack of a therapeutic antihypertensive plasma vitamin C concentration via oral administration may be due to its renal threshold at doses between 60 and 100 mg/day. The steady-state concentration of vitamin C is attained at approximately 80 μmol/L, and plasma is completely saturated at daily doses of over 400 mg [114]. Pharmacokinetic modeling indicates that, with oral administration, even at very large and frequent doses of vitamin C, plasma concentrations will only be increased modestly, from 70 μmol/L to a maximum of 220 μmol/L, whereas intravenous administration increases it as high as 14 mmol/L [115]. Thus the antihypertensive effect may only following infusion of high vitamin C doses. Accordingly, intra-arterial administration of vitamin C has been shown to cause a decrease in BP in subjects with essential hypertension [116] The molecular mechanisms underlying the in vivo antioxidant effects of vitamin C related with BP modulation are not fully understood. Nevertheless, it was shown that these effects are mediated in part by the ability of vitamin C to protect BH_4 from oxidation and thereby increase the enzymatic activity of eNOS. It should be noted that BH_4 is a cofactor necessary for NO generation via eNOS, otherwise becoming uncoupled, a form now recognized as an important source of superoxide rather than NO [117] a condition likely to occur under a prooxidant state.

5.2. Vitamin E

Vitamin E is a major lipid-soluble antioxidant that has received considerable attention. Epidemiological data support a role of high dietary vitamin E intake and a reduced incidence of cardiovascular disease [118]. Tocopherols have been shown to increase PGI_2 levels in endothelial cells via opposing effects on phospholipase A_2 and cyclo-oxygenase 2 [119], a potential beneficial effect against endothelial dysfunction as PGI_2 is a prostanoid vasodilator that is important for maintaining normal vascular function. Furthermore, vitamin E can act as a biological modifier independently of its antioxidant activity. Thus, vitamin E is capable to exert a dose-dependent regulation of mitochondrial generation of superoxide and H_2O_2. This effect is reached through the prevention of electron leakage, by mediating the superoxide generation systems directly and/or by scavenging superoxide generated. By down-regulating mitochondrial generation of superoxide and related ROS, vitamin E not only attenuates oxidative damage but also modulates the expression and activation of signal transduction pathways and other redox-sensitive biological modifiers [120]. However, intervention trials have not been convincing, with a number of studies demonstrating no beneficial effect of vitamin E on cardiovascular disease outcomes [121-124]. Most of these studies have generally not reported BP outcomes, although a subset of the Primary Prevention Project (PPP) study [125] did show no effect of vitamin E supplementation on clinic or ambulatory BP in treated hypertensive patients. Moreover, a meta-analysis has highlighted an increase in all-cause mortality with high-dose vitamin E supplementation [126]. In support of this view, other study using supplementation with vitamin E, either as α-tocopherol or mixed tocopherols, showed a significant increase in BP, pulse pressure and heart rate in individuals with type 2 diabetes. These increases were observed despite a reduction in plasma total F2-isoprostanes [127]. It should be noted that although vitamin E can inhibit LDL oxidation in vitro, it is unlikely to achieve sufficiently high concentrations in the vascular microenvironment to interfere effectively with all components of oxidative stress, and has limited activity against superoxide and peroxynitrite driven processes [128]. Therefore, taken together these data support the view that vitamin E alone supplements at daily doses over 400 IU are not effective as antihypertensive agents, may increase all-cause mortality and should be avoided.

5.3. Association of Vitamins C and E

It is of interest to note that the association of vitamins C and E is expected to have an antihypertensive effect probably due to the fact that this combined therapy provides a reinforcement of their individual properties through a complementary effect in improving endothelial dysfunction [129]. Both vitamins C and E not only behave as scavengers of ROS, but also are able to induce the down-regulation of NADPH oxidase and the up-regulation of eNOS [104, 130]. Vitamin C may reduce the α-tocopheroxyl radical, thereby abrogating lipid peroxidation [131] and further supporting an antihypertensive effect for this association. The use of these association aimed to cause an antihypertensive effect is discussed below. Despite the biological effects of both vitamin C and E, as shown by experimental models, long-term clinical trials have failed to consistently support their antihypertensive effects in patients at high cardiovascular risk. Most of clinical studies have looked at all-cause or cardiovascular mortality, rarely focusing on BP as a primary end point [132], but none of the large clinical trials examined the effects of antioxidants specifically on BP [82]. Some short-term trials have shown that supplemental antioxidant vitamin intake lowers BP [110, 133, 134] but the majority of clinical trials did not find any antihypertensive effects of antioxidant vitamins. However, most of these studies lack rigorous exclusion criteria in the selection of subjects to avoid the influence of confounders [89]. It deserves special mention that regarding cohorts included in large trials, most subjects had irreversible cardiovascular disease. Some of these alterations could contribute to perpetuate the increased ROS production by the vascular wall. Thus, in atherosclerotic arteries there is evidence for increased expression of the NADPH oxidase subunit gp91phox and Nox4, both of which may contribute to increased oxidative stress within vascular tissue [135]. In addition, in this setting there is an increase in the expression of the AT_1 receptor, providing evidence for stimulation of the renin angiotensin system and simultaneously for an activation of the NADPH oxidase in the arterial wall [136]. Recently, a randomized double-blind placebo-controlled study was conducted to test the hypothesis that oral administration of vitamins C and E together, by improving the antioxidant status, causes a decrease in BP in patients with mild-to-moderate essential hypertension [137]. The results of this study, performed with newly diagnosed hypertensives, without end-organ damage, showed for the first time a specific association between oxidative-stress-related parameters and BP, thus suggesting a role of oxidative stress in the pathogenesis of essential hypertension. Moreover, the concomitant decrease in BP and oxidative stress raises the possibility that oral administration of vitamins C + E in patients with essential hypertension may be considered as an adjunct therapy for hypertension in those patients. In summary, the available data lead us to think in a beneficial antihypertensive effect of vitamins C and E if administered during the phase of endothelial dysfunction, which precedes an established vascular damage. In this setting it would be more likely to successfully reverse, or at least counteract, the deleterious effects of ROS on the vascular wall. In contrast, it should not be expected an antihypertensive effect in patients having significant cardiovascular disease, in which case chronic damaging effects of oxidative stress may be irreversible.

5.4. N-acetylcysteine

The antioxidant N-acetyl-L-cysteine (NAC), a sulfhydryl group donor, improves renal dysfunction and markedly decreases arterial pressure and renal injury, as shown in an experimental model of Dahl salt-sensitive hypertension [138]. Furthermore, systolic BP was significantly higher in rats with 10% glucose feeding for 20 weeks [139]. This was associated with a higher production of superoxide anion and NADPH oxidase activity in aorta. The therapeutic effects of NAC in rats with established L-NAME hypertension were less pronounced than the preventive effects of NAC on the development of L-NAME hypertension [140]. Similarly, in spontaneously hypertensive rats, chronic administration of NAC partially attenuated the BP increase in young rats, while its effect was negligible in adults with fully developed hypertension. These results suggest that the inhibition of the oxidative stress in hypertensive states contributes to the therapeutic effects of NAC; it seems that ROS play a more important role in the induction than in the maintenance of hypertension. On the other hand, in patients with type 2 diabetes and hypertension, oral supplementation of NAC + L-arginine for 6 months caused a reduction of both systolic and diastolic mean arterial BP [141]. NAC administered intravenously during hemodialysis reduced plasma ADMA levels more significantly than hemodialysis alone [142]. In relation to the mechanisms accounting for these results, the effect of NAC may be mediated by an NO-dependent mechanism, probably through the protective effect of NAC on NO oxidation. In patients with type 2 diabetes NAC improves NO bioavailability both via reduction of oxidative stress and increase of NO production. NAC augments the levels of reduced glutathione and enhances the activity of NOS, probably by protecting its essential cofactor BH_4 from oxidation by the excess superoxide. Moreover, NAC has been shown to protect the sulfhydryl groups of NOS from destruction by free radicals and thus to maintain its activity [143]. These data are consistent with the NAC-induced enhancement of the hypotensive effect of ACEI, as it is an effect at least partially mediated by NO. Therefore, NAC could be considered as an adjuvant in the pharmacology of antihypertensive drugs having antioxidant properties and/or acting through an improvement of NO bioactivity.

5.5. Polyphenols

Polyphenols are the most abundant antioxidant in the diet. Their intake is 10 times higher than vitamin C and 100 times higher than vitamin E or carotenoids. Polyphenols like catechin or quercetin can directly scavenge ROS such as superoxide, hydrogen peroxide or hypochlorous acid, all of which can be deleterious by damaging lipids, proteins and DNA. These compounds might protect the cardiovascular system by improving the endothelial function. The endothelium plays a key role in the control of vascular tone by releasing several vasorelaxing factors, which have been identified later on as NO and EDHF [144]. Endothelial dysfunction results from the imbalanced release of endothelium-derived relaxing and contracting factors, in favor of the latter [145]. Grape derived products, rich in polyphenols, increase the eNOS activity, leading to enhanced formation of NO, which subsequently relaxes the VSMC via the cGMC-mediated pathway, enhancing by this way the endothelial function. In this line, polyphenols also prevent cyclooxygenase-dependent formation of endothelium-derived contracting factors [146], scavenge ROS, and inhibit NADPH and xanthine oxidases and chelate metals, processes altogether aimed to increase the NO bioavailability [147], with an antihypertensive effect as result. Other interesting sources of polyphenols are berries and red fruits, mainly rich in anthocyanins and ellagitannins [148]. Activation of eNOS is mostly dependent upon an increase in the free cytosolic calcium concentration ($[Ca^{2+}]_i$) in endothelial cells [149], except for shear stress. Nevertheless, due to low increase in $[Ca^{2+}]_i$ secondary to polyphenols, compared with physiological agonists [148], it is likely that additional mechanisms contribute to eNOS activation by polyphenols. An important signal pathway that activates the eNOS is the PI3-kinase/Akt pathway, responsible for the response to shear stress. This mechanism is triggered through a phosphorylation of the enzyme at SER 1177 position [150]. It has been shown that low concentrations of resveratrol (a polyphenol found in grapes and wine) and black tea polyphenols, are capable to activate estrogen receptors resulting in activation of p38 mitogen-activated protein kinase (p38 MAPK) and subsequently eNOS in endothelium [151, 152]. In addition, a recent study indicated that green tea polyphenols downregulate caveolin-1 protein expression, a major negative regulator of eNOS, so this effect might contribute to increasing eNOS activation [153]. Together with eNOS activation, polyphenols have been shown to increase the expression level of eNOS [154]. Thus, it has been shown that resveratrol up-regulates the expression of sirtuin-1 (SIRT-1) and induces its enzymatic activation, leading to an up-regulation of eNOS mRNA expression, producing a vasorelaxing effect [155] and to AT_1 receptor suppression in VSMC, the latter attempting to explain resveratrol-BP lowering in Ang-II-induced hypertension models [156]. Sirtuins are a family of conserved proteins with deacetylase and ADP-ribosyltransferase activities. In humans they are coded by seven genes (SIRT1-7). The most widely investigated and best known sirtuin is SIRT1, which can be activated by the natural phytocompound resveratrol and plays a role in several physiologic (apoptosis, autophagy, chromatin integrity, and transcriptional state) and pathologic (cardiovascular disorders, diabetes, cancer, and neurodegeneration) conditions [157]. Moreover, although SIRT1 is not directly involved in glucose metabolism, variability in the gene that encodes for it may modulate the outcome of a lifestyle intervention in diabetic patients and could also be relevant for the risk of cardiovascular mortality or the responsiveness of people to different forms of cardiovascular treatment [158]. Thus, resveratrol could play a key role in counterbalancing these pathophysiological pathways in these patients. Besides sirtuins, eNOS and ciclooxygenase activity, the other component of endothelium-derived relaxations due to polyphenols, has been attributed to EDHF induction [148]. Several mechanisms have been proposed to explain the EDHF vasorelaxing processes; sharing all of them the hyperpolarization-associated relaxation of VSMC. Red wine polyphenols caused relaxation and hyperpolarizations of VSMC in isolated porcine coronary arteries [159]. Moreover, intercellular communication through gap junctions may be involved in red wine polyphenols-induced EDHF-mediated relaxation [160]. This phenomenon may be dependent on endothelial redox-sensitive mechanism involving intracellular formation of superoxide anions [159]; also involves activation of PI3-kinase/Akt pathway [161].

5.6. Diet

There is sufficient evidence to suggest that dietary approaches may help to prevent and control high BP. The incidence and severity of hypertension are affected by nutritional status and intake of many nutrients. Short-term studies indicate that specialized diets may prevent or ameliorate mild hypertension; most notable are the Dietary Approaches to Stop Hypertension (DASH) diet, which is high in fruits, vegetables, and low-fat dairy products, and the DASH low sodium diet; these might reach an appropriate BP partly due to the presence of polyphenol rich foods [162-164]. Moreover, "Mediterranean Diet", which has lead to increased life expectancy and lower BP levels in Mediterranean countries, unlike northern Europe and USA, is related with the elevated presence of polyphenols in form of fruits, vegetables, olive oil and wine [164, 165]. Several studies have assessed the potential role of this diet in preventing or treating essential hypertension [166, 167]. However, this diet includes other antioxidants such as vitamin C, α-tocopherol, β-carotenes and polyunsaturated fatty acids, which could also explain the observed antihypertensive effect. Intake of grape-derived products reduced BP in hypertension models including spontaneously hypertensive rats [168], the N^G-nitro L-arginine-induced hypertension [169], the DOCA salt-induced hypertension [170] and the Ang II-induced hypertension in rats [171]. The administration of purple grape juice in human hypertensive patients increases NO release and reduces superoxide production in the vessels [172], and reduced, given daily for 8 weeks, both systolic and diastolic BP by, respectively, 7.2 and 6.2 mmHg [110]. Furthermore, a regular ingestion of black tea for 4 weeks has been shown to result in a significant increase in endothelium-dependent vasodilatation [173]. In addition, some clinical studies have shown that flavonoid-rich foods can improve endothelial function in patients with hypertension and ischemic heart disease [174], such as chronic intake of dark chocolate, which decreased BP in upper range hypertension or stage-1 hypertension without concomitant risk factors [175, 176], and tea intake, which also reduced levels of hypertension and had a protective effect in the development of the disease [177-179]. Chocolate (containing cocoa) and tea are a rich source of flavonoids, particularly flavan-3-ols in chocolate [180] and catechins in tea (up to 30% of the dry weight in green tea) [181]. Regarding to cocoa, some studies have assessed its relationship with low incidence and/or decrease of BP high levels [182, 183]. Several studies have shown that flavonoids, and especially flavan-3-ol- and procyanidins-rich foods, can inhibit ACE in vitro [184-186]. Consistent with these results, one study with humans showed that the consumption of flavonoid-rich pomegranate juice decreased ACE plasma activity by about 30%, and reduced systolic BP by 5% [187], equaling the effect sought by the ACEI, the cornerstone of hypertension treatment. Another important source of polyphenols is olive oil; 50% of the phenolic compounds contained in olives and virgin olive oil are hydroxytyrosol and derivatives. This polyphenol is well absorbed into plasma [188]. Olive oil consumption, in the context of Mediterranean diet and per se, is related with reduction of BP levels [189], an effect not only related with polyphenols content, but mainly with monounsaturated fatty acids presence in olive oil [190]. Other sources of plant polyphenols are hawthorn, maritime pine bark, honey, propolis and specially wines.

5.7. Wine

Numerous epidemiological studies indicate that light to moderate consumption of alcoholic beverages reduces all-cause mortality [191]. In this line, wine drinkers had a lower age-adjusted risk of coronary heart disease and all-cause mortality than did beer and spirits drinkers, but the wine drinkers also had a better life style. For example, much less smoking [192], the latter possibly being a confounding factor. Specially, red wine has long been thought to have beneficial effects on cardiovascular health, as clearly seen in Mediterranean diet [193] and in the "French Paradox" phenomenon, a protective effect of red wine despite a high-fat diet. Indirect evidence favoring this hypothesis is that the French habitually drink wine with their meals, which are often fatty, and this wine is most often red [194]. Furthermore, Alsace, a white-wine drinking region of France, has a much higher mortality (about 50% higher) than red wine-drinking Mediterranean areas [195], though having a lower mean serum cholesterol level [196]. In addition, several studies show cardiovascular protection induced by red wine but less by white wine [194, 197, 198], likely because the skins, seeds and stems of grape are present during the fermentation of red wine but not white wine [199]. Although the alcohol component of red wine may contribute to the protective effect by increasing the concentration of high density lipoproteins, decreasing the fibrinogen level [200] and producing NADH through alcohol dehydrogenase and aldehyde dehydrogenase mediated reactions [201], cofactor which increases overall antioxidant capacity, several studies suggest also a key role of the polyphenolic component [202, 203]. It is of interest to consider that red wine is one of the most abundant sources of polyphenols [204], extracted from grapes during the process of vinification. Grape is a phenol-rich plant, and these phenolics are mainly distributed in the skin, stem, leaf and seed of grape, rather than their juicy middle sections [205]. Red wine polyphenols include flavonols such as myricetin, kaempferol and the predominant quercetin, the flavan-3-ol monomers catechin and epicatechin, the oligomeric and polymeric flavan-3-ols or proanthocyanidins, various highly coloured anthocyanins, various phenolic acids (gallic acid, caftaric acid, caffeic acid, p-coumaric acid) and the stilbene resveratrol [199]. Some investigations have shown that anthocyanins enriched fractions and oligomeric proanthocyanidins, mainly dimers, trimers, and tetramers were the active compounds responsible for vasorelaxation activity, whereas monomers (catechins) and simple phenols, such as benzoic acid, gallic acid and hydroxycinnamates, were devoid of effect [206-208]. After 2 weeks of daily low to moderate red wine consumption, plasma levels of total phenolic concentrations increased significantly, and trace levels of metabolites, mainly glucuronides and methyl glucuronides of (+)-catechin and (−)-epicatechin, were detected in plasma [209]. Resveratrol remains as the most powerful polyphenol in red wine [210]. Red wine and grapes exhibit endothelium-dependent relaxation of blood vessels via enhanced generation and/or increased biological activity of NO, leading to the elevation of cGMP levels [211, 212]. This effect is not solely by direct stimulation of eNOS, but also due to increase in intracellular Ca^{2+} as it has been seen in several studies [172, 213]. In addition, it occurs an increase of the expression of this enzyme, thus explaining the long-term beneficial effects of red wine intake on the cardiovascular function [154], even using a red wine extract without alcohol. Red wine polyphenols may promote the release of endothelial NO through the redox sensitive PI3K/Akt pathway [159]. In vivo, red wine polyphenols were shown to reduce BP in normo- and hypertensive rats [214, 215], and end-organ damage in hypertensive animals; these effects could be due to reduced oxidative stress and endothelial dysfunction [216]. In humans, 30 min after the consumption of red wine or polyphenols (1 g/kg body weight), circulating NO concentration increases to 30 and 40 nM, respectively. Furthermore, a reduction in BP and an increase in heart rate are observed [217]. The endothelium-dependent vasodilation was improved after acute intake of 500 mL of red wine or red wine without alcohol in men, as determined by ultrasonography of the brachial artery [218]. The amplitude of vasorelaxation changed as a function of the variability of wine constituents according to grape varieties, area of cultivation and vinification methods [203]. Consequently, the vasodilatatory effect does not apply to all wines and the degree of vasorelaxation is correlated to the content and type of phenols [219]. Estrogen receptor α (ERα) has been identified as the key receptor transducing vascular effects exerted by red wine polyphenols, particularly delphinidin with respect to NO production [220] and endothelium-dependent vascular relaxation. Besides NO, red wine affected the formation of other mediators of vascular tone, such as EDHF [159] and prostacyclin [221]. In addition, the synthesis of a potent vasoconstrictor such as ET-1 is reduced by red wine in bovine aortic endothelial cells [222].

5.8. Supplements

Due to the extreme complexity of the polyphenolic composition of food and beverages, crude preparations from dietary components have been used in experimental studies, and their effects have been compared to those of commercially available reference defined compounds [202]. In this line, several studies have reported antihypertensive effects in response to several purified polyphenols from fruits and vegetables, such as quercetin, a flavonol found widely in fruits and vegetables [174]; genistein, an isoflavone found mainly in vegetables [223]; and hesperitin and glucosyl-hesperidin, two flavonones [224]. Supplementation with quercetin significantly reduced systolic BP of individuals with a high-cardiometabolic risk phenotype on established cardiovascular disease risk biomarkers [225]. It was suggested that pure quercetin can improve endothelial function by modulating the circulating concentrations of vasoactive NO products and ET-1 [226]. Additionally, by evidence shown in some studies [227, 228], it may be concluded that a certain degree of hypertension might be required for quercetin to exert a BP-lowering effect. In a rat model of injured aorta, a lower dose of resveratrol (10 mg/kg) enhanced eNOS expression and accelerated the repair of the injured artery; however, a higher dose (50 mg/kg) had minimal effects [229]. Another rat model showed resveratrol to decrease ET-1 and Ang-II concentrations, while increased NO concentration, effects which in conjunction protected against increased BP and subsequent cardiac hypertrophy [230]. This effect, with regards to polyphenols, in general leads to a preponderancy of vasorelaxing factors over vasoconstrictant, resulting in a vasodilating effect. Resveratrol and quercetin have been shown to induce an increase of $[Ca^{2+}]_i$, by activating K^+ channels or inhibition of Ca^{2+}-ATPases of the endoplasmic reticulum in endothelial cells [231, 232]; these mechanisms could explain polyphenols-induced activation of eNOS and subsequent NO production. In addition, the stimulation of NADPH oxidase, a major source of ROS, by oxidized LDL in vascular endothelial cells was inhibited by resveratrol by reducing the membrane association of two of the proteins in the active enzyme complex, gp91 (phox) and Rac1 [233]. However, there is controversy in models of spontaneously hypertensive rats. For instance, a significant drop in mean BP after resveratrol treatment was shown in one of these models [234], opposite to another study with young stroke-prone spontaneously hypertensive rats, where systolic BP was not lowered by resveratrol [235] and quercetin did not delay or lessen the onset or severity of cardiovascular complications, including hypertension [236]. On the other hand, being phase-2-conjugates of resveratrol its predominant forms in vivo after ingestion, there are no reports documenting their relative biological activity [199]. Flavan-3-ols, or the catechins and their oligo- and polymeric derivatives the proanthocyanidins, have also attracted considerable interest due to their ability to improve endothelial function and vascular tone. In particular, ingestion of cocoa flavan-3-ols [237, 238] and acute dietary supplementation with epigallocatechin gallate, a major catechin in tea [239], have been shown, consistently, to improve vascular function. Grape proanthocyanidin supplementation to SHR significantly reduced BP and superoxide production by 23% [168]. Anthocyanins from wine inhibit phosphodiesterase-5 activity, enzyme which degrades cGMP, thus reducing the risk of cardiovascular disease by vasorelaxation [203]. In addition, it has been shown that oligomeric procyanidins inhibit ET-1 synthesis [240] and inhibit ACE activity [184], both in concentrations similar to those found in red wines; also, it stimulates prostacyclin release [241]. On the other hand, quercetin inhibited the release of prostacyclin [241]. In addition, polyphenols can activate DHF-dependent relaxations as it has been observed in response to the extract of Eucommia bark, a traditional Chinese medicinal herb, in the rat mesenteric artery [242, 243] and red wine polyphenols [244]. Thus, at least fruit and vegetable consumption, if not particular supplementation, should be encouraged in order to obtain polyphenolic-derived beneficial effects.

5.9. Inhibition of Arginase

Arginase is a hydrolytic enzyme responsible for converting L-arginine to urea and L-ornithine, the synthesis precursor of polyamines. Mammalian arginases exist in two distinct isoforms type I and type II. Arginase I is a cytosolic enzyme located primarily in the liver, whereas arginase II is located within the mitochondrion and is expressed at high levels in the kidneys [245]. However, both arginase isoforms are also expressed by endothelial and VSMC

[246-248]. Because NOS and arginase use L-arginine as a common substrate, arginase may downregulate NO biosynthesis by competing with NOS for L-arginine degradation. Consistent with this hypothesis, NO production has been inversely correlated to arginase activity in vessels at both physiological [249] and pathological conditions such as hypertension [250], atherosclerosis [251] diabetes [252] erectile dysfunction [253] and aging [254]. A recent study in rats [255], showed that arginase inhibition in SHR with fully developed hypertension reduced systolic BP and target organ damage including artery remodelling, cardiac fibrosis, and changes in vascular compliance. These results suggest that arginase is a promising target to reduce BP and to improve cardiovascular function in patients with essential hypertension. Arginase inhibition might also be useful for reducing cardiovascular risk in hypertensive patient since a large meta-analysis of trials in hypertension reported that antihypertensive drug treatment improves cardiovascular outcome mainly through lowering of SBP [251]. Interestingly, recent clinical studies confirmed the critical role of arginase in the control of BP. More precisely, plasma arginase activity is high in hypertensive pre-eclamptic women and correlates with plasma NO and BP levels [256] Additionally, BP level, risk of myocardial infarction and common intima-media thickness are dependent on arginase I polymorphisms [257, 258].

Conclusion and Perspectives

Oxidative stress can play a pivotal role in the elevation of BP. Therefore, if oxidative stress is indeed a cause of hypertension, it should be expected that antioxidants have beneficial effect on hypertension control; i.e together with inducing a reduction of oxidative damage, antioxidants should result in a reduction in BP. Thus, oxidative stress could be considered a therapeutic target in the management of hypertension. Nevertheless, supplementation treatment with both single or combination antioxidant therapy has not been shown to be consistently effective in improving BP in hypertensive subjects. Some studies reported antihypertensive effects, whereas others found no change in BP following antioxidant exposure. Vitamin E alone supplements at daily are not effective as antihypertensive agents, may increase all-cause mortality and should be avoided. In contrast, the association of vitamins C and E is expected to have an antihypertensive effect probably due to the fact that this combined therapy provides a reinforcement of their individual properties. N-acetylcysteine could be considered as an adjuvant in the pharmacology of antihypertensive drugs having antioxidant properties and/or acting through an improvement of NO bioactivity. The antihypertensive effect of polyphenols may arise from their properties to scavenge ROS, inhibit NADPH and xanthine oxidases and chelate metals, processes altogether aimed to increase the NO bioavailability. The vasodilatatory effect of wines and diet is partly due to their content and type of polyphenols. More studies, including dosing and adverse events assessments, are needed before the use antioxidant supplements could be considered in the treatment of hypertension. In summary, antioxidants could be suitable as an adjunct therapy for hypertension, particularly for new onset hypertension. Nevertheless, it should be expected that this treatment be more efficient in the prevention than in the reduction of established hypertension.

References

[1] Taniyama Y, Griendling KK. Reactive oxygen species in the vasculature: molecular and cellular mechanisms. *Hypertension* 2003;42:1075-1081.

[2] Montezano AC, Touyz RM. Oxidative stress, Noxs, and hypertension: experimental evidence and clinical controversies. *Ann Med* 2012;44:2-16.

[3] Rodrigo R, González J, Paoletto F. The role of oxidative stress in the pathophysiology of hypertension. *Hypertens Res* 2011;34:431-440.

[4] Rodrigo R, Passalacqua W, Araya J, Orellana M, Rivera G. Implications of oxidative stress and homocysteine in the pathophysiology of essential hypertension. *J Cardiovasc Pharmacol* 2003;42:453-461.

[5] Touyz RM, Schiffrin EL. Increased generation of superoxide by angiotensin II in smooth muscle cells from resistance arteries of hypertensive patients: role of phospholipase D-dependent NADPH oxidase-sensitive pathways. *J Hypertens 2001*; 19:1245-1254.

[6] Ghiadoni L, Magagna A, Versari D, Kardasz I Huang Y, Taddei S, Salvetti A. Different effect of antihypertensive drugs on conduit artery endothelial function. *Hypertension* 2003; 41: 1281-1286.

[7] Lassègue B, Clempus RE. Vascular NADPH oxidases: specific features, expression, and regulation. *Am J Physiol Regul Integr Comp Physiol* 2003;285:277-297.

[8] Michel JB, Feron O, Sase K, Prabhakar P, Michel T. Caveolin versus calmodulin. Counterbalancing allosteric modulators of endothelial nitric oxide synthase. *J Biol Chem* 1997;272:25907-25912.

[9] Paravicini TM, Touyz RM. Redox signaling in Hypertension. *Cardiovasc Res* 2006;71: 247-258.

[10] Simko F, Luptak I, Matuskova J, Krajcirovicova K, Sumbalova Z, Kucharska J, Gvozdjakova A, Simko J, Babal P, Pechanova O, Bernatova I. L-arginine fails to protect against myocardial remodeling in L-NAME-induced hypertension. *Eur J Clin Invest* 2005;38:831-838.

[11] Lassègue B, Griendling K. Reactive oxygen species in hypertension, an update. *Am. J Hypertens* 2004;17:852-860.

[12] Schramm A, Matusik P, Osmenda G, Guzik TJ. Targeting NADPH oxidases in vascular pharmacology. *Vascul Pharmacol* 2012;56:216-231.

[13] Touyz RM. Reactive oxygen species in vascular biology: role in arterial hypertension. *Expert Rev Cardiovasc Ther* 2003;1:91-106.

[14] Redon J, Oliva MR, Tormos C, Giner V, Chaves J, Iradi A, Saez GT. Antioxidant activities and oxidative stress byproducts in human hypertension. *Hypertension* 2003;41:1096–1101.

[15] Ward NC, Hodgson JM, Puddey IB, Mori TA, Beilin LJ, Croft KD. Oxidative stress in human hypertension: association with antihypertensive treatment, gender, nutrition, and lifestyle. *Free Radic Biol Med* 2004;36:226-232.

[16] Minuz P, Patrignani P, Gaino S, Seta F, Capone ML, Tacconelli S, Degan M, Faccini G, Fornasiero A, Talamini G, Tommasoli R, Arosio E, Santonastaso CL, Lechi A, Patrono C. Determinants of platelet activation in human essential hypertension. *Hypertension* 2004;43:64-70.

[17] Yasunari K, Maeda K, Nakamura M, Yoshikawa J.Oxidative stress in leukocytes is a possible link between blood pressure, blood glucose, and C-reacting protein. *Hypertension* 2002;39:777-780.

[18] Corry DB, Eslami P, Yamamoto K, Nyby MD, Makino H, Tuck ML. Uric acid stimulates vascular smooth muscle cell proliferation and oxidative stress via the vascular renin-angiotensin system. *J Hypertens* 2008;26:269-275.

[19] Tanito M, Nakamura H, Kwon YW, Teratani A, Masutani H, Shioji K, Kishimoto C, Ohira A, Horie R, Yodoi J. Enhanced oxidative stress and impaired thioredoxin expression in spontaneously hypertensive rats. *Antioxid Redox Signal* 2004;6:89-97.

[20] Hisaki R, Fujita H, Saito F, Kushiro T. Tempol attenuates the development of hypertensive renal injury in Dahl salt-sensitive rats. *Am J Hypertens* 2005;18:707-713.

[21] Touyz RM. Reactive oxygen species, vascular oxidative stress, and redox signaling in hypertension: what is the clinical significance? *Hypertension* 2004; 44:248-252.

[22] Harrison DG, Widder J, Grumbach I, Chen W, Weber M, Searles C. Endothelial: mechanotransduction, nitric oxide and vascular inflammation. *J Intern Med* 2006;259:351–363.

[23] Touyz RM. Reactive oxygen species as mediators of calcium signaling by angiotensin II: implications in vascular physiology and pathophysiology. *Antioxid Redox Signal* 2005;7:1302-1314.

[24] Mueller CF, Laude K, McNally JS, Harrison DG. ATVB in focus: redox mechanisms in blood vessels. *Arterioscler Thromb Vasc Biol* 2005;25:274–278.

[25] San Martin A, Du P, Dikalova A, Lassegue B, Aleman M, Gongora MC, Brown K, Joseph G, Harrison DG, Taylor WR, Jo H, Griendling KK. Reactive oxygen species-selective regulation of aortic inflammatory gene expression in type 2 diabetes. *Am J Physiol Heart Circ Physiol* 2007;292:H2073–H2082.

[26] Pawlak K, Naumnik B, Brzosko S, Pawlak D, Mysliwiec M. Oxidative stress: a link between endothelial injury, coagulation activation, and atherosclerosis in haemodialysis patients. *Am J Nephrol* 2004;24:154–161.

[27] Wattanapitayakul SK, Bauer JA. Oxidative pathways in cardiovascular disease: roles, mechanisms, and therapeutic implications. *Pharmacol Ther* 2001;89:187–206.

[28] Kimura S, Zhang GX, Nishiyama A, Shokoji T, Yao L, Fan YY, Rahman M, Abe Y. Mitochondria-derived reactive oxygen species and vascular MAP kinases: comparison of angiotensin II and diazoxide. *Hypertension* 2005;45:438–444.

[29] Hool LC, Corry B. Redox control of calcium channels: from mechanisms to therapeutic opportunities. *Antioxid Redox Signal* 2007;9:409–435.

[30] Yoshioka J, Schreiter ER, Lee RT. Role of thioredoxin in cell growth through interactions with signaling molecules. *Antioxid Redox Signal* 2006;8:2143–21451.

[31] Landmesser U, Cai H, Dikalov S, McCann L, Hwang J, Jo H, Holland SM, Harrison DG. Role of p47(phox) in vascular oxidative stress and hypertension caused by angiotensin II. *Hypertension* 2002;40:511-515.

[32] Landmesser U, Dikalov S, Price SR, McCann L, Fukai T, Holland SM, Mitch WE, Harrison DG. Oxidation of tetrahydrobiopterin leads to uncoupling of endothelial cell nitric oxide synthase in hypertension. *J Clin Invest* 2003;111:1201-1209.

[33] Cracowski JL, Baguet JP, Ormezzano O, Bessard J, Stanke-Labesque F, Bessard G, Mallion JM. Lipid peroxidation is not increased in patients with untreated mild-to-moderate hypertension. *Hypertension* 2003;41:286–288.

[34] Virdis A, Schiffrin EL. Vascular inflammation: a role in vascular disease in hypertension? *Curr Opin Nephrol Hypertens* 2003;12:181-187.

[35] Ross R. Atherosclerosis is an inflammatory disease. *Am. Heart J.* 1999;138:S419-S420.

[36] Hansson GK, Robertson AK, Söderberg-Nauclér C. Inflammation and atherosclerosis. *Annu. Rev. Pathol.* 2006;1:297-329.

[37] Chae CU, Lee RT, Rifai N, Ridker PM. Blood pressure and inflammation in apparently healthy men. *Hypertension* 2001;38:399–403.

[38] Clinton SK, Underwood R, Hayes L, Sherman ML, Kufe DW, Libby P. Macrophage colony-stimulating factor gene expression in vascular cells and in experimental and human atherosclerosis. *Am. J. Pathol.* 1992;140:301-316.

[39] Xu Q. Role of heat shock proteins in atherosclerosis. Arterioscler. *Thromb. Vasc. Biol.* 2002;22:1547-1559.

[40] Han D, Antunes F, Canali R, Rettori D, Cadenas E. Voltage-dependent anion channels control the release of the superoxide anion from mitochondria to cytosol. *J Biol Chem.* 2003;278:5557-5563

[41] Hink U, Li H, Mollnau H, Oelze M, Matheis E, Hartmann M, Skatchkov M, Thaiss F, Stahl RA, Warnholtz A, Meinertz T, Griendling K, Harrison DG, Forstermann U, Munzel T. Mechanisms underlying endothelial dysfunction in diabetes mellitus. *Circ Res* 2001;88:E14-E22.

[42] Yang Z, Ming XF. Recent advances in understanding endothelial dysfunction in atherosclerosis. *Clin Med Res* 2006;4:53-65.

[43] Endemann DH, Schiffrin EL. Endothelial dysfunction. *J Am Soc Nephrol* 2004;15:1983-1992.

[44] Münzel T, Sinning C, Post F, Warnholtz A, Schulz E. Pathophysiology, diagnosis and prognostic implications of endothelial dysfunction. *Ann Med* 2008;40:180-196.

[45] Lacy F, Kailasam MT, O'Connor DT, Schmid-Schonbein GW, Parmer RJ. Plasma hydrogen peroxide production in human essential hypertension: role of heredity, gender, and ethnicity. *Hypertension* 2000;36:878–884.

[46] Stojiljkovic MP, Lopes HF, Zhang D, Morrow JD, Goodfriend TL, Egan BM. Increasing plasma fatty acids elevates F2-isoprostanes in humans: implications for the cardiovascular risk factor cluster. *J Hypertens* 2002;201:1215–1221.

[47] Kashyap MK, Yadav V, Sherawat BS, Jain S, Kumari S, Khullar M, Sharma PC, Nath R. Different antioxidants status, total antioxidant power and free radicals in essential hypertension. *Mol Cell Biochem* 2005;277:89–99.

[48] Bengtsson SH, Gulluyan LM, Dusting GJ, Drummond GR. Novel isoforms of NADPH oxidase in vascular physiology and pathophysiology. *Clin. Exp. Pharmacol. Physiol* 2003;30:849–854.

[49] Savoia C, Schiffrin EL. Inflammation in hypertension. *Curr Opin Nephrol Hypertens* 2006;15:152-158.

[50] Boos CJ, Lip Gregory YH. Is Hypertension an Inflammatory Process? *Current Pharmaceutical Design* 2006; 12:1623-1635.

[51] Rodrigo R, Parra M, Bosco C, Fernández V, Barja P, Guajardo J, Messina R. Pathophysiological basis for the prophylaxis of preeclampsia through early supplementation with antioxidant vitamins. *Pharmacol Ther.* 2005;107:177-197.

[52] Ashworth JR, Warren AY, Baker PN, Johnson IR. Loss of endotheliumdependent relaxation in myometrial resistance arteries in pre-eclampsia. *BJOG* 1997; 104:1152–1158.

[53] Ashworth JR, Baker PN, Warren AY, Phil M, Johnson IR. Mechanisms of endothelium-dependent relaxation in myometrial resistance vessels and their alteration in preeclampsia. *Hypertens Pregnancy* 1999; 18:57–71.

[54] Wimalasundera RC, Thom SAM, Regan L, Hughes AD. Effects ofvasoactive agents on intracellular calcium and force in myometrial and subcutaneous resistance arteries isolated from preeclamptic, pregnant, and nonpregnant woman. *Am J Obstet Gynecol* 2005; 192:625–632.

[55] Wareing M, Myers JE, O'Hara M, Kenny LC, Warren AY, Taggart MJ, Skillern L, Machin I, Baker PN. Effects of a phosphodiesterase-5 (PDE5) inhibitor on endothelium-dependent relaxation of myometrial small arteries. *Am J Obstet Gynecol* 2004; 190:1283–1290.

[56] Kenny LC, Baker PN, Kendall DA, Randall MD, Dunn WR. Differential mechanisms of endothelium-dependent vasodilator responses in human myometrial small arteries in normal pregnancy and pre-eclampsia. *Clin Sci* 2002; 103:67–73.

[57] Cockell AP, Poston L. Flow-mediated vasodilatation is enhanced in normal pregnancy but reduced in preeclampsia. *Hypertension* 1997; 30: 247–251.

[58] Knock GA, Poston L. Bradykinin-mediated relaxation of isolated maternal resistance arteries in normal pregnancy and preeclampsia. *Am J Obstet Gynecol* 1996; 175:1668–1674.

[59] Suzuki Y, Kajikuri J, Suzumori K, Itoh T. Mechanisms underlying the reduced endothelium-dependent relaxation in human omental resistance artery in pre-eclampsia. *J Physiol* 2000; 527:163–174.

[60] Suzuki Y, Hattori T, Kajikuri J, Yamamoto T, Suzumori K, Itoh T. Reduced function of endothelial prostacyclin in human omental resistance arteries in pre-eclampsia. *J Physiol* 2002; 545:269–277.

[61] McCarthy AL, Woolfson RG, Raju SK, Poston L. Abnormal endothelial cell function of resistance arteries from women with preeclampsia. *Am J Obstet Gynecol* 1993; 168:1323–1330.

[62] Luksha L, Nisell H, Luksha N, Kublickas M, Hultenby K, Kublickiene K. Endothelium-derived hyperpolarizing factor in preeclampsia: heterogeneous contribution, mechanisms, and morphological prerequisites. *Am J Physiol Regul Integr Comp Physiol* 2008; 294:R510–R519.

[63] Luksha L, Agewall S, Kublickiene K. Endothelium-derived hyperpolarizing factor in vascular physiology and cardiovascular disease. *Atherosclerosis* 2009; 202:330–344.

[64] Feletou M, Vanhoutte PM. EDHF: an update. *Clin Sci* 2009; 117:139–155.

[65] Luksha L, Nisell H, Kublickiene K. The mechanism of EDHF-mediated responses in subcutaneous small arteries from healthy pregnant women. *Am J Physiol Regul Integr Comp Physiol* 2004; 286:R1102–R1109.

[66] Dechend R, Homuth V, Wallukat G, Kreuzer J, Park JK, Theuer J, Juepner A, Gulba DC, Mackman N, Haller H, Luft FC. AT(1) receptor agonistic antibodies from preeclamptic patients cause vascular cells to express tissue factor. *Circulation* 2000; 101:2382–2387.

[67] Dechend R, Viedt C, Muller DN, Ugele B, Brandes RP, Wallukat G, Park JK, Janke J, Barta P, Theuer J, Fiebeler A, Homuth V, Dietz R, Haller H, Kreuzer J, Luft FC. AT1 receptor agonistic antibodies from preeclamptic patients stimulate NADPH oxidase. *Circulation* 2003; 107:1632–1639.

[68] Dechend R, Müller DN, Wallukat G, Homuth V, Krause M, Dudenhausen J, Luft FC. Activating auto-antibodies against the AT1 receptor in preeclampsia. *Autoimmun Rev* 2005; 4:61–65.

[69] Dechend R, Homuth V, Wallukat G, Müller DN, Krause M, Dudenhausen J, Haller H, Luft FC. Agonistic antibodies directed at the angiotensin II, AT1 receptor in preeclampsia. *J Soc Gynecol Investig* 2006; 13:79–86.

[70] Xia Y, Ramin SM, Kellems RE. Potential roles of angiotensin receptor-activating autoantibody in the pathophysiology of preeclampsia. *Hypertension* 2007; 50:269–275.

[71] Dechend R, Gratze P, Wallukat G, Shagdarsuren E, Plehm R, Bräsen JH, Fiebeler A, Schneider W, Caluwaerts S, Vercruysse L, Pijnenborg R, Luft FC, Müller DN. Agonistic autoantibodies to the AT1 receptor in a transgenic rat model of preeclampsia. *Hypertension* 2005; 45:742–746.

[72] LaMarca BB, Wallukat G, Llinas M, Herse F, Dechend R, Granger JP. Elevated agonistic autoantibodies to the angiotensin type 1 (AT1-AA) receptor in responseto placental ischemia and TNFα in pregnant rats. *Hypertension* 2008; 52:7–11.

[73] LaMarca B, Parrish M, Ray LF, Murphy SR, Roberts L, Glover P, Wallukat G, Wenzel K, Cockrell K, Martin JN Jr, Ryan MJ, Dechend R. Hypertension in response to autoantibodies to the angiotensin II type I receptor (AT1-AA) in pregnant rats: role of endothelin-1. *Hypertension* 2009; 54:905–909.

[74] Parrish MR, Murphy SR, Rutland S, Wallace K, Wenzel K, Wallukat G, Keiser S, Ray LF, Dechend R, Martin JN, Granger JP, LaMarca B. The effect of immune factors, tumor necrosis factor-α, and agonistic autoantibodies to the angiotensin II type I receptor on soluble fms-like tyrosine-1 and soluble endoglin production in response to hypertension during pregnancy. *Am J Hypertens* 2010; 23:911–916.

[75] Irani RA, Zhang Y, Zhou CC, Blackwell SC, Hicks MJ, Ramin SM, Kellems RE, Xia Y. Autoantibody-mediated angiotensin receptor activation contributes to preeclampsia through tumor necrosis factor-α signaling. *Hypertension* 2010; 55:1246–1253.

[76] Surdacki A, Nowicki M, Sandmann J, Tsikas D, Boeger RH., Bode- Boeger SM. Kruszelnicka-Kwiatkowska O, Kokot F, Dubiel JS, Froelich JC. Reduced urinary excretion of nitric oxide metabolites and increased plasma levels of asymmetric dimethylarginine in men with essential hypertension. *J Cardiovasc Pharmacol* 1999; 33: 652– 658.

[77] Böger RH, Bode-Böger SM, Szuba A, Tsao PS, Chan JR, Tangphao O, Blaschke TF, Cooke JP. Asymmetric dimethylarginine (ADMA): a novel risk factor for endothelial dysfunction: its role in hypercholesterolemia. *Circulation* 1998;98:1842-1847.

[78] Sydow K, Schwedhelm E, Arakawa N, Bode-Böger SM, Tsikas D, Hornig B, Frölich JC, Böger RH. ADMA and oxidative stress are responsible for endothelial dysfunction in hyperhomocyst(e)inemia: effects of L-arginine and B vitamins. *Cardiovasc Res.* 2003;57:244-252.

[79] Stühlinger MC, Oka RK, Graf EE, Schmölzer I, Upson BM, Kapoor O, Szuba A, Malinow MR, Wascher TC, Pachinger O, Cooke JP. Endothelial dysfunction induced

by hyperhomocyst(e)inemia: role of asymmetric dimethylarginine. *Circulation.* 2003;108:933-938.

[80] Holden DP, Fickling SA, Whitley GS, Nussey SS. Plasma concentrations of asymmetric dimethylarginine, a natural inhibitor of nitric oxide synthase, in normal pregnancy and preeclampsia. *Am J Obstet Gynecol.* 1998;178:551-556.

[81] Pettersson A, Hedner T, Milsom I. Increased circulating concentrations of asymmetric dimethyl arginine (ADMA), an endogenous inhibitor of nitric oxide synthesis, in preeclampsia. *Acta Obstet Gynecol Scand.* 1998;77:808-813.

[82] Touyz RM, Schiffrin EL. Reactive oxygen species in vascular biology: implications in hypertension. *Histochem Cell Biol* 2004; 122: 339– 352.

[83] Savvidou MD, Hingorani AD, Tsikas D, Frölich JC, Vallance P, Nicolaides KH.Endothelial dysfunction and raised plasma concentrations of asymmetric dimethylarginine in pregnant women who subsequently develop pre-eclampsia. *Lancet* 2003;361:1511-1517.

[84] Delles C, Schneider MP, John S, Gekle M, Schmieder RE. Angiotensin converting enzyme inhibition and angiotensin II AT1-receptor blockade reduce the levels of asymmetrical N(G), N(G)-dimethylarginine in human essential hypertension. *Am J Hypertens.* 2002;15:590-593

[85] Maas R, Böger RH, Schwedhelm E, Casas JP, López-Jaramillo P, Serrano N, Díaz LA.Plasma concentrations of asymmetric dimethylarginine (ADMA) in Colombian women with pre-eclampsia. *JAMA.* 2004;291:823-824.

[86] Tojo A, Onozato ML, Kobayashi N, Goto A, Matsuoka H, Fujita T. Angiotensin II and oxidative stress in Dahl Salt-sensitive rat with heart failure. *Hypertension.* 2002;40:834-8339.

[87] Feng D, Yang C, Geurts AM, Kurth T, Liang M, Lazar J, Mattson DL, O'Connor PM, Cowley AW Jr. Increased expression of NAD(P)H oxidase subunit p67(phox) in the renal medulla contributes to excess oxidative stress and salt-sensitive hypertension. *Cell Metab.* 2012;15:201-208.

[88] Kosaka S, Pelisch N, Rahman M, Nakano D, Hitomi H, Kobori H, Fukuoka N, Kobara H, Mori H, Masaki T, Cervenka L, Matsumura Y, Houchi H, Nishiyama A. Effects of angiotensin II AT_1-receptor blockade on high fat diet-induced vascular oxidative stress and endothelial dysfunction in Dahl salt-sensitive rats. *J Pharmacol Sci.* 2013;121:95-102.

[89] Rodrigo R, Guichard C, Charles R. Clinical pharmacology and therapeutic use of antioxidant vitamins. *Fundam Clin Pharmacol.* 2007;21:111-127.

[90] Zicha J., Dobesova Z., Kunes J. Relative deficiency of nitric oxide-dependent vasodilation in salt- hypertensive Dahl rats: the possible role of superoxide anions. *J Hypertens* 2001;19:247 254.

[91] Piccoli C, Quarato G, D'Aprile A, Montemurno E, Scrima R, Ripoli M, Gomaraschi M, Cirillo P, Boffoli D, Calabresi L, Gesualdo L, Capitanio N. Native LDL-induced oxidative stress in human proximal tubular cells: multiple players involved. *J Cell Mol Med.* 2011 ;15:375-95.

[92] Klahr S. Urinary tract obstruction. *Semin Nephrol* 2001; 21: 133–145.

[93] Grande MT, Pe´rez-Barriocanal F, Lo´pez-Novoa JM. Role of inflammation in tubulointerstitial damage associated to obstructive nephropathy. *J Inflamm (Lond)* 2010; 22: 7–19.

[94] Sachse A, Wolf G. Angiotensin II-induced reactive oxygen species and the kidney. *J Am Soc Nephrol* 2007; 18: 2439–2446.

[95] Chung S, Park CW, Shin SJ, Lim JH, Chung HW, Youn DY, Kim HW, Kim BS, Lee JH, Kim GH, Chang YS. Tempol or candesartan prevents high-fat diet-induced hypertension and renal damage in spontaneously hypertensive rats. *Nephrol Dial Transplant* 2010; 25: 389–399.

[96] Grassi G. Assessment of sympathetic cardiovascular drive in human hypertension: achievements and perspectives. *Hypertension* 2009; 54: 690–697.

[97] Guyenet PG. The sympathetic control of blood pressure. *Nat Rev Neurosci* 2006; 7: 335–346.

[98] Kishi T, Hirooka Y, Kimura Y, Ito K, Shimokawa H, Takeshita A. Increased reactive oxygen species in rostral ventrolateral medulla contribute to neural mechanisms of hypertension in stroke-prone spontaneously hypertensive rats. *Circulation* 2004; 109: 2357–2362.

[99] Hirooka Y, Sagara Y, Kishi T, Sunagawa K. Oxidative stress and central cardiovascular regulation. Pathogenesis of hypertension and therapeutic aspects. *Circ J* 2010; 74: 827–835.

[100] Sved AF, Ito S, Sved JC. Brainstem mechanisms of hypertension: role of the rostral ventrolateral medulla. *Curr Hypertens Rep* 2003; 5: 262–268.

[101] Campos RR, Oliveira-Sales EB, Nishi EE, Boim MA, Dolnikoff MS, Bergamaschi CT. The role of oxidative stress in renovascular hypertension. *Clin Exp Pharmacol Physiol.* 2011;38:144-152.

[102] Oliveira-Sales EB, Nishi EE, Carillo BA, Boim MA, Dolnikoff MS, Bergamaschi CT, Campos RR. Oxidative stress in the sympathetic promotor neurons contributes to sympathetic activation in renovascular hypertension. *Am J Hypertens* 2009; 22: 484–492.

[103] Zimmerman MC, Lazartigues E, Sharma RV, Davisson RL. Hypertension caused by angiotensin II infusion involves increased superoxide production in the central nervous system. *Circ Res* 2004; 95: 210–216.

[104] Ulker S, McKeown PP, Bayraktutan U. Vitamins reverse endothelial dysfunction through regulation of eNOS and NAD(P)H oxidase activities. *Hypertension* 2003;41:534–539.

[105] Böhm F, Settergren M, Pernow J. Vitamin C blocks vascular dysfunction and release of interleukin-6 induced by endothelin-1 in humans in vivo. *Atherosclerosis* 2007;190:408-415.

[106] Houston MC. Nutraceuticals, vitamins, antioxidants, and minerals in the prevention and treatment of hypertension. *Prog Cardiovasc Dis* 2005;47:396–449

[107] Czernichow S, Bertrais S, Blacher J, Galan P, Briançon S, Favier A, Safar M, Hercberg S. Effect of supplementation with antioxidants upon long-term risk of hypertension in the SU.VI.MAX study: association with plasma antioxidant levels. *J Hypertens* 2005;23:2013-2018.

[108] Duffy SJ, Gokce N, Holbrook M, Huang A, Frei B, Keaney JF Jr, Vita JA. Treatment of hypertension with ascorbic acid. *Lancet* 1999;354:2048–2049.

[109] Bates CJ, Walmsley CM, Prentice A, Finch S. Does vitamin C reduce blood pressure? Results of a large study of people aged 65 or older. *J Hypertens* 1998;16:925–932.

[110] Fotherby MD, Williams JC, Forster LA, Craner P, Ferns GA. Effect of vitamin C on ambulatory blood pressure and plasma lipids in older persons. *J Hypertens* 2000;18:411–415.

[111] Block G, Mangels AR, Norkus EP, Patterson BH, Levander OA, Taylor PR. Ascorbic acid status and subsequent diastolic and systolic blood pressure. *Hypertension* 2001;37:261–267.

[112] Ghosh SK, Ekpo EB, Shah IU, Girling AJ, Jenkins C, Sinclair AJ. A double-blind, placebo-controlled parallel trial of vitamin C treatment in elderly patients with hypertension. *Gerontology* 1994;40:268–272.

[113] Pryor WA, Squadrito GL. The chemistry of peroxynitrite: a product from the reaction of nitric oxide with superoxide. *Am J Physiol* 1995;268:L699–L722.

[114] Padayatty SJ, Katz A, Wang Y, Eck P, Kwon O, Lee JH, Chen S, Corpe C, Dutta A, Dutta SK, Levine M. Vitamin C as an antioxidant: evaluation of its role in disease prevention. *J Am Coll Nutr* 2003;22:18–35.

[115] Padayatty SJ, Sun H, Wang Y, Riordan HD, Hewitt SM, Katz A, Wesley RA, Levine M. Vitamin C pharmacokinetics: implications for oral and intravenous use. *Ann Intern Med* 2004;140:533–537.

[116] Schneider MP, Delles C, Schmidt BM, Oehmer S, Schwarz TK, Schmieder RE, John S. Superoxide scavenging effects of N-acetylcysteine and vitamin C in subjects with essential hypertension. *Am J Hypertens* 2005;18:1111–1117.

[117] Forstermann U. Endothelial NO synthase as a source of NO and superoxide. *Eur J Clin Pharmacol* 2006;62:5–12.

[118] Meydani M. Vitamin E modulation of cardiovascular disease. *Ann NY Acad Sci* 2004; 1031:271–279.

[119] Wu D, Liu L, Meydani M, Meydani SN. Vitamin E increases production of vasodilator prostanoids in human aortic endothelial cells through opposing effects on cyclooxygenase-2 and phospholipase A2. *J Nutr* 2005;135:1847–1853.

[120] Chow CK. Vitamin E regulation of mitochondrial superoxide generation. *Biol Signals Recept* 2001;10:112-124

[121] Rapola JM, Virtamo J, Ripatti S, Huttunen JK, Albanes D, Taylor PR, Heinonen OP. Randomised trial of a-tocopherol and b-carotene supplements on incidence of major coronary events in men with previous myocardial infarction. *Lancet* 1997; 349:1715–1720.

[122] GISSI-Prevenzione Investigators. Dietary supplementation with n-3 polyunsaturated fatty acids and vitamin E after myocardial infarction: results of the GISSI-Prevenzione Trial. *Lancet* 1999; 354:447–455.

[123] Lonn E, Bosch J, Yusuf S, Sheridan P, Pogue J, Arnold JM, Ross C, Arnold A, Sleight P, Probstfield J, Dagenais GR; HOPE and HOPE-TOO Trial Investigators. Effects of long-term vitamin E supplementation on cardiovascular events and cancer: a randomized controlled trial. *JAMA* 2005; 293:1338–1347.

[124] Lee IM, Cook NR, Gaziano JM, Gordon D, Ridker PM, Manson JE, Hennekens CH, Buring JE. Vitamin E in the primary prevention of cardiovascular disease and cancer: the Women's Health Study: a randomized controlled trial. *JAMA* 2005;294:56-65.

[125] Palumbo G, Avanzini F, Alli C, Roncaglioni MC, Ronchi E, Cristofari M, Capra A, Rossi S, Nosotti L, Costantini C, Cavalera C. Effects of vitamin E on clinic and ambulatory blood pressure in treated hypertensive patients. Collaborative Group of the

Primary Prevention Project (PPP)--Hypertension study. *Am J Hypertens* 2000;13:564-567.

[126] Miller ER III, Pastor-Barriuso R, Dalal D, Riemersma RA, Appel LJ, Guallar E. Meta-analysis: high-dosage vitamin E supplementation may increase all-cause mortality. *Ann Intern Med* 2005;142:37–46.

[127] Ward NC, Wu JH, Clarke MW, Puddey IB, Burke V, Croft KD, Hodgson JM. The effect of vitamin E on blood pressure in individuals with type 2 diabetes: a randomized, double-blind, placebo-controlled trial. *J Hypertens* 2007;25:227-234.

[128] Münzel T, Keaney JF Jr. Are ACE inhibitors a "magic bullet" against oxidative stress? *Circulation* 2001;104:1571–1574.

[129] Bilodeau JF, Hubel CA. Current concepts in the use of antioxidants for the treatment of preeclampsia. *J Obstet Gynaecol Can* 2003;25:742–750.

[130] Attia DM, Verhagen AM, Stroes ES, van Faassen EE, Gröne HJ, De Kimpe SJ, Koomans HA, Braam B, Joles JA. Vitamin E alleviates renal injury, but not hypertension, during chronic nitric oxide synthase inhibition in rats. *J Am Soc Nephrol* 2001;12:2585–2593.

[131] Heller R, Werner-Felmayer G, Werner ER. Antioxidants and endothelial nitric oxide synthesis. *Eur J Clin Pharmacol* 2006;62:21–28.

[132] Ward NC, Croft KD. Hypertension and oxidative stress. *Clin Exp Pharmacol Physiol.* 2006;33:872-876.

[133] Mullan B, Young IS, Fee H, McCance DR. Ascorbic acid reduces blood pressure and arterial stiffness in type 2 diabetes. *Hypertension.* 2002;40:804–809.

[134] Galley HF, Thornton J, Howdle PD, Walker BE, Webster NR. Combination oral antioxidant supplementation reduces blood pressure. *Clin Sci* 1997;92:361–365.

[135] Sorescu D, Weiss D, Lassègue B, Clempus RE, Szöcs K, Sorescu GP, Valppu L, Quinn MT, Lambeth JD, Vega JD, Taylor WR, Griendling KK. Superoxide production and expression of nox family proteins in human atherosclerosis. *Circulation* 2002;105:1429–1435.

[136] Nickenig G, Bäumer AT, Temur Y, Kebben D, Jockenhövel F, Böhm M. Statin-sensitive dysregulated AT1 receptor function and density in hypercholesterolemic men. *Circulation* 1999;100:2131–2134.

[137] Rodrigo R, Prat H, Passalacqua W, Araya J, Bächler JP. Decrease in oxidative stress through supplementation of vitamins C and E is associated with a reduction in blood pressure in patients with essential hypertension. *Clin Sci* 2008;114:625-634.

[138] Tian N, Rose RA, Jordan S, Dwyer TM, Hughson MD, Manning RD Jr. N-Acetylcystcine improves renal dysfunction, ameliorates kidney damage and decreases blood pressure in salt-sensitive hypertension. *J Hypertens* 2006;24:2263-2270.

[139] El Midaoui A, Ismael MA, Lu H, Fantus IG, de Champlain J, Couture R. Comparative effects of N-acetylcysteine and ramipril on arterial hypertension, insulin resistance, and oxidative stress in chronically glucose-fed rats. *Can J Physiol Pharmacol* 2008;86:752-760.

[140] Rauchová H, Pechánová O, Kunes J, Vokurková M, Dobesová Z, Zicha J. Chronic N-acetylcysteine administration prevents development of hypertension in N(omega)-nitro-L-arginine methyl ester-treated rats: the role of reactive oxygen species. *Hypertens Res* 2005;28:475-482.

[141] Martina V, Masha A, Gigliardi VR, Brocato L, Manzato E, Berchio A, Massarenti P, Settanni F, Della Casa L, Bergamini S, Iannone A. Long-term N-acetylcysteine and L-arginine administration reduces endothelial activation and systolic blood pressure in hypertensive patients with type 2 diabetes. *Diabetes Care* 2008;31:940-944.

[142] Thaha M, Widodo, Pranawa W, Yogiantoro M, Tomino Y. Intravenous N-acetylcysteine during hemodialysis reduces asymmetric dimethylarginine level in end-stage renal disease patients. *Clin Nephrol* 2008;69:24-32.

[143] Zembowicz A, Hatchett RJ, Radziszewski W, Gryglewski RJ. Inhibition of endothelial nitric oxide synthase by ebselen. Prevention by thiols suggests the inactivation by ebselen of a critical thiol essential for the catalytic activity of nitric oxide synthase. *J Pharmacol Exp Ther* 1993;267:1112-1118

[144] Schini-Kerth VB, Auger C, Etienne-Selloum N, Chataigneau T. Polyphenol-induced endothelium-dependent relaxations role of NO and EDHF. *Adv Pharmacol.* 2010;60:133-175.

[145] Tang EH, Vanhoutte PM. Endothelial dysfunction: a strategic target in the treatment of hypertension? *Pflugers Arch.* 2010;459:995-1004.

[146] Kane MO, Etienne-Selloum N, Madeira SV, Sarr M, Walter A, Dal-Ros S, Schott C, Chataigneau T, Schini-Kerth VB. Endothelium-derived contracting factors mediate the Ang II-induced endothelial dysfunction in the rat aorta: preventive effect of red wine polyphenols. *Pflugers Arch.* 2010;459:671-679.

[147] Nijveldt RJ, van Nood E, van Hoorn DE, Boelens PG, van Norren K, van Leeuwen PA. Flavonoids: a review of probable mechanisms of action and potential applications. *Am J Clin Nutr.* 2001;74:418-425

[148] Schini-Kerth VB, Auger C, Kim JH, Etienne-Selloum N, Chataigneau T. Nutritional improvement of the endothelial control of vascular tone by polyphenols: role of NO and EDHF. *Pflugers Arch* 2010 ;459:853-862

[149] Mombouli JV, Vanhoutte PM. Endothelial dysfunction: from physiology to therapy. *J Mol Cell Cardiol* 1999;31:61-74.

[150] Dimmeler S, Fleming I, Fisslthaler B, Hermann C, Busse R, Zeiher AM. Activation of nitric oxide synthase in endothelial cells by Akt-dependent phosphorylation. *Nature* 1999;399:601-605.

[151] Klinge CM, Blankenship KA, Risinger KE, Bhatnagar S, Noisin EL, Sumanasekera WK, Zhao L, Brey DM, Keynton RS. Resveratrol and estradiol rapidly activate MAPK signaling through estrogen receptors alpha and beta in endothelial cells. *J Biol Chem* 2005;280:7460-7468.

[152] Anter E, Chen K, Shapira OM, Karas RH, Keaney JF Jr. p38 mitogen-activated protein kinase activates eNOS in endothelial cells by an estrogen receptor alpha-dependent pathway in response to black tea polyphenols. *Circ Res* 2005;96:1072-1078.

[153] Li Y, Ying C, Zuo X, Yi H, Yi W, Meng Y, Ikeda K, Ye X, Yamori Y, Sun X. Green tea polyphenols down-regulate caveolin-1 expression via ERK1/2 and p38MAPK in endothelial cells. *J Nutr Biochem* 2009;20:1021-1027.

[154] Leikert JF, Räthel TR, Wohlfart P, Cheynier V, Vollmar AM, Dirsch VM. Red wine polyphenols enhance endothelial nitric oxide synthase expression and subsequent nitric oxide release from endothelial cells. *Circulation* 2002;106:1614-1617.

[155] Mattagajasingh I, Kim CS, Naqvi A, Yamamori T, Hoffman TA, Jung SB, DeRicco J, Kasuno K, Irani K. SIRT1 promotes endothelium-dependent vascular relaxation by

activating endothelial nitric oxide synthase. *Proc Natl Acad Sci U S A* 2007;104:14855-14860.

[156] Miyazaki R, Ichiki T, Hashimoto T, Inanaga K, Imayama I, Sadoshima J, Sunagawa K. SIRT1, a longevity gene, downregulates angiotensin II type 1 receptor expression in vascular smooth muscle cells. *Arterioscler Thromb Vasc Biol* 2008;28:1263-1269.

[157] Albani D, Polito L, Forloni G. Sirtuins as novel targets for Alzheimer's disease and other neurodegenerative disorders: experimental and genetic evidence. *J Alzheimers Dis.* 2010;19:11-26.

[158] Polito L, Kehoe PG, Forloni G, Albani D. The molecular genetics of sirtuins: association with human longevity and age-related diseases. *Int J Mol Epidemiol Genet.* 2010;1:214-225.

[159] Ndiaye M, Chataigneau T, Chataigneau M, Schini-Kerth VB. Red wine polyphenols induce EDHF-mediated relaxations in porcine coronary arteries through the redox-sensitive activation of the PI3-kinase/Akt pathway. *Br J Pharmacol* 2004;142:1131-1136.

[160] Dal-Ros S, Bronner C, Schott C, Kane MO, Chataigneau M, Schini-Kerth VB, Chataigneau T. Angiotensin II-induced hypertension is associated with a selective inhibition of endothelium-derived hyperpolarizing factor-mediated responses in the rat mesenteric artery. *J Pharmacol Exp Ther* 2009;328:478-486.

[161] Ndiaye M, Chataigneau M, Lobysheva I, Chataigneau T, Schini-Kerth VB. Red wine polyphenol-induced, endothelium-dependent NO-mediated relaxation is due to the redox-sensitive PI3-kinase/Akt-dependent phosphorylation of endothelial NO-synthase in the isolated porcine coronary artery. *Faseb J* 2005;19:455–457.

[162] Alonso A, de la Fuente C, Martín-Arnau AM, de Irala J, Martínez JA, Martínez-González MA. Fruit and vegetable consumption is inversely associated with blood pressure in a Mediterranean population with a high vegetable-fat intake: the Seguimiento Universidad de Navarra (SUN) Study. *Br J Nutr* 2004;92:311-319.

[163] Estruch R, Martínez-González MA, Corella D, Salas-Salvadó J, Ruiz-Gutiérrez V, Covas MI, Fiol M, Gómez-Gracia E, López-Sabater MC, Vinyoles E, Arós F, Conde M, Lahoz C, Lapetra J, Sáez G, Ros E; PREDIMED Study Investigators. Effects of a Mediterranean-style diet on cardiovascular risk factors: a randomized trial. *Ann Intern Med.* 2006;145:1-11.

[164] Medina-Remón A, Zamora-Ros R, Rotchés-Ribalta M, Andres-Lacueva C, Martínez-González MA, Covas MI, Corella D, Salas-Salvadó J, Gómez-Gracia E, Ruiz-Gutiérrez V, García de la Corte FJ, Fiol M, Pena MA, Saez GT, Ros E, Serra-Majem L, Pinto X, Warnberg J, Estruch R, Lamuela-Raventos RM; on behalf of the PREDIMED Study Investigators. Total polyphenol excretion and blood pressure in subjects at high cardiovascular risk. *Nutr Metab Cardiovasc Dis.* 2011;21:323-331.

[165] Panagiotakos DB, Pitsavos CH, Chrysohoou C, Skoumas J, Papadimitriou L, Stefanadis C, Toutouzas PK. Status and management of hypertension in Greece: role of the adoption of a Mediterranean diet: the Attica study. *J Hypertens* 2003;21:1483-1489.

[166] Martínez-González MA, Fernández-Jarne E, Serrano-Martínez M, Marti A, Martinez JA, Martín-Moreno JM. Mediterranean diet and reduction in the risk of a first acute myocardial infarction: an operational healthy dietary score. *Eur J Nutr* 2002 ;41:153-160.

[167] Schroder H, Schmelz E, Marrugat J. Relationship between diet and blood pressure in a representative Mediterranean population. *Eur J Nutr* 2002;41:161–167.

[168] Peng N, Clark JT, Prasain J, Kim H, White CR, Wyss JM. Antihypertensive and cognitive effects of grape polyphenols in estrogen-depleted, female, spontaneously hypertensive rats. *Am J Physiol Regul Integr Comp Physiol.* 2005;289:771-775.

[169] Bernátová I, Pechánová O, Babál P, Kyselá S, Stvrtina S, Andriantsitohaina R. Wine polyphenols improve cardiovascular remodeling and vascular function in NO-deficient hypertension. *Am J Physiol Heart Circ Physiol.* 2002;282:942-948.

[170] Jiménez R, López-Sepúlveda R, Kadmiri M, Romero M, Vera R, Sánchez M, Vargas F, O'Valle F, Zarzuelo A, Dueñas M, Santos-Buelga C, Duarte J. Polyphenols restore endothelial function in DOCA-salt hypertension: role of endothelin-1 and NADPH oxidase. *Free Radic Biol Med* 2007;43:462-473.

[171] Sarr M, Chataigneau M, Martins S, Schott C, El Bedoui J, Oak MH, Muller B, Chataigneau T, Schini-Kerth VB. Red wine polyphenols prevent angiotensin II-induced hypertension and endothelial dysfunction in rats: role of NADPH oxidase. *Cardiovasc Res* 2006;71:794-802.

[172] Zenebe W, Pechánová O, Andriantsitohaina R. Red wine polyphenols induce vasorelaxation by increased nitric oxide bioactivity. *Physiol Res* 2003;52:425–432.

[173] Hodgson JM, Puddey IB, Burke V, Watts GF, Beilin LJ. Regular ingestion of black tea improves brachial artery vasodilator function. *Clin Sci* 2002;102:195-201.

[174] Perez-Vizcaino F, Duarte J, Andriantsitohaina R. Endothelial function and cardiovascular disease: effects of quercetin and wine polyphenols. *Free Radic Res* 2006;40:1054–1065.

[175] Grassi D, Necozione S, Lippi C, Croce G, Valeri L, Pasqualetti P, Desideri G, Blumberg JB, Ferri C. Cocoa reduces blood pressure and insulin resistance and improves endothelium-dependent vasodilation in hypertensives. *Hypertension* 2005;46:398-405.

[176] Taubert D, Berkels R, Roesen R, Klaus W. Chocolate and blood pressure in elderly individuals with isolated systolic hypertension. *JAMA* 2003;290:1029-1030.

[177] Duffy SJ, Keaney JF Jr, Holbrook M, Gokce N, Swerdloff PL, Frei B, Vita JA. Short- and long-term black tea consumption reverses endothelial dysfunction in patients with coronary artery disease. *Circulation* 2001;104:151-156.

[178] Hodgson JM, Devine A, Puddey IB, Chan SY, Beilin LJ, Prince RL. Tea intake is inversely related to blood pressure in older women. *J Nutr* 2003;133:2883 2886.

[179] Yang YC, Lu FH, Wu JS, Wu CH, Chang CJ. The protective effect of habitual tea consumption on hypertension. *Arch Intern Med* 2004;164.1534-1540.

[180] Wollgast J, Pallaroni L, Agazzi ME, Anklam E. Analysis of procyanidins in chocolate by reversed-phase high-performance liquid chromatography with electrospray ionisation mass spectrometric and tandem mass spectrometric detection. *J Chromatogr A* 2001;926:211-220.

[181] Arts IC, Hollman PC, Feskens EJ, Bueno de Mesquita HB, Kromhout D. Catechin intake might explain the inverse relation between tea consumption and ischemic heart disease: the Zutphen Elderly Study. *Am J Clin Nutr* 2001;74:227-232.

[182] Buijsse B, Feskens EJ, Kok FJ, Kromhout D. Cocoa intake, blood pressure, and cardiovascular mortality: the Zutphen Elderly Study. *Arch Intern Med* 2006;166:411-417.

[183] McCullough ML, Chevaux K, Jackson L, Preston M, Martinez G, Schmitz HH, Coletti C, Campos H, Hollenberg NK. Hypertension, the Kuna, and the epidemiology of flavanols. *J Cardiovasc Pharmacol* 2006;47:S103-S109.

[184] Actis-Goretta L, Ottaviani JI, Keen CL, Fraga CG. Inhibition of angiotensin converting enzyme (ACE) activity by flavan-3-ols and procyanidins. *FEBS Lett* 2003;555:597–600.

[185] Actis-Goretta L, Ottaviani JI, Fraga CG. Inhibition of angiotensin converting enzyme activity by flavanol-rich foods. *J Agric Food Chem* 2006;54:229-234.

[186] Ottaviani JI, Actis-Goretta L, Villordo JJ, Fraga CG. Procyanidin structure defines the extent and specificity of angiotensin I converting enzyme inhibition. *Biochimie* 2006;88:359-365.

[187] Stowe CB. The effects of pomegranate juice consumption on blood pressure and cardiovascular health. *Complement Ther Clin Pract* 2011;17:113-115.

[188] Raederstorff D. Antioxidant activity of olive polyphenols in humans: a review. *Int J Vitam Nutr Res* 2009;79:152-165.

[189] Psaltopoulou T, Naska A, Orfanos P, Trichopoulos D, Mountokalakis T, Trichopoulou A. Olive oil, the Mediterranean diet, and arterial blood pressure: the Greek European Prospective Investigation into Cancer and Nutrition (EPIC) study. *Am J Clin Nutr* 2004;80:1012-1018.

[190] Alonso A, Martínez-González MA. Olive oil consumption and reduced incidence of hypertension: the SUN study. *Lipids* 2004b;39: 1233-1238.

[191] de Lorimier AA. Alcohol, wine and health. *Am J Surg* 2000;180:357-361.

[192] Wannamethee SG, Shaper AG. Type of alcoholic drink and risk of major coronary heart disease events and all-cause mortality. *Am J Publ Health* 1999;89:685–690.

[193] De Lorgeril M, Salen P, Martin JL, Mamelle N, Monjaud I, Touboul P, Delaye J. Effect of a mediterranean type of diet on the rate of cardiovascular complications in patients with coronary artery disease. Insights into the cardioprotective effect of certain nutriments. *J Am Coll Cardiol.* 1996;28:1103-1108.

[194] Opie LH, Lecour S. The red wine hypothesis: from concepts to protective signalling molecules. *Eur Heart J* 2007;28:1683-1693.

[195] de Lorgeril M, Salen P, Paillard F, Laporte F, Boucher F, de Leiris J. Mediterranean diet and the French paradox: two distinct biogeographic concepts for one consolidated scientific theory on the role of nutrition in coronary heart disease. *Cardiovasc Res* 2002;54:503–515.

[196] Renaud S, de Lorgeril M. Wine, alcohol, platelets, and the French paradox for coronary heart disease. *Lancet* 1992;339:1523–1526.

[197] Karatzi KN, Papamichael CM, Karatzis EN, Papaioannou TG, Aznaouridis KA, Katsichti PP, Stamatelopoulos KS, Zampelas A, Lekakis JP, Mavrikakis ME. Red wine acutely induces favorable effects on wave reflections and central pressures in coronary artery disease patients. *Am J Hypertens* 2005;18:1161–1167.

[198] Papamichael C, Karatzi K, Karatzis E, Papaioannou TG, Katsichti P, Zampelas A, Lekakis J. Combined acute effects of red wine consumption and cigarette smoking on haemodynamics of young smokers. *J Hypertens* 2006;24:1287–1292.

[199] Brown L, Kroon PA, Das DK, Das S, Tosaki A, Chan V, Singer MV, Feick P. The biological responses to resveratrol and other polyphenols from alcoholic beverages. *Alcohol Clin Exp Res.* 2009;33:1513-1523.

[200] Rimm EB, Williams P, Fosher K, Criqui M, Stampfer MJ. Moderate alcohol intake and lower risk of coronary heart disease: metaanalysis of effects on lipids and haemostatic factors. *BMJ* 1999;319:1523–1528.

[201] Bello AT, Bora NS, Lange LG, Bora PS. Cardioprotective effects of alcohol: mediation by human vascular alcohol dehydrogenase. *Biochem Biophys Res Commun.* 1994;203:1858-64.

[202] Stoclet JC, Chataigneau T, Ndiaye M, Oak MH, El Bedoui J, Chataigneau M, Schini-Kerth VB. Vascular protection by dietary polyphenols. *Eur J Pharmacol* 2004;500:299–313.

[203] Dell'Agli M, Galli GV, Vrhovsek U, Mattivi F, Bosisio E. In vitro inhibition of human cGMP-specific phosphodiesterase-5 by polyphenols from red grapes. *J Agric Food Chem* 2005;53:1960–1965.

[204] Medić-Šarić M, Rastija V, Bojić M, Males Z. From functional food to medicinal product: systematic approach in analysis of polyphenolics from propolis and wine. *Nutr J* 2009;8:33.

[205] Rodrigo R, Miranda A, Vergara L. Modulation of endogenous antioxidant system by wine polyphenols in human disease. *Clin Chim Acta* 2011;412:410-424

[206] Andriambeloson E, Kleschyov AL, Muller B, Beretz A, Stoclet JC, Andriantsitohaina R. Nitric oxide production and endothelium-dependent vasorelaxation induced by wine polyphenols in rat aorta. *Br J Pharmacol* 1997;120:1053-1058.

[207] Andriambeloson E, Magnier C, Haan-Archipoff G, Lobstein A, Anton R, Beretz A, Stoclet JC, Andriantsitohaina R. Natural dietary polyphenolic compounds cause endotheliumdependent vasorelaxation in rat thoracic aorta. *J Nutr* 1998;128:2324-2333.

[208] Fitzpatrick DF, Bing B, Maggi DA, Fleming RC, O'Malley RM. Vasodilating procyanidins derived from grape seeds. *Ann N Y Acad Sci* 2002;957:78-89.

[209] Tsang C, Higgins S, Duthie GG, Duthie SJ, Howie M, Mullen W, Lean ME, Crozier A. The influence of moderate red wine consumption on antioxidant status and indices of oxidative stress associated with CHD in healthy volunteers. *Br J Nutr.* 2005;93:233-240.

[210] Soleas GJ, Grass L, Josephy PD, Goldberg DM, Diamandis EP. A comparison of the anticarcinogenic properties of four red wine polyphenols. *Clin Biochem* 2006;39:492–497.

[211] Fitzpatrick D, Hirschfield SL, Coffey RG. Endothelium dependent relaxing activity of wine and other grape products. *Am J Physiol* 1993;265:H774-H778.

[212] Flesch M, Schwarz A, Böhm M. Effects of red wine on endothelium-dependent vasorelaxatin of rat aorta and human coronary arteries. *Am J Physiol* 1998;275:H1183-H1190.

[213] Martin S, Andriambeloson E, Takeda K, Andriantsitohaina R. Red wine polyphenols increase calcium in bovine aortic endothelial cells: a basis to elucidate signalling pathways leading to nitric oxide production. *Br J Pharmacol* 2002;135:1579 –1587.

[214] Mizutani K, Ikeda K, Kawai Y, Yamori Y. Extract of wine phenolics improves aortic biomechanical properties in stroke-prone spontaneously hypertensive rats (SHRSP). *J Nutr Sci Vitaminol* 1999;45:95 – 106.

[215] Diebolt M, Bucher B, Andriantsitohaina R. Wine polyphenols decrease blood pressure, improve NO vasodilatation, and induce gene expression. *Hypertension* 2001;38:159–165.

[216] Perez-Vizcaino F, Duarte J, Jimenez R, Santos-Buelga C, Osuna A. Antihypertensive effects of the flavonoid quercetin. *Pharmacol Rep* 2009;61:67-75.

[217] Matsuo S, Nakamura Y, Takahashi M, Ouchi Y, Hosoda K, Nozawa M, Kinoshita M. Effect of red wine and ethanol on production of nitric oxide in healthy subjects. *Am J Cardiol* 2001;87:1029–1031.

[218] Hashimoto M, Kim S, Eto M, Iijima K, Ako J, Yoshizumi M, Akishita M, Kondo K, Itakura H, Hosoda K, Toba K, Ouchi Y. Effect of acute intake of red wine on flow-mediated vasodilatation of the brachial artery. *Am J Cardiol* 2001;88:1457-1460.

[219] Burns J, Gardner PT, O'Neil J, Crawford S, Morecroft I, McPhail DB, Lister C, Matthews D, MacLean MR, Lean ME, Duthie GG, Crozier A. Relationship among antioxidant activity, vasodilation capacity, and phenolic content of red wines. *J Agric Food Chem* 2000;48:220-230.

[220] Chalopin M, Tesse A, Martínez MC, Rognan D, Arnal JF, Andriantsitohaina R. Estrogen receptor alpha as a key target of red wine polyphenols action on the endothelium. *PLoS ONE* 2010;5:e8554.

[221] Derek D, Pearson DA, German JB. Endothelial cell basal PGI2 release is stimulated by wine in vitro: one mechanism that may mediate the vasoprotective effects of wine. *J Nutr Biochem* 1997;8:647 – 651.

[222] Corder R, Douthwaite JA, Lees DM, Khan NQ, Viseu Dos Santos AC, Wood EG, Carrier MJ. Endothelin-1 synthesis reduced by red wine. *Nature.* 2001;414:863-864.

[223] Vera R, Sánchez M, Galisteo M, Villar IC, Jimenez R, Zarzuelo A, Pérez-Vizcaíno F, Duarte J. Chronic administration of genistein improves endothelial dysfunction in spontaneously hypertensive rats: involvement of eNOS, caveolin and calmodulin expression and NADPH oxidase activity. *Clin Sci* 2007;112:183-191.

[224] Yamamoto M, Suzuki A, Hase T. Short-term effects of glucosyl hesperidin and hesperetin on blood pressure and vascular endothelial function in spontaneously hypertensive rats. *J Nutr Sci Vitaminol* 2008;54:95-98.

[225] Egert S, Boesch-Saadatmandi C, Wolffram S, Rimbach G, Müller MJ. Serum lipid and blood pressure responses to quercetin vary in overweight patients by apolipoprotein E genotype. *J Nutr* 2010;140:278–284.

[226] Loke WM, Hodgson JM, Proudfoot JM, McKinley AJ, Puddey IB, Croft KD. Pure dietary flavonoids quercetin and (-)-epicatechin augment nitric oxide products and reduce endothelin-1 acutely in healthy men. *Am J Clin Nutr.* 2008;88:1018-1025.

[227] Conquer JA, Maiani G, Azzini E, Raguzzini A, Holub BJ.Supplementation with quercetin markedly increases plasma quercetin concentration without effect on selected risk factors for heart disease in healthy subjects. *J Nutr.* 1998;128:593-597.

[228] Edwards RL, Lyon T, Litwin SE, Rabovsky A, Symons JD, Jalili T.Quercetin reduces blood pressure in hypertensive subjects. *J Nutr.* 2007;137:2405-2411.

[229] Gu J, Wang CQ, Fan HH, Ding HY, Xie XL, Xu YM, Wang BY, Huang DJ. Effects of resveratrol on endothelial progenitor cells and their contributions to reendothelialization in intima-injured rats. *J Cardiovasc Pharmacol* 2006;47:711–721.

[230] Liu Z, Song Y, Zhang X, Liu Z, Zhang W, Mao W, Wang W, Cui W, Zhang X, Jia X, Li N, Han C, Liu C. Effects of trans-resveratrol on hypertension-induced cardiac

hypertrophy using the partially nephrectomized rat model. *Clin Exp Pharmacol Physiol* 2005;32:1049-1054.

[231] Li HF, Chen SA, Wu SN. Evidence for the stimulatory effect of resveratrol on Ca(2+)-activated K+ current in vascular endothelial cells. *Cardiovasc Res* 2000;45:1035–1045.

[232] McKenna E, Smith JS, Coll KE, Mazack EK, Mayer EJ, Antanavage J, Wiedmann RT, Johnson RG Jr. Dissociation of phospholamban regulation of cardiac sarcoplasmic reticulum Ca2+-ATPase by quercetin. *J Biol Chem* 1996;271:24517–24525.

[233] Chow SE, Hshu YC, Wang JS, Chen JK. Resveratrol attenuates ox-LDL-stimulated NADPH oxidase activity and protects endothelial cells from oxidative functional damages. *J Appl Physiol* 2007;102:1520–1527.

[234] Miatello R, Vázquez M, Renna N, Cruzado M, Zumino AP, Risler N. Chronic administration of resveratrol prevents biochemical cardiovascular changes in fructose-fed rats. *Am J Hypertens* 2005;18:864-870.

[235] Mizutani K, Ikeda K, Kawai Y, Yamori Y. Protective effect of resveratrol on oxidative damage in male and female stroke-prone spontaneously hypertensive rats. *Clin Exp Pharmacol Physiol* 2001;28:55–59.

[236] Carlstrom J, Symons JD, Wu TC, Bruno RS, Litwin SE, Jalili T. A quercetin supplemented diet does not prevent cardiovascular complications in spontaneously hypertensive rats. *J Nutr* 2007;137:628–633.

[237] Schroeter H, Heiss C, Balzer J, Kleinbongard P, Keen CL, Hollenberg NK, Sies H, Kwik-Uribe C, Schmitz HH, Kelm M. (−)-Epicatechin mediates beneficial effects of flavanol-rich cocoa on vascular function in humans. *Proc Natl Acad Sci* U S A 2006;103:1024–1029.

[238] Heiss C, Finis D, Kleinbongard P, Hoffmann A, Rassaf T, Kelm M, Sies H. Sustained increase in flow-mediated dilation after daily intake of high-flavanol cocoa drink over 1 week. *J Cardiovasc Pharmacol* 2007;49:74–80.

[239] Widlansky ME, Hamburg NM, Anter E, Holbrook M, Kahn DF, Elliott JG, Keaney JF Jr, Vita JA. Acute EGCG supplementation reverses endothelial dysfunction in patients with coronary artery disease. *J Am Coll Nutr* 2007;26:95-102.

[240] Corder R, Mullen W, Khan NQ, Marks SC, Wood EG, Carrier MJ, Crozier A. Oenology: red wine procyanidins and vascular health. *Nature* 2006;444:566.

[241] Zhao X, Gu Z, Attele AS, Yuan CS. Effects of quercetin on the release of endothelin, prostacyclin and tissue plasminogen activator from human endothelial cells in culture. *J Ethnopharmacol* 1999;67:279-285.

[242] Deyama T, Nishibe S, Nakazawa Y. Constituents and pharmacological effects of Eucommia and Siberian ginseng. *Acta Pharmacol Sin* 2001;22:1057-1070.

[243] Kwan CY, Zhang WB, Deyama T, Nishibe S. Endothelium-dependent vascular relaxation induced by Eucommia ulmoides Oliv. bark extract is mediated by NO and EDHF in small vessels. *Naunyn Schmiedebergs Arch Pharmacol* 2004;369:206-211.

[244] Dal-Ros S, Bronner C, Schott C, Kane MO, Chataigneau M, Schini-Kerth VB, Chataigneau T. Angiotensin II-induced hypertension is associated with a selective inhibition of endothelium-derived hyperpolarizing factor-mediated responses in the rat mesenteric artery. *J Pharmacol Exp Ther.* 2009;328:478-486.

[245] Jenkinson CP, Grody WW, Cederbaum SD. Comparative properties of arginases. *Comp Biochem Phys* 1996;114:107–132.

[247] Buga GM, Singh R, Pervin S, Rogers NE, Schmitz DA, Jenkinson CP, Cederbaum SD, Ignarro LJ. Arginase activity in endothelial cells: inhibition by NG-hydroxy-L-arginine during high-output NO production. *Am J Physiol.* 1996;271:H1988-1998.

[248] Ignarro LJ, Buga G, Wie LH, Bauer PM, Wu G, del Soldato P. Role of arginine-nitric oxide pathway in the regulation of vascular smooth muscle cell proliferation. *Proc Natl Acad Sci* USA 2001;98:4202–4208.

[249] Zhang C, Hein TW, Wang W, Miller MW, Chang CI, Kuo L. Constitutive expression of arginase in microvascular endothelial cells counteracts nitric-oxide-mediated vasodilatory function. *FASEB J* 2001;15:1264–1266.

[250] Demougeot C, Prigent-Tessier A, Marie C, Berthelot A. Arginase inhibition reduces endothelial dysfunction and blood pressure rising in spontaneously hypertensive rats. *J Hypertens* 2005;25:971–978.

[251] Ryoo S, Gupta G, Benjo A, Lim HK, Camara A, Sikka G, Lim HK, Sohi J, Santhanam L, Soucy K, Tuday E, Baraban E, Ilies M, Gerstenblith G, Nyhan D, Shoukas A, Christianson DW, Alp NJ, Champion HC, Huso D, Berkowitz DE. Endothelial arginase II: a novel target for the treatment of atherosclerosis. *Circ Res.* 2008;102:923-932.

[252] Kashyap SR, Lara A, Zhang R, Park YM, DeFronzo RA. Insulin reduces plasma arginase activity in type 2 diabetic patients. *Diabetes Care* 2008;31:134–139.

[253] Masuda H. Significance of nitric oxide and its modulation mechanisms by endogenous nitric oxide synthase inhibitors and arginase in the micturition disorders and erectile dysfunction. *Int J Urol* 2008;15:128–134.

[254] Berkowitz DE, White R, Li D, Minhas KM, Cernetich A, Kim S, Burke S, Shoukas AA, Nyhan D, Champion HC, Hare JM. Arginase reciprocally regulates nitric oxide synthase activity and contributes to endothelial dysfunction in aging blood vessels. *Circulation.* 2003;108:2000-2006.

[255] Bagnost T, Ma L, da Silva RF, Rezakhaniha R, Houdayer C, Stergiopulos N, André C, Guillaume Y, Berthelot A, Demougeot C. Cardiovascular effects of arginase inhibition in spontaneously hypertensive rats with fully developed hypertension. *Cardiovasc Res* 2010;87:569-577.

[256] Bernardi F, Constantino L, Machado R, Petronilho F, Dal-Pizzol F. Plasma nitric oxide, endothelin-1, arginase and superoxide dismutase in pre-eclamptic women. *J Obste Gynaecol Res* 2008;34:957–963.

[257] Meroufel D, Dumont J, Médiène-Benchekor S, Benhammamouch S, Ducimetière P, Cottel D, Montaye M, Amouyel P, Brousseau T. Characterization of arginase 1 gene polymorphisms in the Algerian population and association with blood pressure. *Clin Biochem* 2009;42:1178-1182.

[258] Dumont J, Zureik M, Cottel D, Montaye M, Ducimetière P, Amouyel P, Brousseau T. Association of arginase 1 gene polymorphisms with the risk of myocardial infarction and common carotid intima media thickness. *J Med Genet* 2007;44: 526-531.

In: Advances in Hypertension Research
Editor: Ramón Rodrigo

ISBN: 978-1-62948-857-8

Chapter 2

Endothelial Dysfunction and Hypertension*

Felipe Feliú*† *and Daniel Hasson
[1]Molecular and Clinical Pharmacology Program, Institute of Biomedical Sciences, Faculty of Medicine, University of Chile, Chile

Abstract

The endothelial layer of blood vessels is critical to vascular health and plays an important role in the pathophysiology of hypertension. Endothelial dysfunction is characterized by a switch on endothelial function to a proinflammatory, prothrombotic, vasoconstricting state. Oxidative stress is a common denominator in many pathologies and an integrative model for endothelial dysfunction through an inhibiting effect on the nitric oxide, prostacyclin, and endothelial-derived hyperpolarizing factor pathways, which are the major endothelium-dependent vasodilator pathways. There is currently no "gold standard" method for the evaluation of endothelial dysfunction and existing ones are very varied, but can be roughly divided in functional and biochemical methods. Functional ones measure endothelium-dependent vasodilation whereas biochemical methods assess circulating endothelial-derived molecules. Current established antihypertensive therapies have diverse effects on endothelial function while therapies targeting endothelial dysfunction as a primary endpoint, although they are well underway, currently show a modest effect on blood pressure and do not have clinical expression. The nature of these therapies is diverse and goes from lifestyle changes to molecules acting as transcription enhancers. This chapter presents a synthesis of the current knowledge in endothelial dysfunction, approaching its pathophysiology, diagnosis and treatment, in order to be a solid basis for clinical practice.

Keywords: Endothelial dysfunction, brachial flow mediated dilation, pulse amplitude tonometry, hypertension treatment, cNOS modulators

---

* Supported by FONDECYT, grant 1120594.
† Corresponding author: Lic. Felipe Feliú. Molecular and Clinical Pharmacology Program, Institute of Biomedical Sciences, Faculty of Medicine, University of Chile, Independencia 1027, C.P 8380453, Santiago 7, Chile. Telephone: 56-2-29786126 Fax: 56-2-29786126; E-mail: afeliusoto@gmail.com.

Abbreviations

ADMA	asymmetric dimethyl arginine
AT-II	angiotensin II
CAD	coronary artery disease
CNP	C-natriuretic peptide
COX	cyclooxygenase
BH_2	dihydrobiopterin
BH_4	tetrahydrobiopterin
EC	epicatechin
EDCF	endothelium-derived contracting factor
EDHF	endothelial-derived hyperpolarizing factor
EETs	epoxyeicosatrienoic acids
eNOS	endothelial nitric oxide synthase
EPC	endothelial progenitor cells
ET	endothelin
ET-1	endothelin-1
FMD	flow mediated dilation
H_2O_2	hydrogen peroxide
L-NAME	Nω-nitro-L-arginine methyl ester
L-NMMA	NG-monomethyl L-arginine
NO	nitric oxide
O_2•–	superoxide anion
ONOO–	peroxynitrite
PAT	pulse amplitude tonometry
PGI2	prostacyclin
SHR	spontaneously hypertensive rat
SHRSP	stroke-prone spontaneously hypertensive rat
VSMC	vascular smooth muscle cell
WKY	Wistar-Kyoto rats

1. Introduction

Although the endothelium forms a single layer of cells, the total volume of the endothelial cells of the human body is comparable to that of the liver [1]. The endothelium is a major regulator of local vascular homeostasis through several actions: maintenance of the balance between vasodilation and vasoconstriction; inhibition and promotion of the proliferation and migration of smooth muscle cells; prevention and stimulation of the adhesion and aggregation of platelets and participating in thrombogenesis and fibrinolysis [2]. The endothelium achieves these tasks by sensing mechanical and hormonal stimuli to which it responds, in the case of vascular tone, by releasing agents that regulate vasomotor function. [Table 2.1] [3].

Table 2.1. Endothelium mediators of vascular tone

Endothelium relaxing factors	Endothelium contracting factors
Adenosine prostacyclin (PGI2) nitric oxide (NO) hydrogen peroxide (H_2O_2) epoxyeicosatrienoic acids (EETs) C-natriuretic peptide (CNP)	thromboxane A2 isoprostanes 20-hydroxyeicosatetraenoic acid superoxide anion ($O_2^{\bullet-}$) H_2O_2 endothelin-1(ET-1) angiotensin II (AT-II) uridine adenosine tetraphosphate

Under physiological conditions the endothelium shows a predominantly vasorelaxant activity, nevertheless, under some pathophysiological circumstances it switches to a prothrombotic, proinflammatory and vasoconstricting phenotype, characterized by a higher release of ET-1, AT-II, urotensin II, superoxide anions, vasoconstrictor prostaglandins and thromboxane A2 and a paradoxical vasoconstricting response to acethylcoline [4].

The term "endothelial dysfunction" was coined in the mid-eighties, following the major breakthrough by Furchgott and Zawadzki [5] who discovered that acetylcholine requires the presence of endothelial cells to relax the underlying vascular smooth muscle. The factor that was released by acetylcholine, first termed as endothelium-derived relaxing factor (EDRF), was identified later by Palmer, Ferrige and Moncada as nitric oxide (NO) [6]. On the other hand, it had already been observed that the endothelium-dependent relaxations in the aorta of hypertensive rats were impaired [7]; [8]. Since then, this "endothelial dysfunction" has been associated not only with hypertension, but also with physiological and pathophysiological processes, including aging, heart and renal failure, preeclampsia, type 1 and type 2 diabetes mellitus, atherosclerosis, inflammation, among others [3]. This suggests an underlying mechanism connecting these phenotypes that could explain their association with endothelial dysfunction.

Endothelial dysfunction is considered a hallmark of hypertension and may reflect the premature aging of the intima exposed to chronic blood pressure increase [9]. Characteristic findings in essential hypertension are an impaired vasomotor response, vascular smooth muscle cell (VSMC) proliferation and migration, extracellular matrix protein deposition, platelet activation, vascular permeability, and a proinflammatory and prothrombotic phenotype [10-12]. In essential hypertension, endothelial dysfunction is present in both resistance and conduit arteries and has shown to be an early independent predictor of cardiovascular events [13-15]. Moreover, it has proved to predict long-term cardiovascular events in coronary disease [16-19], heart failure [20] and atherosclerosis [21]. However, whether or not endothelial dysfunction is a true independent predictor, a risk factor, a risk marker, or a surrogate end point is still a matter of debate [22-24].

This chapter aims to present an overview of the current knowledge on endothelial dysfunction, in order to generate a solid basis for clinical practice. The first part addresses the pathophysiology of endothelial dysfunction, emphasizing the role of oxidative stress and the mechanisms underlying the progression of endothelial dysfunction. The second part deals with diagnostic techniques for endothelial dysfunction, comparing several criteria amongst them in order to show advantages and disadvantages of each technique. Finally, this chapter reviews current therapies that have shown improvement or reversion of endothelial dysfunction, ranging from diet and physical exercise to specific transcription enhancers. A brief explanation of the mechanism of action of each therapy is provided, with an emphasis on the antioxidant effects of these therapies.

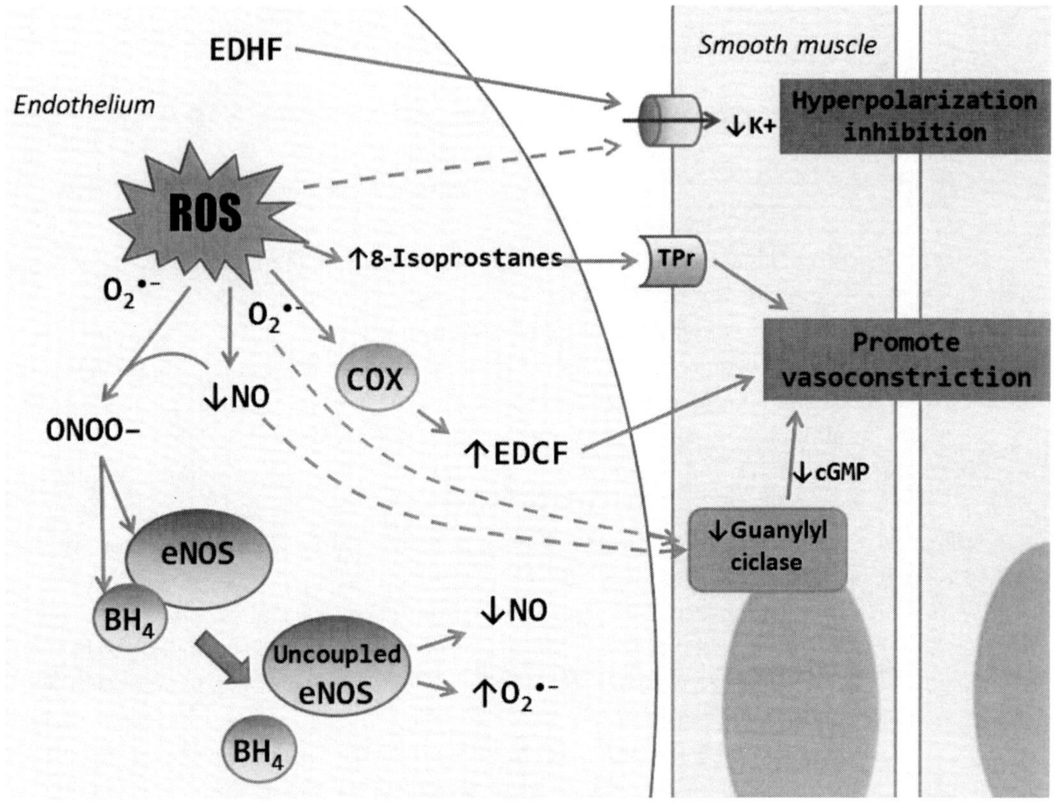

Figure 2.1. Role of oxidative stress in endothelial dysfunction. Superoxide anions (O2•–) interact with nitric oxide (NO) to form peroxynitrite (ONOO–), reducing NO bioavailability, thus diminishing guanilate cyclase production of GMPc. NO interaction with O_2•– also decreases the NO production through eNOS uncoupling. Oxidative stress mediated by reactive oxygen species (ROS) increases isoprostane levels, thus increasing their interaction with the thromboxane-prostanoid receptor (TPr) which mediates a vasoconstricting response. Superoxide anion activates ciclooxygenase (COX) producing endothelial derived contracting factors (EDCF). ROS decrease the calcium activated potasium channel activity involved in endothelial derived hyperpolarising (EDHF) factor response. Continous arrows represent promoted pathways or positive regulation; discontinuous arrows represent inhibited pathway or negative regulation.

2. Pathophysiology

2.1. Oxidative Stress and Endothelial Dysfunction

Although endothelial dysfunction occurs in many different disease processes, oxidative stress can be identified as a common denominator in them [25, 26]. In the pathogenesis of endothelial dysfunction, reactive oxygen species can inhibit the three major endothelium-dependent vasodilator pathways, i.e., NO, prostacyclin and endothelial-derived hyperpolarizing factor (EDHF) [Figure 2.1] [3]. Starting with the NO pathway, superoxide anions not only reduce the bioavailability of NO but also directly inhibit its main target, soluble guanylyl cyclase [27-29]. Furthermore, superoxide anions can react with NO leading to the formation of peroxynitrite ($ONOO^-$) which uncouples NO synthase by oxidizing in one hand the Zn-thiolate complexes within the enzyme [30] and on the other hand the essential cofactor tetrahydrobiopterin (BH_4) [31]. When endothelial nitric oxide synthase (eNOS) becomes unstable and uncoupled, it leads to subsequent less NO production and more superoxide generation [32]. Additionally, $ONOO^-$ inhibits guanylyl cyclase, inactivates the prostacyclin synthase by tyrosine nitration, and further enhances oxidative stress by inhibiting superoxide dismutase [27, 33].

The activity of calcium-activated potassium channels involved in EDHF-mediated response is decreased by the chronic action of superoxide anion [34], and oxidative stress decreases the electrotonic signaling by means of myoendothelial and smooth muscle gap junctions by interacting with connexins 37, 40, and 43 [35]. In addition, reactive oxygen species promote the contraction of VSMC by facilitating the mobilization of calcium and increasing the sensitivity of the contractile proteins to calcium ions [36, 37]. Furthermore, superoxide anions can also activate endothelial enzymes, including cyclooxygenases, which produce endothelium-derived contracting factors [38]. Besides, isoprostanes are not only markers of oxidative stress [39] but are also bioactive molecules that produce vasoconstriction by activating thromboxane-prostanoid receptors on vascular smooth muscle [40]. Hydrogen peroxide (H_2O_2), which is produced by both the endothelium and the smooth muscle cells, is not only a relaxing and a hyperpolarizing factor [41], but depending on the species, the artery, and local concentration, it can also cause smooth muscle depolarization and vasoconstriction [42].

2.2. Animal Models

In the spontaneously hypertensive rat (SHR), plasma endothelin (ET) levels are similar or slightly elevated compared with those of normotensive Wistar-Kyoto (WKY) rats [43-46]. ET-1 is one of the most potent known vasoconstrictor peptides produced and released mainly by endothelial cells. This peptide is also involved in proliferation and hypertrophy of VSMC [47, 48]. In stroke-prone spontaneously hypertensive rat (SHRSP), a more severe model of genetic hypertension, an increase in the circulating level of the peptide is consistently observed [43]. In this latter strain, ET contributes to end-organ damage, vascular remodeling but only moderately to the increase in blood pressure [47].

In the aorta of SHR, the endothelium-dependent relaxations are impaired and are associated with the generation of endothelium-derived contracting factor (EDCF) with no or little alteration in the production of NO. The release of cyclooxygenase-derived contractile prostanoids, but not that of ET, is responsible for these endothelium-dependent contractions [38, 49]. Inhibitors of thromboxane synthase do not affect the endothelium-dependent contraction to acetylcholine, indicating that thromboxane A2 is not the EDCF released following muscarinic receptor activation [50-60]. The massive release of prostacyclin, which in the SHR aorta paradoxically is not a relaxing but a contracting prostaglandin, and also that of the endoperoxide Prostaglandin H2, accounts for the biological activity of EDCF [51, 52, 61].

In the aorta of young SHRSP, in the developmental stage of hypertension, the endothelium-dependent relaxations and the production of NO in response to cholinergic agonists are enhanced paradoxically, although the so-called "basal release" of NO is already impaired [62-64]. Endothelial dysfunction develops later involving both a decrease in NO bioavailability (with no changes in the expression of NO synthase) and the cyclooxygenase-dependent production of an EDCF associated with an enhanced production of prostacyclin and thromboxane A2 [65-67].

2.3. Human Hypertension

In humans, reactive oxygen species are elevated in many cardiovascular diseases, including essential, renovascular, and malignant hypertension as well as preeclampsia. An increased production of reactive oxygen species, a decreased antioxidant activity, and a reduced ability to scavenge oxygen-derived free radicals all contribute to oxidative stress [68]. The renin-angiotensin system is likely to play a major role in the generation of reactive oxygen species through the activation of nicotinamide adenine dinucleotide phosphate (NADPH) oxidase [69].

The involvement of the ET system possibly further exacerbates oxidative stress [70]. Human ET plasma levels are not correlated with blood pressure and in most patients with essential hypertension these levels are not elevated [71]. However, ET_A and mixed ET_A-ET_B receptor antagonists decrease blood pressure in mild to moderately hypertensive patients [72; 73]. Furthermore, in patients with essential hypertension, but not in normotensive controls, the combined blockade of ET_A and ET_B receptors or, but to a lesser extent, the selective blockade of the ET_A receptor in and by itself increases the forearm blood flow and potentiates the endothelium-dependent vasodilations to acetylcholine[74-76].

Endothelium-dependent vasodilations to physical (shear stress) and/or pharmacological (acetylcholine, bradykinin, substance P, etc.) stimuli are impaired in the forearm, coronary, and renal vasculature as well as in various microcirculatory beds of patients with essential or secondary hypertension [77-82]. In patients with essential hypertension, but not in those with secondary (primary aldosteronism or renovascular hypertension) hypertension, nonspecific cyclooxygenase (COX) inhibitors partially restore the acetylcholine-induced forearm vasodilation, suggesting in the former the release of EDCF [79, 83]. By contrast, selective COX-2 inhibitors worsen the endothelium dysfunction in patients with essential hypertension [84], indicating that it is the COX-1 isoform that is associated with the generation of EDCF. Inhibition of cyclooxygenase also enhances the bioavailability of NO because the vasoconstriction evoked by the administration of an inhibitor of NO synthase is restored [83].

Vitamin C normalizes the impaired endothelium-dependent vasodilation in the forearm and the coronary circulation in patients with essential hypertension, confirming that the generation of reactive oxygen species partially explains the substantial decrease of NO [85, 86]. Additionally, the production of NO can be impaired because of polymorphisms of the eNOS gene [87], deficiency in the essential cofactor tetrahydrobiopterin [88], impairment of the L-arginine transport system [89], and increased serum levels of asymmetric dimethyl-arginine (an endogenous inhibitor of NO synthase) [90-92]. In patients with essential hypertension, vasodilations of the forearm vascular bed to bradykinin are resistant to an inhibitor of NO synthase. In the presence of this inhibitor they are of comparable amplitude in normotensive and hypertensive subjects [93, 94]. In the latter, they become sensitive to ouabain, an inhibitor of Na-K-ATPase, suggesting that an uncharacterized EDHF-mediated component partially compensates for the reduced importance of NO mediated vasodilation in hypertensive patients [95].

A nontraditional cardiovascular risk factor that leads to endothelial dysfunction is hyperhomocysteinemia. Normotensive patients with hyperhomocysteinemia display endothelial dysfunction [96]. Folic acid supplementation was able to reduce homocysteine levels and improve endothelial dysfunction in children with chronic renal failure [97]. Cellular [98], animal [99], and human studies [96] suggest that homocysteine reduces NO bioavailability by oxidative excess. There is now also evidence that homocysteine may cause asymmetric dimethyl arginine (ADMA) accumulation by inhibition of dimethylarginine dimethylaminohydrolase [100]. Experimental studies in humans have confirmed that hyperhomocysteinemia may lead to endothelial dysfunction via accumulation of ADMA [101, 102]. However, not all studies support this link [103]. These mechanisms may explain the increased cardiovascular risk of patients with hyperhomocysteinemia. This is of special importance for patients with chronic renal failure, who often have increased homocysteine levels, which were shown to predict cardiovascular outcomes in a recent study [104].

In secondary hypertensive patients, the normalization of arterial blood pressure restores endothelium-dependent vasodilations, indicating that the endothelial dysfunction is a consequence of the high arterial blood pressure [82]. In human isolated arterioles, a transient increase in intravascular pressure directly and specifically impairs endothelium-dependent vasodilation [105]. However, in essential hypertension, endothelial dysfunction is believed to precede the onset of the high arterial blood pressure, because in young genetically predisposed normotensive offspring of essential hypertensive patients, the response to acetylcholine is already reduced [106].

Antihypertensive agents do not have the same impact on endothelial function despite similar reduction of arterial blood pressure [107, 108]. In patients with essential hypertension, diuretics given in monotherapy do not affect endothelial function [109, 110], and β-adrenergic blockers have minimal or even deleterious effects of endothelium-dependent vasodilation [111-113]. Exceptions are nebivolol and cardevilol, possibly because of their NO donor and antioxidant properties, respectively [114]. Calcium channel blockers, especially dihydropyridines, improve endothelial function, a phenomenon associated with a reduction in oxidative stress [81, 112].Certain dihydropyridines can evoke endothelium-dependent, NO-dependent relaxations, a property that is not linked to the calcium-blocking properties of these compounds [115, 116] and which involves bradykinin B2 receptor activation and/or eNOS phosphorylation [117, 118]. In most of the studies involving acetylcholine-induced forearm vasodilation, the angiotensin converting enzyme inhibitors did not affect the response to acetylcholine [119-122]. However, these inhibitors improve endothelial function in subcutaneous and coronary arteries [111, 123].

Table 2.2. Comparison of functional techniques for endothelial dysfunction assessment

Functional	Technique summary	Invasive	Advantages	Disadvantages	Cardiovascular event predictor
Intracoronary agonist infusion with quantitative coronary angiography	Vasomotor substance (usually acetylcholine) is infused selectively into the coronary circulation then measured with intracoronary Doppler wires.	Yes	Measures endothelial function in the coronary vascular bed. Allows for mapping dose-response relationships of endothelial agonists and antagonists [129].	Expensive Carries risks inherent with coronary artery catheterization (stroke, MI, infection, vascular injury) [129].	Yes, strong evidence [129].
Brachial artery catheterization with venous occlusive plethysmography	Measurement of limb blood flow changes before and after direct intraarterial infusions of vasoactive substances through strain-gauge or electrically calibrated plethysmography.	Yes	Highly reproducible. Easier application than coronary angiography. Can perform acute repeated measurements Allows for mapping dose-response relationships of endothelial agonists and antagonists [129].	Risk of median nerve injury, infection, vascular injury. [129]	Yes, strong evidence [130].
Brachial artery flow-mediated dilation assessment (FMD)	Imaging of flow-mediated dilation of the brachial artery using vascular ultrasound.	No	Safer and faster than invasive methods. Regularly reproducible [128].	Requires extensive sonographer training [131]. Highly operator dependent [128]. High variability between centers. [132] Requires excellent patient cooperation. [128]	Yes, strong evidence [21;133].
Positron emission tomography (PET)	Quantitative assessment of myocardial blood flow and its metabolic activity before and after cold pressor test and/or sympathetic stress test.	No	Measures endothelial function in the coronary vascular bed. Highly reproducible. Can perform acute repeated measurements [134].	Expensive Limited to a few laboratories [135].	Yes [134].
Digital pulse amplitude tonometry (PAT)	Measurement of volumetric changes in the fingertip through a probe that quantifies pulse amplitude in response to reactive hyperemia.	No	Very simple to perform. May be used for large scale ambulatory testing. Computerized analysis minimizes operator dependency and interobserver variability [131]. Reproducible [136].	Current results may not reflect in ambulatory settings [136]. Most research has been done on European ethnicity patients [136].	Yes, weak evidence [137].

3. Assessment

In healthy vessels, acetylcholine evokes an NO-mediated vasodilatory response. After Ludmer et al. showed the paradoxical response to acetylcholine in the coronary arteries of patients with mild atherosclerosis [124], the measurement of endothelial-dependent vasodilation through angiography and intracoronary Doppler for the direct calculation of changes in coronary blood flow and coronary vascular resistance [12] became the "gold standard" for endothelial dysfunction assessment and was considered as such for a long time. [12, 125, 126]. The gold standard status of this technique is now a contentious issue [127] due to the drawbacks it presents, such as a greater variability than conduit vessel assessment and its disadvantages, such as being invasive and expensive, with the risks of coronary catheterization, and that it cannot be used as a screening test in the general population [128]. Due to this and the multi-faceted nature of endothelial dysfunction, multiple methods for its assessment have emerged. These methods can be divided in functional, by measuring endothelium-dependent dilation in vitro or in vivo or biochemical, by measurement of biomarkers in the blood. A summary of functional methods is presented in Table 2.2.

Functional assessments in vascular beds different from coronary arteries are supported by the notion that the endothelial dysfunction process is systemic, and, as such, may be measured in any place in the body; however, the picture may be more complex. While on one hand, brachial flow mediated dilation (FMD) and coronary angiographic assessment have been shown to be moderately correlated [138], and strain-gauge plethysmography and FMD seem to be highly correlated [139], on the other hand pulse amplitude tonometry (PAT) and coronary angiography, and PAT and brachial FMD have shown a weak correlation at best, and differing patterns in risk factor associations [140].These results support the notion that the measurement of macrovascular conduit artery vasodilator capacity and microvascular function in a terminal vascular bed are nonequivalent, yet valuable indexes of endothelial health. For example, the closer association of glycemic parameters with PAT may reflect microvascular impairment in early phases of metabolic vascular disease [141] which suggests that different stages of disease processes may have disparate effects on different vascular beds [142]. Nevertheless, the clinical significance of these results is yet unclear.

4. Therapies

4.1. Exercise Training

Aerobic exercise reduces blood pressure in both hypertensive and normotensive individuals [142]. Thus, an increase in aerobic physical activity should be considered an important component of lifestyle modification for prevention and treatment of high blood pressure. According to the current knowledge, regular exercise is a non-pharmacological therapeutic modality that enhances endothelial function in subjects with cardiovascular risk factors, including hypertension [143], metabolic syndrome [144], and type 2 diabetes mellitus [145], among others. Beck et al. [146] reported a prospective randomized and controlled study that both resistance exercise training and endurance exercise training had beneficial effects reducing mean blood pressure in association with improving endothelial function assessed by brachial artery FMD and endothelial function biomarkers.

The effects of exercise over endothelial dysfunction have been tested on animal, *in vitro* and human models. Studies using animal models [147, 148] and cultured endothelial cells [149; 150] suggested that shear stress increases eNOS expression and activity, probably due to the stabilization of eNOS mRNA [149] or the presence of transcription factors in the promoter region of eNOS gene enhancing the synthesis of mRNA [151]. Hambrecht et al., in 2003 [152], performed the first study demonstrating the positive effects of exercise training on vascular function and eNOS expression in the human vascular system. The authors found a 2-fold increase in eNOS mRNA expression and a 3.2 increase in the phosphorylation of eNOS on serine 1177 residue after 4 weeks of regular exercise training in coronary artery disease (CAD) patients. This led to a rise in the enzymatic activity of eNOS and consequently to an enhanced NO production.

Furthermore, regular exercise tends to increase the antioxidant defenses and through this mechanism reduce NO degradation [153]. This was attributed to an increase of antioxidant defenses, such as the enhanced activity of superoxide dismutase and glutathione peroxidase [154]. Moreover, *in vitro* studies showed that the application of laminar shear stress to cultured endothelial cells activates eNOS as well as the cytosolic copper/zinc-containing Superoxide Dismutase pathway [155-158]. This increase in the antioxidant defenses, observed both in myocardium and endothelial cells [159], seems to result from repetitive exposure to increased laminar shear stress during acute bouts of exercise training. However, it should be noted that exercise intensity seems to be a crucial variable in this response. It is well established that moderate-intensity aerobic exercise augments endothelium-dependent vasodilation in subjects with impaired endothelial function [160, 161]. Nevertheless, recent studies have shown that high-intensity aerobic interval exercise was better than moderate-intensity aerobic exercise to increase endothelial function and NO availability [162, 163]. This suggests that the superior effect of aerobic interval training could be elicited by higher shear stress during the acute bouts of exercise, which triggers larger responses at the cellular and molecular level.

Additionally, exercise training has been reported to chronically increase the number of circulating endothelial progenitor cells (EPC) in healthy subjects [164]. In animal models, in response to hypertension, the amount of peripheral blood-EPC and number of colonies are decreased in comparison with control levels. Nevertheless, exercise training normalized EPC levels and their function [165]. Laufs et al. [164] reported an average increase of 280% in the circulating EPC after 4 weeks of regular exercise training. Such an increase could be partially explained by the stimulation of bone marrow as a result of local increase in the bioavailability of NO [166], in turn favoring the mobilization of EPC. Another hypothesis about the positive impact of exercise training on the survival, differentiation, and function of EPC is that it could be indirectly related to the reduction of circulating levels of C-reactive protein [167]. However, a meta-analysis of randomized controlled trials showed no association between exercise and C-reactive protein [168].

4.2. Cocoa Derived Products

Cocoa derived products have been thoroughly studied and demonstrated to be efficient in improving endothelial function and decreasing blood pressure [169-172]. Cocoa, and cocoa-derived foods and beverages contain important amounts of flavan-3-ols or flavanols, a subfamily of flavonoids [173]. Flavonols could be responsible for this improvement in endothelial dysfunction and decreasing blood pressure through: i) their free radical scavenging action [174] ii) a decrease in superoxide anion concentration in the cell by diminishing NADPH oxidase expression and/or activity; iii) an increase in NO production by augmentation of eNOS expression and/or activity; iv) the modulation of enzymes and receptors associated with reactive oxygen species production, e.g., AT-II-mediated pathways, [175, 176] and v) the protection from oxidative loss of tetrahydrobiopterin to avoid eNOS uncoupling [177]. Intervention trials with cocoa and cocoa products have included different groups of subjects: normotensive (young, old, overweight, hypercholesterolemic), pre-hypertensive, hypertensive stage 1, and hypertensive with impaired glucose tolerance. Most of the studies showed that cocoa consumption was associated with a decrease in blood pressure [178].

A recent meta-analysis evaluating the effect of cocoa rich-foods on the blood pressure of hypertensive and normotensive individuals concluded that dark chocolate is superior to placebo in reducing systolic hypertension or diastolic prehypertension [172].

The blood pressure lowering effect of cocoa-rich products has been correlated with increases in plasma and urine NO-derived species, improvement in NO-mediated FMD, and reduced oxidative stress. Plasma NO metabolites (measured as S-nitrosothiols) were increased in prehypertensive and hypertensive patients after 18 weeks of daily consumption of 6.3 g of chocolate (30 mg of polyphenols) [169]. Moreover, a commercially available natural flavonoid-enriched cocoa powder was tested in SHR. A single oral administration of different doses of the product (50–600 mg/kg) produced an antihypertensive effect in SHR without modifications in the blood pressure of normotensive WKY rats. The maximum effect on blood pressure, caused by 300 mg/kg of powder, produced a blood pressure decrease similar to the one obtained with 50 mg/kg captopril [179]. Nevertheless, an important factor to be considered when an integrative conclusion is to be drawn from all these investigations is the composition of the chocolate used. Unfortunately, there is not a standardized chocolate or a consistent standardization (qualitative and/or quantitative) of the chocolate components through the different studies. In contrast to studies using chocolate or cocoa preparations, only few studies have been developed on human subjects by using purified flavanols. Being epicatechin (EC) the most abundant flavanol in cocoa, the potential of this compound as responsible for the cocoa and chocolate BP-lowering effect is of singular relevance. Sprague-Dawley rats were pre-treated with the NO-synthase inhibitor Nω-nitro-L-arginine methyl ester (L-NAME) in the drinking water during 6 days. After that period, an increase of 25 mm Hg to 122 ± 6 mm Hg was observed. From that day, the rats were maintained during 8 days under the same L-NAME treatment, but receiving different diets: one group was fed with a control diet (L-NAME group) and the second group with an EC-enriched diet (0.4 g EC/100 g diet) (L-NAME + EC group). Systolic blood pressure was measured during the following 8 days in both dietary groups. At the end of that period, the group receiving control diet showed an additional increase in blood pressure. Meanwhile, the group receiving the diet supplemented with EC maintained the initial blood pressure values. These results suggest that the presence of EC in the diet can prevent the sustained BP increase induced by a deficiency in NO production associated to the L-NAME treatment [171].

The basic chemical features of EC, shared with most of the flavonoids, allow them to act as classic antioxidants, i.e., free radical scavengers and/or redox-active metal chelators. Even though those antioxidant reactions are thermodynamically favored, the actual concentration of flavonoids reached in the vasculature makes quantitatively unfeasible these direct antioxidant mechanisms [180]. Then, other biochemical mechanisms, probably related to more specific interactions with proteins or lipids, should be responsible for the *in vivo* effects of flavanols decreasing oxidative stress. These mechanisms should be attained at the low flavanol concentration estimated to occur in most human and animal tissues.

4.3. Nitrate/Nitrite Reduction to Nitric Oxide

While nitrate and nitrite were long thought of as stable end-products of NO metabolism, recent evidence supports nitrate and nitrite as potential sources of NO under appropriate conditions [181-185]. As opposed to the NOS enzymes, which require oxygen as a substrate for NO generation, nitrite-generated production of NO has been shown to occur more readily under acidic and hypoxic conditions [186-189]. Nitrate/nitrite reduction has been shown to occur via deoxygenated hemoglobin, myoglobin, enzymatic, and non-enzymatic means [190-194]. A class of molybdenum-containing enzymes, including xanthine oxidoreductase, aldehyde oxidase, and sulfite oxidase, have been identified as enzymes that may facilitate the reduction of nitrate and nitrite to NO at the molybdenum-containing site [195]. Due to its relative stability, nitrite then has the ability to circulate to other areas in the body and undergo reduction to NO under acidic and hypoxic conditions [190]. Acting in this way, circulating nitrite has been described as a "storage pool" for NO within the body [183].

4.4. Effects of Antihypertensive Treatment on Endothelial Function

4.4.1. β-Blockers

Classic β-adrenoceptor antagonists, especially atenolol, have been employed as the control arm in several studies assessing the impact of other antihypertensive compounds on endothelial function. The totality of these studies indicated that chronic treatment with atenolol was not able to produce endothelium-dependent relaxation, an effect observed in different vascular districts [112, 196]. However, a different effectiveness has been proposed for the so-called third-generation β-blockers, such as nebivolol and carvedilol.

Nebivolol is a selective β1-receptor blocker that has vasodilating properties that are attributable to its ability to increase NO bioactivity, as demonstrated in animals and human volunteers [197, 198]. In a double-blind, crossover trial comparing the effects of nebivolol and atenolol on vascular NO bioactivity in patients with essential hypertension, it was demonstrated that nebivolol/bendrofluazide treatment lowered blood pressure and reversed endothelial dysfunction in patients with essential hypertension as assessed by an increase in the vasodilating effect of acetylcholine. Atenolol/bendrofluazide treatment similarly lowered blood pressure but did not alter endothelial function [114]. Intra-arterial infusion of elevated concentrations of nebivolol in the forearm microcirculation of healthy volunteers caused vasodilation, an effect inhibited by NG-monomethyl L-arginine (L-NMMA), thus indicating that, acutely, nebivolol evokes NO-dependent vasodilation [198]. It was hypothesized that nebivolol may be able to increase NO synthase, but such a result is unlikely to have a beneficial effect on endothelial function in essential hypertension, considering that the oxidant excess characterizing this clinical condition rapidly abrogates the NO activity. However, a more recent experimental report demonstrated that nebivolol inhibits NADPH oxidase activity [199]. Such an interesting effect, which may reduce an important source of oxidative stress in hypertension [68], needs clarification in human studies.

Carvedilol, a nonselective β-blocker with additional α1-adrenoceptor antagonist activity, has also been shown to exert important beneficial actions on endothelial dysfunction via an elevated antioxidant effect [200]. Recent results indicated that carvedilol was able to improve endothelial function, assessed by noninvasive flow-mediated dilation (FMD), in a group of hypertensive patients with diabetes mellitus [201]. More recently, this beneficial effect has been confirmed in the forearm microcirculation of patients with dilated cardiomyopathy [202]. Further studies are needed to clarify the molecular mechanisms whereby carvedilol exerts its antioxidant activity leading to the reversal of endothelial dysfunction.

4.4.2. Calcium Channel Antagonists

Calcium channel antagonists increase endothelium dependent relaxations in different vascular districts [107]. A year of treatment with nifedipine showed an improved relaxation to acetylcholine in subcutaneous resistance small arteries of hypertensive patients [196] along with improved coronary endothelial function [203]. Concerning peripheral macrocirculation, one study showed that a 6 month treatment with nifedipine in patients with essential hypertension did not improve FMD of the brachial artery [119], while other study showed an improvement in FMD after a two-month therapy with nifedipine [204]. This difference could be explained by sample size. Subsequent assessment of the effect of calcium channel antagonists on endothelial function in the forearm microcirculation provided further positive results [205, 206]. Moreover, verapamil, a diphenylalkylamine, ameliorates the vasodilation to acetylcholine and restores the inhibiting activity exerted by L-NMMA on acetylcholine in the forearm circulation of patients with essential hypertension [207].

Experimental evidence suggests that calcium antagonists exert their beneficial activity by an antioxidant effect [208]. It is likely that the beneficial effect of calcium channel antagonists on NO availability is secondary to an antioxidant property, which likely originates from a class effect, as human evidence suggests.

4.4.3. Therapeutic Effects of eNOS Modulators

Tetrahydrobiopterin BH_4

Since uncoupled eNOS can increase the production of reactive oxygen species, promote BH_4 oxidation, and self-limit its NO biosynthesis, modulating eNOS uncoupling is an attractive therapeutic approach in endothelial dysfunction. The most straightforward way to modulate eNOS is administration of its essential cofactor BH_4 [209]. Supplementation with BH_4 increases NOS activity by recoupling uncoupled eNOS in mice with hypertension-induced heart failure with subsequent reversal of cardiac hypertrophy and fibrosis [210]. Chronic oral administration of BH_4 has been reported to improve endothelium function [211,

212], decrease vascular superoxide production, and increase vascular NO production. As a result, it blunts the increase in blood pressure in a hypertensive mice model [212]. Porkert et al. [213] demonstrated in subjects with poorly controlled hypertension that orally administering (400 mg or higher) BH_4 daily has a significant and sustained antihypertensive effect. Importantly, this effect is associated with reversing the uncoupling of NOS and improving NO bioavailability [214].

Although studies suggest that BH_4 administration shows beneficial results for endothelial dysfunction, it may have limited long-term benefit in improving eNOS coupling [215]. Chronic BH_4 administration may result in endothelial dihydrobiopterin (BH_2) accumulation and consequent eNOS uncoupling because BH_2 can replace eNOS-bound BH_4 competitively [215, 216]. Recently, Moens et al. [217] studied the therapeutic efficacy of BH_4 in hypertension-induced heart failure in a mouse model of pressure overload, demonstrating a bimodal dose-dependent relationship, first rising and then declining at higher doses. Importantly, this study indicates that, at higher doses of exogenous BH_4 (and thus BH_2), the intrinsic capacity to maintain BH_4:BH_2 ratios may become compromised, limiting net efficacy. These results expose a potential limitation for the clinical use of BH_4 in diseases characterized by oxidative stress.

l-Arginine

L-Arginine, a semiessential amino acid found in large quantities in fish, chicken, and beans, is the substrate for the production of NO. L-Arginine deficiency or the presence of its endogenous inhibitors, i.e., ADMA, may lead to eNOS uncoupling [218]. L-Arginine activates oxygen uptake by eNOS [219] and prevents superoxide generation within uncoupled eNOS by electron interaction with heme-bound oxygen [220]. In addition, L-arginine may be able to restore the physiological status by normalizing the extracellular L-arginine: ADMA ratio [221]. Although L-arginine improves both endothelium-dependent vasodilation and abnormal interactions of vascular cells, platelets, and monocytes, clinical studies with L-arginine have shown inconsistent effects on endothelial function [32]. Despite L-arginine could be the key to future treatment of cardiovascular disorders, it has not been possible to draw any general conclusion supporting the use of L-arginine for improving the clinical treatment in patients with endothelial dysfunction.

eNOS Transcription Enhancers

The novel small molecules AVE9488 and AVE3085 are eNOS transcription enhancers. AVE9488 has proven *in vivo* effects improving left ventricular remodeling in a rat model of myocardial infarction [222] and a mouse model of cardiac ischemia/reperfusion injury [223]. Wolfhart et al. [224] demonstrated in a model of experimental atherosclerosis that both AVE9488 and AVE3085 have vasoprotective properties, i.e., the increased endothelial NO generation associated with reduced cuff-induced neointima formation and reduced formation of atherosclerotic plaques in apoE−/− mice. This study indicates that both compounds showed the concomitant increase in eNOS transcription and eNOS protein levels; BH4 levels also increased, although GTPCH mRNA levels did not. In addition, the mechanisms for the increase in BH4 by these eNOS enhancers still remain unknown. Recently, Yang et al. [225] demonstrated that AVE3085 restored impaired endothelial function in a hypertensive model by upregulated expression of eNOS protein and mRNA, enhanced eNOS phosphorylation, and decreased formation of nitrotyrosine. While these preclinical data are very promising, no clinical studies have been initiated at the moment.

Research into arginase, a competing enzyme of eNOS for the substrate l-arginine and arginase inhibition therapies is addressed in chapter 1, "Oxidative Stress and Hypertension".

Conclusion and Perspectives

Endothelial dysfunction triggers a chain of undesired responses, including increased platelet aggregation, expression of adhesion molecules, vasoconstriction and vascular muscle growth and through these responses seems to play a central role in cardiovascular disease progression. In essential hypertension, endothelial dysfunction has shown to be an independent predictor of cardiovascular events, therefore, endothelial dysfunction should be considered as a central target in the treatment of hypertension. Although the pathophysiology of endothelial dysfunction has not been completely elucidated, a central role of oxidative stress is consistently observed. A reduced bioavailability of NO, an alteration in prostanoid production, an impairment of endothelium-dependent hyperpolarizations, as well as an increased release of ET-1 can individually, or in association, contribute to endothelial dysfunction. Therapeutic interventions do not necessarily restore a proper endothelial function and, when they do, may improve only part of these variables. Additionally, there seems to be a major role of eNOS uncoupling in this process, turning it into a promising therapeutic target.

Assessment of endothelial dysfunction is an important target in research, since an easy-to-perform, safe, cost-effective, reproducible, non-invasive technique could provide with an overall marker of endothelial health to be used in ambulatory settings, providing a valuable tool in clinical practice. Early detection could be of high clinical value due to the natural history of endothelial dysfunction. An etiology-oriented treatment could be aimed towards stopping or reversing the pathological process of endothelial dysfunction before the induction of the structural damage which eventually leads to atherosclerosis. Brachial artery FMD assessment and pulse amplitude tonometry show promise towards becoming the technique of choice, but brachial artery FMD assessment has drawbacks intrinsic to the technique that make its large scale application unlikely, while pulse amplitude tonometry is still lacking in reproducibility and strong cardiovascular event association. Further research is required to propose either brachial artery FMD assessment, pulse amplitude tonometry or other technique as an endothelial health marker to be used in clinical settings.

Non-pharmacologic therapies for hypertension such as physical exercise have been proven to reduce blood pressure and an improvement in endothelial function. Diet recommendations that include a high intake of polyphenols, as in the case of cocoa derived products, improve endothelial dysfunction and decrease blood pressure in hypertensive patients. Next generation pharmacological hypertension therapy should have as a secondary endpoint an improvement in endothelial dysfunction while current therapy should privilege drugs that improve endothelial dysfunction. Pharmacological therapy for the reversal of endothelial dysfunction still requires more research to show relevant clinical endpoint changes, such as a decrease in cardiovascular events or overall mortality.

References

[1] Chong AY, Blann AD, Lip GY. Assessment of endothelial damage and dysfunction: observations in relation to heart failure. *QJM.* 2003; 96: 253-267.

[2] Davignon J, Ganz P. Role of endothelial dysfunction in atherosclerosis. *Circulation.* 2004; 109: III27-32.

[3] Félétou M, Vanhoutte PM. Endothelial dysfunction: a multifaceted disorder (The Wiggers Award Lecture). *Am J Physiol Heart Circ Physiol.* 2006; 291: H985-1002.

[4] Rodrigo R, González J, Paoletto F. The role of oxidative stress in the pathophysiology of hypertension. *Hypertens Res.* 2011; 34: 431-40.

[5] Furchgott RF, Zawadzki JV. The obligatory role of endothelial cells in the relaxation of arterial smooth muscle by acetylcholine. *Nature.* 1980; 288: 373-376.

[6] Palmer RM, Ferrige AG, Moncada S. Nitric oxide release accounts for the biological activity of endothelium-derived relaxing factor. *Nature.* 1987; 327: 524-526.

[7] Lockette W, Otsuka Y, Carretero O. The loss of endothelium-dependent vascular relaxation in hypertension. *Hypertension.* 1986; 8: II61-66.

[8] Winquist RJ, Bunting PB, Baskin EP, Wallace AA. Decreased endothelium-dependent relaxation in New Zealand genetic hypertensive rats. J Hypertens. 1984; 2: 541-545.

[9] Félétou M, Köhler R, Vanhoutte PM. Endothelium-derived vasoactive factors and hypertension: possible roles in pathogenesis and as treatment targets. *Curr Hypertens Rep.* 2010; 12: 267-275.

[10] Savoia C, Burger D, Nishigaki N, Montezano A, Touyz RM. Angiotensin II and the vascular phenotype in hypertension. *Expert Rev Mol Med.* 2011; 13: e11.

[11] Schiffrin EL; Canadian Institutes of Health Research Multidisciplinary Research Group on Hypertension. Beyond blood pressure: the endothelium and atherosclerosis progression. *Am J Hypertens.* 2002; 15: 115S-122S.

[12] Endemann DH, Schiffrin EL. Endothelial dysfunction. *J Am Soc Nephrol.* 2004; 15: 1983-1992.

[13] Bellien J, Joannides R, Richard V, Thuillez C. Modulation of cytochrome-derived epoxyeicosatrienoic acids pathway: a promising pharmacological approach to prevent endothelial dysfunction in cardiovascular diseases? *Pharmacol Ther.* 2011; 131: 1-17.

[14] Modena MG, Bonetti L, Coppi F, Bursi F, Rossi R. Prognostic role of reversible endothelial dysfunction in hypertensive postmenopausal women. *J Am Coll Cardiol.* 2002; 40: 505-510

[15] Perticone F, Ceravolo R, Pujia A, Ventura G, Iacopino S, Scozzafava A, Ferraro A, Chello M, Mastroroberto P, Verdecchia P, Schillaci G. Prognostic significance of endothelial dysfunction in hypertensive patients. *Circulation.* 2001; 104: 191-196.

[16] Chan SY, Mancini GB, Kuramoto L, Schulzer M, Frohlich J, Ignaszewski A. The prognostic importance of endothelial dysfunction and carotid atheroma burden in patients with coronary artery disease. *J Am Coll Cardiol.* 2003; 42: 1037-1043.

[17] Fichtlscherer S, Breuer S, Zeiher AM. Prognostic value of systemic endothelial dysfunction in patients with acute coronary syndromes: further evidence for the existence of the "vulnerable" patient. *Circulation.* 2004; 110: 1926-1932.

[18] Schächinger V, Britten MB, Zeiher AM. Prognostic impact of coronary vasodilator dysfunction on adverse long-term outcome of coronary heart disease. *Circulation.* 2000; 101: 1899-1906.

[19] Suwaidi JA, Hamasaki S, Higano ST, Nishimura RA, Holmes DR Jr, Lerman A. Long-term follow-up of patients with mild coronary artery disease and endothelial dysfunction. *Circulation.* 2000; 101: 948-954.

[20] Heitzer T, Baldus S, von Kodolitsch Y, Rudolph V, Meinertz T. Systemic endothelial dysfunction as an early predictor of adverse outcome in heart failure. *Arterioscler Thromb Vasc Biol.* 2005; 25: 1174-1779.

[21] Gokce N, Keaney JF Jr, Hunter LM, Watkins MT, Nedeljkovic ZS, Menzoian JO, Vita JA. Predictive value of noninvasively determined endothelial dysfunction for long-term cardiovascular events in patients with peripheral vascular disease. *J Am Coll Cardiol.* 2003; 41: 1769-1775.

[22] Elliott HL. Endothelial dysfunction in cardiovascular disease: risk factor, risk marker, or surrogate end point? *J Cardiovasc Pharmacol.* 1998; 32 Suppl 3: S74-77.

[23] Fathi R, Haluska B, Isbel N, Short L, Marwick TH. The relative importance of vascular structure and function in predicting cardiovascular events. *J Am Coll Cardiol.* 2004; 43: 616-623.

[24] Mancini GB. Vascular structure versus function: is endothelial dysfunction of independent prognostic importance or not? J Am Coll Cardiol. 2004; 43: 624-628.

[25] Griendling KK, FitzGerald GA. Oxidative stress and cardiovascular injury: Part I: basic mechanisms and in vivo monitoring of ROS. Circulation. 2003; 108: 1912-1916.

[26] Griendling KK, FitzGerald GA. Oxidative stress and cardiovascular injury: Part II: animal and human studies. Circulation. 2003; 108: 2034-2040.

[27] Münzel T, Daiber A, Ullrich V, Mülsch A. Vascular consequences of endothelial nitric oxide synthase uncoupling for the activity and expression of the soluble guanylyl cyclase and the cGMP-dependent protein kinase. Arterioscler Thromb Vasc Biol. 2005; 25: 1551-1557.

[28] Price DT, Vita JA, Keaney JF Jr. Redox control of vascular nitric oxide bioavailability. Antioxid Redox Signal. 2000; 2: 919-935.

[29] Rubanyi GM, Vanhoutte PM. Superoxide anions and hyperoxia inactivate endothelium-derived relaxing factor. Am J Physiol. 1986; 250: H822-827.

[30] Zou MH, Shi C, Cohen RA. Oxidation of the zinc-thiolate complex and uncoupling of endothelial nitric oxide synthase by peroxynitrite. J Clin Invest. 2002; 109: 817-826.

[31] Chen W, Druhan LJ, Chen CA, Hemann C, Chen YR, Berka V, Tsai AL, Zweier JL. Peroxynitrite induces destruction of the tetrahydrobiopterin and heme in endothelial nitric oxide synthase: transition from reversible to irreversible enzyme inhibition. Biochemistry. 2010; 49: 3129-3137.

[32] Kietadisorn R, Juni RP, Moens AL. Tackling endothelial dysfunction by modulating NOS uncoupling: new insights into its pathogenesis and therapeutic possibilities. Am J Physiol Endocrinol Metab. 2012; 302: E481-495.

[33] Zou MH, Cohen R, Ullrich V. Peroxynitrite and vascular endothelial dysfunction in diabetes mellitus. *Endothelium.* 2004; 11: 89-97.

[34] Kusama N, Kajikuri J, Yamamoto T, Watanabe Y, Suzuki Y, Katsuya H, Itoh T. Reduced hyperpolarization in endothelial cells of rabbit aortic valve following chronic nitroglycerine administration. *Br J Pharmacol.* 2005; 146: 487-497.

[35] Griffith TM, Chaytor AT, Bakker LM, Edwards DH. 5-Methyltetrahydrofolate and tetrahydrobiopterin can modulate electrotonically mediated endothelium-dependent vascular relaxation. *Proc Natl Acad Sci U S A*. 2005; 102: 7008-7013.

[36] Jin N, Packer CS, Rhoades RA. Reactive oxygen-mediated contraction in pulmonary arterial smooth muscle: cellular mechanisms. *Can J Physiol Pharmacol.* 1991; 69: 383-388.

[37] Suzuki YJ, Ford GD. Superoxide stimulates IP3-induced Ca2+ release from vascular smooth muscle sarcoplasmic reticulum. *Am J Physiol.* 1992; 262: H114-116.

[38] Vanhoutte PM, Feletou M, Taddei S. Endothelium-dependent contractions in hypertension. *Br J Pharmacol.* 2005; 144: 449-458.

[39] Praticò D, Lawson JA, Rokach J, FitzGerald GA.The isoprostanes in biology and medicine. *Trends Endocrinol Metab.* 2001; 12: 243-247.

[40] Yang D, Gluais P, Zhang JN, Vanhoutte PM, Félétou M. Nitric oxide and inactivation of the endothelium-dependent contracting factor released by acetylcholine in spontaneously hypertensive rat. *J Cardiovasc Pharmacol.* 2004; 43: 815-820.

[41] Shimokawa H, Matoba T.Hydrogen peroxide as an endothelium-derived hyperpolarizing factor. *Pharmacol Res.* 2004; 49: 543-549.

[42] Félétou M and Vanhoutte PM. *EDHF: the complete story*. Boca Raton, FL: Taylor & Francis CRC, 2006, p. 1–278.

[43] Abdel-Sayed S, Nussberger J, Aubert JF, Gohlke P, Brunner HR, Brakch N. Measurement of plasma endothelin-1 in experimental hypertension and in healthy subjects. *Am J Hypertens.* 2003; 16: 515-521.

[44] Bolterman RJ, Manriquez MC, Ortiz Ruiz MC, Juncos LA, Romero JC. Effects of captopril on the renin angiotensin system, oxidative stress, and endothelin in normal and hypertensive rats. *Hypertension.* 2005; 46: 943-947.

[45] Iyer RS, Singh G, Rebello S, Roy S, Bhat R, Vidyasagar D, Gulati A. Changes in the concentration of endothelin-1 during development of hypertensive rats. *Pharmacology.* 1995; 51: 96-104.

[46] Suzuki N, Miyauchi T, Tomobe Y, Matsumoto H, Goto K, Masaki T, Fujino M.Plasma concentrations of endothelin-1 in spontaneously hypertensive rats and DOCA-salt hypertensive rats. *Biochem Biophys Res Commun.* 1990; 167: 941-947.

[47] Schiffrin EL. State-of-the-Art lecture. Role of endothelin-1 in hypertension. *Hypertension.* 1999; 34: 876-881.

[48] Yanagisawa M, Kurihara H, Kimura S, Tomobe Y, Kobayashi M, Mitsui Y, Yazaki Y, Goto K, Masaki T.A novel potent vasoconstrictor peptide produced by vascular endothelial cells. *Nature.* 1988; 332: 411-415.

[49] Lüscher TF, Vanhoutte PM. Endothelium-dependent contractions to acetylcholine in the aorta of the spontaneously hypertensive rat. *Hypertension.* 1986; 8: 344-348.

[50] Auch-Schwelk W, Katusic ZS, Vanhoutte PM. Thromboxane A2 receptor antagonists inhibit endothelium-dependent contractions. *Hypertension.* 1990; 15: 699-703.

[51] Ge T, Hughes H, Junquero DC, Wu KK, Vanhoutte PM, Boulanger CM. Endothelium-dependent contractions are associated with both augmented expression of prostaglandin H synthase-1 and hypersensitivity to prostaglandin H2 in the SHR aorta. *Circ Res.* 1995; 76: 1003-1010.

[52] Gluais P, Lonchampt M, Morrow JD, Vanhoutte PM, Feletou M. Acetylcholine-induced endothelium-dependent contractions in the SHR aorta: the Janus face of prostacyclin. *Br J Pharmacol.* 2005; 146: 834-845.

[53] Kato T, Iwama Y, Okumura K, Hashimoto H, Ito T, Satake T. Prostaglandin H2 may be the endothelium-derived contracting factor released by acetylcholine in the aorta of the rat. *Hypertension.* 1990; 15: 475-481.

[54] Koga T, Takata Y, Kobayashi K, Takishita S, Yamashita Y, Fujishima M. Ageing suppresses endothelium-dependent relaxation and generates contraction mediated by the muscarinic receptors in vascular smooth muscle of normotensive Wistar- Kyoto and spontaneously hypertensive rats. *J Hypertens Suppl. 1988*; 6: S243-245.

[55] Koga T, Takata Y, Kobayashi K, Takishita S, Yamashita Y, Fujishima M. Age and hypertension promote endothelium-dependent contractions to acetylcholine in the aorta of the rat. *Hypertension.* 1989; 14: 542-548.

[56] Tang EH, Ku DD, Tipoe GL, Feletou M, Man RY, Vanhoutte PM. Endothelium-dependent contractions occur in the aorta of wild-type and COX2-/- knockout but not COX1-/- knockout mice. *J Cardiovasc Pharmacol.* 2005; 46: 761-765.

[57] Tesfamariam B, Ogletree ML. Dissociation of endothelial cell dysfunction and blood pressure in SHR. *Am J Physiol.* 1995; 269: H189-194.

[58] Yang D, Félétou M, Boulanger CM, Wu HF, Levens N, Zhang JN, Vanhoutte PM.Oxygen-derived free radicals mediate endothelium-dependent contractions to acetylcholine in aortas from spontaneously hypertensive rats. *Br J Pharmacol.* 2002; 136: 104-110.

[59] Yang D, Félétou M, Levens N, Zhang JN, Vanhoutte PM. A diffusible substance(s) mediates endothelium-dependent contractions in the aorta of SHR. *Hypertension.* 2003; 41: 143-148.

[60] Yang D, Levens N, Zhang JN, Vanhoutte PM, Félétou M. Specific potentiation of endothelium-dependent contractions in SHR by tetrahydrobiopterin. *Hypertension.* 2003; 41: 136-142.

[61] Rapoport RM, Williams SP. Role of prostaglandins in acetylcholine-induced contraction of aorta from spontaneously hypertensive and Wistar-Kyoto rats. *Hypertension.* 1996; 28: 64-75.

[62] Dowell FJ, Martin W, Dominiczak AF, Hamilton CA. Decreased basal despite enhanced agonist-stimulated effects of nitric oxide in 12-week-old stroke-prone spontaneously hypertensive rat. *Eur J Pharmacol.* 1999; 379: 175-182.

[63] Onda T, Mashiko S, Hamano M, Tomita I, Tomita T. Enhancement of endothelium-dependent relaxation in the aorta from stroke-prone spontaneously hypertensive rats at developmental stages of hypertension. *Clin Exp Pharmacol Physiol.* 1994; 21: 857-863.

[64] Tomita T, Onda T, Mashiko S, Hamano M, Tomita I. Blood pressure-related changes of endothelium-dependent relaxation in the aorta from SHRSP at developmental ages of hypertension. *Clin Exp Pharmacol Physiol Suppl.* 1995; 22: S139-141.

[65] Nishikawa M, Kubo Y, Kido H, Nakayama T, Nakamura N. Protection against endothelial abnormalities by a novel calcium channel blocker, AE0047, in stroke-prone spontaneously hypertensive rats. *Gen Pharmacol.* 1999; 32: 299-305.

[66] Novosel D, Lang MG, Noll G, Lüscher TF. Endothelial dysfunction in aorta of the spontaneously hypertensive, stroke-prone rat: effects of therapy with verapamil and trandolapril alone and in combination. *J Cardiovasc Pharmacol.* 1994; 24: 979-985.

[67] Shimamura K, Sekiguchi F, Matsuda K, Ozaki M, Noguchi K, Yamamoto K, Shibano T, Tanaka M, Sunano S. Effect of chronic treatment with perindopril on endothelium-dependent relaxation of aorta and carotid artery in SHRSP. *J Smooth Muscle Res.* 2000; 36: 33-46.

[68] Touyz RM. Reactive oxygen species, vascular oxidative stress, and redox signaling in hypertension: what is the clinical significance? *Hypertension.* 2004; 44: 248-252.

[69] Lassègue B, Griendling KK. Reactive oxygen species in hypertension; *An update. Am J Hypertens.* 2004; 17: 852-860.

[70] Pollock DM. Endothelin, angiotensin, and oxidative stress in hypertension. *Hypertension.* 2005; 45: 477-480.

[71] Schiffrin EL. Vascular endothelin in hypertension. *Vascul Pharmacol.* 2005; 43:19-29.

[72] Krum H, Viskoper RJ, Lacourciere Y, Budde M, Charlon V. The effect of an endothelin-receptor antagonist, bosentan, on blood pressure in patients with essential hypertension. Bosentan Hypertension Investigators. *N Engl J Med.* 1998; 338: 784-790.

[73] Nakov R, Pfarr E, Eberle S; HEAT Investigators. Darusentan: an effective endothelinA receptor antagonist for treatment of hypertension. *Am J Hypertens.* 2002; 15: 583-589.

[74] Cardillo C, Campia U, Kilcoyne CM, Bryant MB, Panza JA. Improved endothelium-dependent vasodilation after blockade of endothelin receptors in patients with essential hypertension. *Circulation.* 2002; 105: 452-456.

[75] Cardillo C, Kilcoyne CM, Waclawiw M, Cannon RO 3rd, Panza JA. Role of endothelin in the increased vascular tone of patients with essential hypertension. *Hypertension.* 1999; 33: 753-758.

[76] Ghiadoni L, Virdis A, Magagna A, Taddei S, Salvetti A. Effect of the angiotensin II type 1 receptor blocker candesartan on endothelial function in patients with essential hypertension. *Hypertension.* 2000; 35: 501-506.

[77] Linder L, Kiowski W, Bühler FR, Lüscher TF. Indirect evidence for release of endothelium-derived relaxing factor in human forearm circulation in vivo. Blunted response in essential hypertension. *Circulation.* 1990; 81: 1762-1767.

[78] Panza JA, Quyyumi AA, Brush JE Jr, Epstein SE. Abnormal endothelium-dependent vascular relaxation in patients with essential hypertension. *N Engl J Med.* 1990; 323: 22-27.

[79] Taddei S, Virdis A, Mattei P, Salvetti A. Vasodilation to acetylcholine in primary and secondary forms of human hypertension. *Hypertension.* 1993; 21: 929-933.

[80] Taddei S, Virdis A, Mattei P, Ghiadoni L, Gennari A, Fasolo CB, Sudano I, Salvetti A. Aging and endothelial function in normotensive subjects and patients with essential hypertension. *Circulation.* 1995; 91: 1981-1987.

[81] Taddei S, Virdis A, Ghiadoni L, Uleri S, Magagna A, Salvetti A. Lacidipine restores endothelium-dependent vasodilation in essential hypertensive patients. *Hypertension.* 1997; 30: 1606-1612.

[82] Taddei S, Virdis A, Ghiadoni L, Salvetti G, Salvetti A. Endothelial dysfunction in hypertension. *J Nephrol.* 2000; 13: 205-210.

[83] Taddei S, Virdis A, Ghiadoni L, Magagna A, Salvetti A. Cyclooxygenase inhibition restores nitric oxide activity in essential hypertension. *Hypertension.* 1997; 29: 274-279.

[84] Bulut D, Liaghat S, Hanefeld C, Koll R, Miebach T, Mügge A.Selective cyclo-oxygenase-2 inhibition with parecoxib acutely impairs endothelium-dependent

vasodilatation in patients with essential hypertension. *J Hypertens.* 2003; 21: 1663-1667.

[85] Solzbach U, Hornig B, Jeserich M, Just H. Vitamin C improves endothelial dysfunction of epicardial coronary arteries in hypertensive patients. *Circulation.* 1997; 96: 1513-1519.

[86] Taddei S, Virdis A, Ghiadoni L, Magagna A, Salvetti A. Vitamin C improves endothelium-dependent vasodilation by restoring nitric oxide activity in essential hypertension. *Circulation. 1998*; 97: 2222-9.

[87] Rossi GP, Taddei S, Virdis A, Cavallin M, Ghiadoni L, Favilla S, Versari D, Sudano I, Pessina AC, Salvetti A. The T-786C and Glu298Asp polymorphisms of the endothelial nitric oxide gene affect the forearm blood flow responses of Caucasian hypertensive patients. *J Am Coll Cardiol.* 2003; 41: 938-945.

[88] Higashi Y, Sasaki S, Nakagawa K, Fukuda Y, Matsuura H, Oshima T, Chayama K. Tetrahydrobiopterin enhances forearm vascular response to acetylcholine in both normotensive and hypertensive individuals. *Am J Hypertens.* 2002; 15: 326-332.

[89] Schlaich MP, Parnell MM, Ahlers BA, Finch S, Marshall T, Zhang WZ, Kaye DM. Impaired L-arginine transport and endothelial function in hypertensive and genetically predisposed normotensive subjects. *Circulation.* 2004; 110: 3680-3686.

[90] Perticone F, Sciacqua A, Maio R, Perticone M, Maas R, Boger RH, Tripepi G, Sesti G, Zoccali C. Asymmetric dimethylarginine, L-arginine, and endothelial dysfunction in essential hypertension. *J Am Coll Cardiol.* 2005; 46: 518-523.

[91] Takiuchi S, Fujii H, Kamide K, Horio T, Nakatani S, Hiuge A, Rakugi H, Ogihara T, Kawano Y. Plasma asymmetric dimethylarginine and coronary and peripheral endothelial dysfunction in hypertensive patients. *Am J Hypertens.* 2004; 17: 802-808.

[92] Vallance P, Leone A, Calver A, Collier J, Moncada S. Accumulation of an endogenous inhibitor of nitric oxide synthesis in chronic renal failure. *Lancet.* 1992; 339: 572-575.

[93] Panza JA, Casino PR, Kilcoyne CM, Quyyumi AA. Impaired endothelium-dependent vasodilation in patients with essential hypertension: evidence that the abnormality is not at the muscarinic receptor level. *J Am Coll Cardiol.* 1994; 23: 1610-1616.

[94] Panza JA, García CE, Kilcoyne CM, Quyyumi AA, Cannon RO 3rd. Impaired endothelium-dependent vasodilation in patients with essential hypertension. Evidence that nitric oxide abnormality is not localized to a single signal transduction pathway. *Circulation.* 1995; 91:1732-1738.

[95] Taddei S, Ghiadoni L, Virdis A, Buralli S, Salvetti A. Vasodilation to bradykinin is mediated by an ouabain-sensitive pathway as a compensatory mechanism for impaired nitric oxide availability in essential hypertensive patients. *Circulation.* 1999; 100: 1400-1405.

[96] Virdis A, Ghiadoni L, Cardinal H, Favilla S, Duranti P, Birindelli R, Magagna A, Bernini G, Salvetti G, Taddei S, Salvetti A. Mechanisms responsible for endothelial dysfunction induced by fasting hyperhomocystinemia in normotensive subjects and patients with essential hypertension. *J Am Coll Cardiol.* 2001; 38: 1106-1115.

[97] Bennett-Richards K, Kattenhorn M, Donald A, Oakley G, Varghese Z, Rees L, Deanfield JE. Does oral folic acid lower total homocysteine levels and improve endothelial function in children with chronic renal failure? *Circulation.* 2002; 105: 1810-1815.

[98] Zhang X, Li H, Jin H, Ebin Z, Brodsky S, Goligorsky MS. Effects of homocysteine on endothelial nitric oxide production. *Am J Physiol Renal Physiol.* 2000; 279: F671-678.

[99] Virdis A, Iglarz M, Neves MF, Amiri F, Touyz RM, Rozen R, Schiffrin EL. Effect of hyperhomocystinemia and hypertension on endothelial function in methylenetetrahydrofolate reductase-deficient mice. *Arterioscler Thromb Vasc Biol.* 2003; 23: 1352-1357.

[100] Stühlinger MC, Tsao PS, Her JH, Kimoto M, Balint RF, Cooke JP. Homocysteine impairs the nitric oxide synthase pathway: role of asymmetric dimethylarginine. *Circulation.* 2001; 104: 2569-2575.

[101] Stühlinger MC, Oka RK, Graf EE, Schmölzer I, Upson BM, Kapoor O, Szuba A, Malinow MR, Wascher TC, Pachinger O, Cooke JP. Endothelial dysfunction induced by hyperhomocyst(e)inemia: role of asymmetric dimethylarginine. *Circulation.* 2003; 108: 933-938.

[102] Böger RH, Lentz SR, Bode-Böger SM, Knapp HR, Haynes WG. Elevation of asymmetrical dimethylarginine may mediate endothelial dysfunction during experimental hyperhomocyst(e)inaemia in humans. *Clin Sci (Lond).* 2001; 100: 161-167.

[103] Wanby P, Brattström L, Brudin L, Hultberg B, Teerlink T. Asymmetric dimethylarginine and total homocysteine in plasma after oral methionine loading. *Scand J Clin Lab Invest.* 2003; 63: 347-353.

[104] Mallamaci F, Zoccali C, Tripepi G, Fermo I, Benedetto FA, Cataliotti A, Bellanuova I, Malatino LS, Soldarini A; CREED Investigators. Hyperhomocysteinemia predicts cardiovascular outcomes in hemodialysis patients. *Kidney Int.* 2002; 61: 609-614.

[105] Paniagua OA, Bryant MB, Panza JA. Transient hypertension directly impairs endothelium-dependent vasodilation of the human microvasculature. *Hypertension.* 2000; 36: 941-944.

[106] Taddei S, Virdis A, Mattei P, Ghiadoni L, Sudano I, Salvetti A. Defective L-arginine-nitric oxide pathway in offspring of essential hypertensive patients. *Circulation.* 1996; 94: 1298-1303.

[107] Taddei S, Virdis A, Ghiadoni L, Sudano I, Salvetti A. Effects of antihypertensive drugs on endothelial dysfunction: clinical implications. *Drugs.* 2002; 62: 265-284.

[108] Thuillez C, Richard V. Targeting endothelial dysfunction in hypertensive subjects. *J Hum Hypertens.* 2005; 19 Suppl 1: S21-25.

[109] Klingbeil AU, John S, Schneider MP, Jacobi J, Handrock R, Schmieder RE. Effect of AT1 receptor blockade on endothelial function in essential hypertension. *Am J Hypertens.* 2003; 16: 123-128.

[110] Mulder HJ, Bal ET, Jukema JW, Zwinderman AH, Schalij MJ, van Boven AJ, Bruschke AV. Pravastatin reduces restenosis two years after percutaneous transluminal coronary angioplasty (REGRESS trial). *Am J Cardiol.* 2000;86:742-746.

[111] Schiffrin EL, Deng LY. Comparison of effects of angiotensin I-converting enzyme inhibition and beta-blockade for 2 years on function of small arteries from hypertensive patients. *Hypertension.* 1995; 25: 699-703.

[112] Taddei S, Virdis A, Ghiadoni L, Magagna A, Pasini AF, Garbin U, Cominacini L, Salvetti A. Effect of calcium antagonist or beta blockade treatment on nitric oxide-dependent vasodilation and oxidative stress in essential hypertensive patients. *J Hypertens.* 2001; 19: 1379-1386.

[113] von zur Mühlen B, Kahan T, Hägg A, Millgård J, Lind L. Treatment with irbesartan or atenolol improves endothelial function in essential hypertension. *J Hypertens.* 2001; 19: 1813-1818.

[114] Tzemos N, Lim PO, MacDonald TM. Nebivolol reverses endothelial dysfunction in essential hypertension: a randomized, double-blind, crossover study. *Circulation.* 2001; 104: 511-514.

[115] Boulanger CM, Nakashima M, Olmos L, Joly G, Vanhoutte PM. Effects of the Ca2+ antagonist RO 40-5967 on endothelium-dependent responses of isolated arteries. *J Cardiovasc Pharmacol.* 1994; 23: 869-876.

[116] Vilaine JP, Biondi ML, Villeneuve N, Feletou M, Peglion JL, Vanhoutte PM. The calcium channel antagonist S 11568 causes endothelium-dependent relaxation in canine arteries. *Eur J Pharmacol.* 1991; 197: 41-48.

[117] Lenasi H, Kohlstedt K, Fichtlscherer B, Mülsch A, Busse R, Fleming I. Amlodipine activates the endothelial nitric oxide synthase by altering phosphorylation on Ser1177 and Thr495. *Cardiovasc Res.* 2003; 59: 844-853.

[118] Zhang L, Fujii S, Igarashi J, Kosaka H. Effects of thiol antioxidant on reduced nicotinamide adenine dinucleotide phosphate oxidase in hypertensive Dahl salt-sensitive rats. *Free Radic Biol Med.* 2004; 37: 1813-1820.

[119] Ghiadoni L, Magagna A, Versari D, Kardasz I, Huang Y, Taddei S, Salvetti A. Different effect of antihypertensive drugs on conduit artery endothelial function. *Hypertension. 2003*; 41: 1281-1286.

[120] Hirooka Y, Imaizumi T, Masaki H, Ando S, Harada S, Momohara M, Takeshita A. Captopril improves impaired endothelium-dependent vasodilation in hypertensive patients. *Hypertension.* 1992; 20: 175-180.

[121] Pitt B. Effect of ACE inhibitors on endothelial dysfunction: unanswered questions and implications for further investigation and therapy. *Cardiovasc Drugs Ther.* 1996; 10: 469-473.

[122] Taddei S, Virdis A, Ghiadoni L, Mattei P, Salvetti A. Effects of angiotensin converting enzyme inhibition on endothelium-dependent vasodilatation in essential hypertensive patients. *J Hypertens.* 1998; 16: 447-456.

[123] Antony I, Lerebours G, Nitenberg A. Angiotensin-converting enzyme inhibition restores flow-dependent and cold pressor test-induced dilations in coronary arteries of hypertensive patients. *Circulation.* 1996; 94: 3115-3122.

[124] Ludmer PL, Selwyn AP, Shook TL, Wayne RR, Mudge GH, Alexander RW, Ganz P.Paradoxical vasoconstriction induced by acetylcholine in atherosclerotic coronary arteries. *N Engl J Med.* 1986; 315: 1046-1051.

[125] Lerman A, Zeiher AM.Endothelial function: cardiac events. *Circulation.* 2005; 111: 363-368.

[126] Ganz P, Vita JA.Testing endothelial vasomotor function: nitric oxide, a multipotent molecule. *Circulation.* 2003; 108: 2049-2053.

[127] Anderson TJ. Arterial stiffness or endothelial dysfunction as a surrogate marker of vascular risk. *Can J Cardiol.* 2006; 22 Suppl B: 72B-80B

[128] Tousoulis D, Antoniades C, Stefanadis C. Evaluating endothelial function in humans: a guide to invasive and non-invasive techniques. *Heart.* 2005; 91: 553-8.

[129] Widlansky ME, Gokce N, Keaney JF Jr, Vita JA. The clinical implications of endothelial dysfunction. *J Am Coll Cardiol.* 2003; 42: 1149-1160.

[130] Heitzer T, Schlinzig T, Krohn K, Meinertz T, Münzel T. Endothelial dysfunction, oxidative stress, and risk of cardiovascular events in patients with coronary artery disease. *Circulation.* 2001; 104: 2673-2678.

[131] Gokce N. Clinical assessment of endothelial function: ready for prime time? *Circ Cardiovasc Imaging.* 2011; 4: 348-350.

[132] Stoner L, Young JM, Fryer S. Assessments of arterial stiffness and endothelial function using pulse wave analysis. *Int J Vasc Med.* 2012; 2012: 903107.

[133] Hijmering ML, Stroes ES, Pasterkamp G, Sierevogel M, Banga JD, Rabelink TJ. Variability of flow mediated dilation: consequences for clinical application. *Atherosclerosis.* 2001; 157: 369-373.

[134] Yoshinaga K, Manabe O, Tamaki N. Assessment of coronary endothelial function using PET. *J Nucl Cardiol.* 2011; 18: 486-500.

[135] Anderson TJ. Assessment and treatment of endothelial dysfunction in humans. *J Am Coll Cardiol.* 1999; 34: 631-638.

[136] Hamburg NM, Benjamin EJ. Assessment of endothelial function using digital pulse amplitude tonometry. *Trends Cardiovasc Med.* 2009; 19: 6-11.

[137] Schwartz BG, Economides C, Mayeda GS, Burstein S, Kloner RA.The endothelial cell in health and disease: its function, dysfunction, measurement and therapy. *Int J Impot Res.* 2010; 22: 77-90.

[138] Anderson TJ, Uehata A, Gerhard MD, Meredith IT, Knab S, Delagrange D, Lieberman EH, Ganz P, Creager MA, Yeung AC, et al.Close relation of endothelial function in the human coronary and peripheral circulations. *J Am Coll Cardiol.* 1995; 26: 1235-41.

[139] Irace C, Ceravolo R, Notarangelo L, Crescenzo A, Ventura G, Tamburrini O, Perticone F, Gnasso A. Comparison of endothelial function evaluated by strain gauge plethysmography and brachial artery ultrasound. *Atherosclerosis.* 2001; 158: 53-59.

[140] Hamburg NM, Palmisano J, Larson MG, Sullivan LM, Lehman BT, Vasan RS, Levy D, Mitchell GF, Vita JA, Benjamin EJ. Relation of brachial and digital measures of vascular function in the community: the Framingham heart study. *Hypertension.* 2011; 57: 390-396.

[141] Hamburg NM, Keyes MJ, Larson MG, Vasan RS, Schnabel R, Pryde MM, Mitchell GF, Sheffy J, Vita JA, Benjamin EJ. Cross-sectional relations of digital vascular function to cardiovascular risk factors in the Framingham Heart Study. *Circulation.* 2008; 117: 2467-2474.

[142] Whelton SP, Chin A, Xin X, He J. Effect of aerobic exercise on blood pressure: a meta-analysis of randomized, controlled trials. *Ann Intern Med.* 2002; 136: 493-503.

[143] Higashi Y, Sasaki S, Kurisu S, Yoshimizu A, Sasaki N, Matsuura H, Kajiyama G, Oshima T. Regular aerobic exercise augments endothelium-dependent vascular relaxation in normotensive as well as hypertensive subjects: role of endothelium-derived nitric oxide. *Circulation.* 1999; 100: 1194-1202.

[144] Lavrencic A, Salobir BG, Keber I. Physical training improves flow-mediated dilation in patients with the polymetabolic syndrome. *Arterioscler Thromb Vasc Biol.* 2000; 20: 551-555.

[145] Maiorana A, O'Driscoll G, Cheetham C, Dembo L, Stanton K, Goodman C, Taylor R, Green D. The effect of combined aerobic and resistance exercise training on vascular function in type 2 diabetes. *J Am Coll Cardiol.* 2001; 38: 860-866.

[146] Beck DT, Casey DP, Martin JS, Emerson BD, Braith RW. Exercise training improves endothelial function in young prehypertensives. *Exp Biol Med (Maywood).* 2013; 238: 433-441.

[147] Sessa WC, Pritchard K, Seyedi N, Wang J, Hintze TH. Chronic exercise in dogs increases coronary vascular nitric oxide production and endothelial cell nitric oxide synthase gene expression. *Circ Res.* 1994; 74: 349-353.

[148] Woodman CR, Muller JM, Laughlin MH, Price EM. Induction of nitric oxide synthase mRNA in coronary resistance arteries isolated from exercise-trained pigs. *Am J Physiol.* 1997; 273: H2575-2579.

[149] Davis ME, Cai H, Drummond GR, Harrison DG. Shear stress regulates endothelial nitric oxide synthase expression through c-Src by divergent signaling pathways. *Circ Res.* 2001; 89: 1073-1080.

[150] Ranjan V, Xiao Z, Diamond SL. Constitutive NOS expression in cultured endothelial cells is elevated by fluid shear stress. *Am J Physiol.* 1995;269:H550-555.

[151] Venema RC, Nishida K, Alexander RW, Harrison DG, Murphy TJ. Organization of the bovine gene encoding the endothelial nitric oxide synthase. *Biochim Biophys Acta.* 1994; 1218: 413-420.

[152] Hambrecht R, Adams V, Erbs S, Linke A, Kränkel N, Shu Y, Baither Y, Gielen S, Thiele H, Gummert JF, Mohr FW, Schuler G. Regular physical activity improves endothelial function in patients with coronary artery disease by increasing phosphorylation of endothelial nitric oxide synthase. *Circulation.* 2003; 107: 3152-3158.

[153] Fukai T, Siegfried MR, Ushio-Fukai M, Cheng Y, Kojda G, Harrison DG. Regulation of the vascular extracellular superoxide dismutase by nitric oxide and exercise training. *J Clin Invest.* 2000; 105: 1631-1639.

[154] Ennezat PV, Malendowicz SL, Testa M, Colombo PC, Cohen-Solal A, Evans T, LeJemtel TH. Physical training in patients with chronic heart failure enhances the expression of genes encoding antioxidative enzymes. *J Am Coll Cardiol.* 2001; 38: 194-198.

[155] Dimmeler S, Haendeler J, Rippmann V, Nehls M, Zeiher AM. Shear stress inhibits apoptosis of human endothelial cells. *FEBS Lett.* 1996; 399: 71-4.

[156] Dimmeler S, Hermann C, Galle J, Zeiher AM. Upregulation of superoxide dismutase and nitric oxide synthase mediates the apoptosis-suppressive effects of shear stress on endothelial cells. *Arterioscler Thromb Vasc Biol.* 1999; 19: 656-664.

[157] Inoue N, Ramasamy S, Fukai T, Nerem RM, Harrison DG. Shear stress modulates expression of Cu/Zn superoxide dismutase in human aortic endothelial cells. *Circ Res.* 1996; 79: 32-37.

[158] Takeshita S, Inoue N, Rikitake Y, Kawashima S, Yokoyama M. Mechanical stress modulates glutathione peroxidase expression in cultured bovine aortic endothelial cells. *Ann N Y Acad Sci.* 2000; 902: 298-301.

[159] Rush JW, Turk JR, Laughlin MH. Exercise training regulates SOD-1 and oxidative stress in porcine aortic endothelium. *Am J Physiol Heart Circ Physiol.* 2003; 284: H1378-1387.

[160] Green DJ, Maiorana A, O'Driscoll G, Taylor R. Effect of exercise training on endothelium-derived nitric oxide function in humans. *J Physiol.* 2004;561:1-25.

[161] Maiorana A, O'Driscoll G, Taylor R, Green D. Exercise and the nitric oxide vasodilator system. *Sports Med.* 2003; 33: 1013-1035.

[162] Tjønna AE, Lee SJ, Rognmo Ø, Stølen TO, Bye A, Haram PM, Loennechen JP, Al-Share QY, Skogvoll E, Slørdahl SA, Kemi OJ, Najjar SM, Wisløff U. Aerobic interval training versus continuous moderate exercise as a treatment for the metabolic syndrome: a pilot study. *Circulation.* 2008; 118: 346-354.

[163] Wisløff U, Støylen A, Loennechen JP, Bruvold M, Rognmo Ø, Haram PM, Tjønna AE, Helgerud J, Slørdahl SA, Lee SJ, Videm V, Bye A, Smith GL, Najjar SM, Ellingsen Ø, Skjaerpe T. Superior cardiovascular effect of aerobic interval training versus moderate continuous training in heart failure patients: a randomized study. *Circulation.* 2007; 115: 3086-3094.

[164] Laufs U, Werner N, Link A, Endres M, Wassmann S, Jürgens K, Miche E, Böhm M, Nickenig G. Physical training increases endothelial progenitor cells, inhibits neointima formation, and enhances angiogenesis. *Circulation.* 2004; 109: 220-226.

[165] Fernandes T, Nakamuta JS, Magalhães FC, Roque FR, Lavini-Ramos C, Schettert IT, Coelho V, Krieger JE, Oliveira EM. Exercise training restores the endothelial progenitor cells number and function in hypertension: implications for angiogenesis. *J Hypertens.* 2012; 30: 2133-2143.

[166] Aicher A, Heeschen C, Mildner-Rihm C, Urbich C, Ihling C, Technau-Ihling K, Zeiher AM, Dimmeler S. Essential role of endothelial nitric oxide synthase for mobilization of stem and progenitor cells. *Nat Med.* 2003; 9: 1370-6.

[167] Verma S, Kuliszewski MA, Li SH, Szmitko PE, Zucco L, Wang CH, Badiwala MV, Mickle DA, Weisel RD, Fedak PW, Stewart DJ, Kutryk MJ. C-reactive protein attenuates endothelial progenitor cell survival, differentiation, and function: further evidence of a mechanistic link between C-reactive protein and cardiovascular disease. *Circulation.* 2004; 109: 2058-2067.

[168] Kelley GA, Kelley KS. Effects of aerobic exercise on C-reactive protein, body composition, and maximum oxygen consumption in adults: a meta-analysis of randomized controlled trials. *Metabolism.* 2006; 55: 1500-1507.

[169] Taubert D, Roesen R, Lehmann C, Jung N, Schömig E. Effects of low habitual cocoa intake on blood pressure and bioactive nitric oxide: a randomized controlled trial. *JAMA.* 2007; 298: 49-60.

[170] Hooper L, Kroon PA, Rimm EB, Cohn JS, Harvey I, Le Cornu KA, Ryder JJ, Hall WL, Cassidy A. Flavonoids, flavonoid-rich foods, and cardiovascular risk: a meta-analysis of randomized controlled trials. *Am J Clin Nutr. 2008*; 88: 38-50.

[171] Fraga CG, Litterio MC, Prince PD, Calabró V, Piotrkowski B, Galleano M. Cocoa flavanols: effects on vascular nitric oxide and blood pressure. *J Clin Biochem Nutr.* 2011; 48: 63-67.

[172] Ried K, Sullivan T, Fakler P, Frank OR, Stocks NP. Does chocolate reduce blood pressure? *A meta-analysis. BMC Med.* 2010; 8: 39.

[173] Jaganath I, Crozier A. Dietary flavonoids and phenolic compounds. In: Fraga CG, editor. *Plant Phenolics and Human Health: Biochemistry, Nutrition and Pharmacology Hoboken.* New Jersey: John Wiley & Sons; 2010. pp. 1–49.

[174] Steffen Y, Gruber C, Schewe T, Sies H. Mono-O-methylated flavanols and other flavonoids as inhibitors of endothelial NADPH oxidase. *Arch Biochem Biophys.* 2008; 469: 209-219.

[175] Zhang H, Du Y, Cohen RA, Chobanian AV, Brecher P. Adventitia as a source of inducible nitric oxide synthase in the rat aorta. *Am J Hypertens.* 1999; 12: 467–475.

[176] Brewster UC, Setaro JF, Perazella MA. The renin-angiotensin-aldosterone system: cardiorenal effects and implications for renal and cardiovascular disease states. *Am J Med Sci.* 2003; 326: 15–24.

[177] Paravicini TM, Touyz RM. Redox signaling in hypertension. *Cardiovasc Res.* 2006; 71: 247–258.

[178] Galleano M, Pechanova O, Fraga CG. Hypertension, nitric oxide, oxidants, and dietary plant polyphenol. *Curr Pharm Biotechnol.* 2010; 11: 837–848.

[179] Cienfuegos-Jovellanos E, Quiñones Mdel, Muguerza B, Moulay L, Miguel M, Aleixandre A. Antihypertensive effect of a polyphenol-rich cocoa powder industrially processed to preserve the original flavonoids of the cocoa beans. *J Agric Food Chem.* 2009; 57: 6156–6162.

[180] Fraga CG. Plant polyphenols: how to translate their in vitro antioxidant actions to in vivo conditions. *IUBMB Life.* 2007; 59: 308–315.

[181] Alef MJ, Tzeng E, Zuckerbraun BS. Nitric oxide and nitrite-based therapeutic opportunities in intimal hyperplasia. *Nitric Oxide.* 2012; 26: 285-294.

[182] Reshma S Baliga, Alexandra B Milsom, Suborno M Ghosh, Sarah L Trinder, Raymond J MacAllister, Amrita Ahluwalia, Adrian J Hobbs. Dietary nitrate ameliorates pulmonary hypertension: cytoprotective role for endothelial nitric oxide synthase and xanthine oxidoreductase. *Circulation.* 2012; 125: 2922–2932.

[183] Dejam A, Hunter CJ, Schechter AN, Gladwin MT. Emerging role of nitrite in human biology. *Blood Cells Mol Dis.* 2004; 32: 423-429.

[184] Gladwin MT, Raat NJ, Shiva S, Dezfulian C, Hogg N, Kim-Shapiro DB, Patel RP. Nitrite as a vascular endocrine nitric oxide reservoir that contributes to hypoxic signaling, cytoprotection, and vasodilation. *Am J Physiol Heart Circ Physiol.* 2006; 291: H2026-2035.

[185] Murata I, Nozaki R, Ooi K, Ohtake K, Kimura S, Ueda H, Nakano G, Sonoda K, Inoue Y, Uchida H, Kanamoto I, Morimoto Y, Kobayashi J. Nitrite reduces ischemia/reperfusion-induced muscle damage and improves survival rates in rat crush injury model. *J Trauma Acute Care Surg. 2012*; 72: 1548-54.

[186] Huang Z, Shiva S, Kim-Shapiro DB, Patel RP, Ringwood LA, Irby CE, Huang KT, Ho C, Hogg N, Schechter AN, Gladwin MT. Enzymatic function of hemoglobin as a nitrite reductase that produces NO under allosteric control. *J Clin Invest.* 2005; 115: 2099-2107.

[187] Li H, Cui H, Kundu TK, Alzawahra W, Zweier JL. Nitric oxide production from nitrite occurs primarily in tissues not in the blood: critical role of xanthine oxidase and aldehyde oxidase. *J Biol Chem.* 2008; 283: 17855-17863.

[188] Li H, Samouilov A, Liu X, Zweier JL. Characterization of the magnitude and kinetics of xanthine oxidase-catalyzed nitrite reduction. Evaluation of its role in nitric oxide generation in anoxic tissues. *J Biol Chem.* 2001; 276: 24482-24489.

[189] Godber BL, Doel JJ, Sapkota GP, Blake DR, Stevens CR, Eisenthal R, Harrison R. Reduction of nitrite to nitric oxide catalyzed by xanthine oxidoreductase. *J Biol Chem.* 2000; 275: 7757-7763.

[190] Cosby K, Partovi KS, Crawford JH, Patel RP, Reiter CD, Martyr S, Yang BK, Waclawiw MA, Zalos G, Xu X, Huang KT, Shields H, Kim-Shapiro DB, Schechter

AN, Cannon RO 3rd, Gladwin MT. Nitrite reduction to nitric oxide by deoxyhemoglobin vasodilates the human circulation. *Nat Med.* 2003; 9: 1498-1505.

[191] Nagababu E, Ramasamy S, Abernethy DR, Rifkind JM. Active nitric oxide produced in the red cell under hypoxic conditions by deoxyhemoglobin-mediated nitrite reduction. *J Biol Chem.* 2003; 278: 46349-46356.

[192] Shiva S, Huang Z, Grubina R, Sun J, Ringwood LA, MacArthur PH, Xu X, Murphy E, Darley-Usmar VM, Gladwin MT. Deoxymyoglobin is a nitrite reductase that generates nitric oxide and regulates mitochondrial respiration. *Circ Res.* 2007; 100: 654-661.

[193] Rassaf T, Flögel U, Drexhage C, Hendgen-Cotta U, Kelm M, Schrader J. Nitrite reductase function of deoxymyoglobin: oxygen sensor and regulator of cardiac energetics and function. *Circ Res.* 2007; 100: 1749-1754.

[194] Zweier JL, Samouilov A, Kuppusamy P. Non-enzymatic nitric oxide synthesis in biological systems. *Biochim Biophys Acta.* 1999; 1411: 250-262.

[195] Maia LB, Moura JJ. Nitrite reduction by xanthine oxidase family enzymes: a new class of nitrite reductases. *J Biol Inorg Chem.* 2011; 16: 443-460.

[196] Schiffrin EL, Deng LY. Structure and function of resistance arteries of hypertensive patients treated with a beta-blocker or a calcium channel antagonist. *J Hypertens.* 1996; 14: 1247-1255.

[197] Gao YS, Nagao T, Bond RA, Janssens WJ, Vanhoutte PM. Nebivolol induces endothelium-dependent relaxations of canine coronary arteries. *J Cardiovasc Pharmacol.* 1991; 17: 964-969.

[198] Cockcroft JR, Chowienczyk PJ, Brett SE, Chen CP, Dupont AG, Van Nueten L, Wooding SJ, Ritter JM. Nebivolol vasodilates human forearm vasculature: evidence for an L-arginine/NO-dependent mechanism. *J Pharmacol Exp Ther.* 1995; 274: 1067-1071.

[199] Mason RP, Kubant R, Jacob RF, Walter MF, Boychuk B, Malinski T. Effect of nebivolol on endothelial nitric oxide and peroxynitrite release in hypertensive animals: Role of antioxidant activity. *J Cardiovasc Pharmacol.* 2006; 48: 862-829.

[200] Feuerstein GZ, Ruffolo RR Jr. Carvedilol, a novel multiple action antihypertensive agent with antioxidant activity and the potential for myocardial and vascular protection. *Eur Heart J.* 1995; 16 Suppl F: 38-42.

[201] Bank AJ, Kelly AS, Thelen AM, Kaiser DR, Gonzalez-Campoy JM. Effects of carvedilol versus metoprolol on endothelial function and oxidative stress in patients with type 2 diabetes mellitus. *Am J Hypertens.* 2007; 20: 777-783.

[202] Nishioka K, Nakagawa K, Umemura T, Jitsuiki D, Ueda K, Goto C, Chayama K, Yoshizumi M, Higashi Y. Carvedilol improves endothelium-dependent vasodilation in patients with dilated cardiomyopathy. *Heart.* 2007; 93: 247-248.

[203] ENCORE Investigators. Effect of nifedipine and cerivastatin on coronary endothelial function in patients with coronary artery disease: the ENCORE I Study (Evaluation of Nifedipine and Cerivastatin On Recovery of coronary Endothelial function). *Circulation.* 2003; 107: 422-428.

[204] Muiesan ML, Salvetti M, Monteduro C, Rizzoni D, Zulli R, Corbellini C, Brun C, Agabiti-Rosei E. Effect of treatment on flow-dependent vasodilation of the brachial artery in essential hypertension. *Hypertension.* 1999; 33: 575-580.

[205] Virdis A, Ghiadoni L, Taddei S.Effects of antihypertensive treatment on endothelial function. *Curr Hypertens Rep.* 2011; 13: 276-81.

[206] Sudano I, Virdis A, Taddei S, Spieker L, Corti R, Noll G, Salvetti A, Luscher TF. Chronic treatment with long-acting nifedipine reduces vasoconstriction to endothelin-1 in essential hypertension. *Hypertension.* 2007; 49: 285-290.

[207] Versari D, Virdis A, Ghiadoni L, Daghini E, Duranti E, Masi S, Magagna A, Taddei S. Effect of verapamil, trandolapril and their combination on vascular function and structure in essential hypertensive patients. *Atherosclerosis.* 2009; 205: 214-220.

[208] Mak IT, Boehme P, Weglicki WB. Antioxidant effects of calcium channel blockers against free radical injury in endothelial cells. Correlation of protection with preservation of glutathione levels. *Circ Res.* 1992; 70: 1099-1103.

[209] Moens AL, Kietadisorn R, Lin JY, Kass D. Targeting endothelial and myocardial dysfunction with tetrahydrobiopterin. *J Mol Cell Cardiol.* 2011; 51: 559-563.

[210] Moens AL, Takimoto E, Tocchetti CG, Chakir K, Bedja D, Cormaci G, Ketner EA, Majmudar M, Gabrielson K, Halushka MK, Mitchell JB, Biswal S, Channon KM, Wolin MS, Alp NJ, Paolocci N, Champion HC, Kass DA. Reversal of cardiac hypertrophy and fibrosis from pressure overload by tetrahydrobiopterin: efficacy of recoupling nitric oxide synthase as a therapeutic strategy. *Circulation.* 2008; 117: 2626-2636.

[211] Cosentino F, Hürlimann D, Delli Gatti C, Chenevard R, Blau N, Alp NJ, Channon KM, Eto M, Lerch P, Enseleit F, Ruschitzka F, Volpe M, Lüscher TF, Noll G. Chronic treatment with tetrahydrobiopterin reverses endothelial dysfunction and oxidative stress in hypercholesterolaemia. *Heart.* 2008; 94: 487-492.

[212] Landmesser U, Dikalov S, Price SR, McCann L, Fukai T, Holland SM, Mitch WE, Harrison DG. Oxidation of tetrahydrobiopterin leads to uncoupling of endothelial cell nitric oxide synthase in hypertension. *J Clin Invest.* 2003; 111: 1201-1209.

[213] Porkert M, Sher S, Reddy U, Cheema F, Niessner C, Kolm P, Jones DP, Hooper C, Taylor WR, Harrison D, Quyyumi AA. Tetrahydrobiopterin: a novel antihypertensive therapy. *J Hum Hypertens.* 2008; 22: 401-407.

[214] Shankar RR, Wu Y, Shen HQ, Zhu JS, Baron AD. Mice with gene disruption of both endothelial and neuronal nitric oxide synthase exhibit insulin resistance. *Diabetes.* 2000; 49: 684-647.

[215] Crabtree MJ, Smith CL, Lam G, Goligorsky MS, Gross SS. Ratio of 5,6,7,8-tetrahydrobiopterin to 7,8-dihydrobiopterin in endothelial cells determines glucose-elicited changes in NO vs. superoxide production by eNOS. *Am J Physiol Heart Circ Physiol.* 2008; 294: H1530-1540.

[216] Vásquez Vivar J, Duquaine D, Whitsett J, Kalyanaraman B, Rajagopalan S. Altered tetrahydrobiopterin metabolism in atherosclerosis: implications for use of oxidized tetrahydrobiopterin analogues and thiol antioxidants. *Arterioscler Thromb Vasc Biol.* 2002; 22: 1655-1661.

[217] Moens AL, Ketner EA, Takimoto E, Schmidt TS, O'Neill CA, Wolin MS, Alp NJ, Channon KM, Kass DA. Bi-modal dose-dependent cardiac response to tetrahydrobiopterin in pressure-overload induced hypertrophy and heart failure. *J Mol Cell Cardiol.* 2011; 51: 564-569.

[218] Sydow K, Münzel T. ADMA and oxidative stress. Atheroscler Suppl. 2003; 4: 41-51.

[219] Gao YT, Roman LJ, Martásek P, Panda SP, Ishimura Y, Masters BS. Oxygen metabolism by endothelial nitric-oxide synthase. *J Biol Chem.* 2007; 282: 28557-28565.

[220] Berka V, Wu G, Yeh HC, Palmer G, Tsai AL. Three different oxygen-induced radical species in endothelial nitric-oxide synthase oxygenase domain under regulation by L-arginine and tetrahydrobiopterin. *J Biol Chem.* 2004; 279: 32243-32251.

[221] Bode-Böger SM, Scalera F, Ignarro LJ. The L-arginine paradox: Importance of the L-arginine/asymmetrical dimethylarginine ratio. *Pharmacol Ther.* 2007; 114: 295-306.

[222] Fraccarollo D, Widder JD, Galuppo P, Thum T, Tsikas D, Hoffmann M, Ruetten H, Ertl G, Bauersachs J. Improvement in left ventricular remodeling by the endothelial nitric oxide synthase enhancer AVE9488 after experimental myocardial infarction. *Circulation.* 2008; 118: 818-827.

[223] Frantz S, Adamek A, Fraccarollo D, Tillmanns J, Widder JD, Dienesch C, Schäfer A, Podolskaya A, Held M, Ruetten H, Ertl G, Bauersachs J.The eNOS enhancer AVE 9488: a novel cardioprotectant against ischemia reperfusion injury. *Basic Res Cardiol.* 2009; 104: 773-779.

[224] Wohlfart P, Xu H, Endlich A, Habermeier A, Closs EI, Hübschle T, Mang C, Strobel H, Suzuki T, Kleinert H, Förstermann U, Ruetten H, Li H. Antiatherosclerotic effects of small-molecular-weight compounds enhancing endothelial nitric-oxide synthase (eNOS) expression and preventing eNOS uncoupling. *J Pharmacol Exp Ther.* 2008; 325: 370-379.

[225] Yang Q, Xue HM, Wong WT, Tian XY, Huang Y, Tsui SK, Ng PK, Wohlfart P, Li H, Xia N, Tobias S, Underwood MJ, He GW.AVE3085, an enhancer of endothelial nitric oxide synthase, restores endothelial function and reduces blood pressure in spontaneously hypertensive rats. *Br J Pharmacol.* 2011; 163: 1078-1085.

In: Advances in Hypertension Research
Editor: Ramón Rodrigo

ISBN: 978-1-62948-857-8

Chapter 3

Hypertension in Preeclampsia

Manuel Rubilar[*] and Sebastián Chávez
Molecular and Clinical Pharmacology Program, Institute of Biomedical Sciences, Faculty of Medicine, University of Chile, Chile

Abstract

Preeclampsia (PE) is a multisystem syndrome of pregnancy characterized by hypertension and proteinuria. It is the principal cause of maternal and foetal mortality. As a syndrome, "the primary event" remains largely unknown, although there are multiple mechanisms contributing to the pathophysiology of this complex obstetric condition. Nevertheless, it is widely accepted that its origin is in the placenta. Accordingly, a deficient invasion of the endometrium by extravillous trophoblast cells during the first trimester of pregnancy is the most widely recognized predisposing factor for preeclampsia. Placental hemodynamics depends mainly on local factors, because it lacks autonomic innervations. Nitric oxide (NO) plays an important role in the maintenance of placental blood flow. It regulates leukocyte adhesion to the endothelium and inhibits vascular smooth muscle cell proliferation and platelet aggregation. In PE, the bioavailability of NO is decreased compared with normal pregnancy. However, less than half of the pregnancies with PE have an altered placentation. A new hypothesis has emerged to postulate that PE is a condition determined by an exacerbated systemic inflammatory response. This systemic inflammatory response is associated with an endothelial dysfunction.

The endothelial dysfunction plays a major role in the underlying pathophysiological mechanism of the disease. Most of the clinical attributes of PE, such as hypertension, proteinuria, and edema, are derived from pathological changes within the maternal vascular endothelium or involve endothelial dysfunction, but "the factors" leading to this syndrome are not clear. Increased production of endothelin, thromboxane and superoxide, as well as an angiogenic imbalance and decreased formation of vasodilators such as nitric oxide, prostacyclin and endothelium derived hyperpolarizing factor are some of the mediators involved in the pathogenesis of preeclampsia. The occurrence of oxidative

* Corresponding author: Lic. Manuel Rubilar, Molecular and Clinical Pharmacology Program, Institute of Biomedical Sciences, Faculty of Medicine, University of Chile, Independencia 1027, C.P 8380453, Santiago 7, Chile, Telephone: 56-2-29786126 Fax: 56-2-29786126, E-mail: m.rubilar.moya@gmail.com.

stress represents a point of convergence for several contributing factors potentially leading to endothelial cell dysfunction and eventually to the clinical manifestations of PE.

This chapter discusses the relevance of endothelial dysfunction in the pathophysiology of PE, and the new evidence about the development of hypertension during the maternal syndrome.

Keywords: Preeclampsia, endothelial dysfunction, hypertension, oxidative stress

Abbreviations

ADMA	Asymmetric dimethylarginine
AT_1-AA	Autoantibodies to angiotensin II type 1 receptor
eNOS	Endothelial nitric oxide synthase
EDHF	Endothelium-derived hyperpolarizing factor
ET-1	Endothelin 1
HIF-1	Hypoxia inducible factor-1
iNOS	Inducible nitric oxide synthase
IL – 6	Interleukin 6
ICAM-1	Intercellular adhesion molecule-1
NO	Nitric oxide
NOS	Nitric oxide synthase
PGI2	Prostacyclin
ROS	Reactive oxygen species
sFlt-1	Soluble fms-like tyrosine kinase-1 factor
TGF-β	Transforming growth factor beta
TNF-α	Tumor necrosis factor-alpha
UT-II	Urotensin II
VEGF	Vascular endothelial growth factor

1. Introduction

Pregnancy is a normal part of the life cycle, but from a medical point of view, it is not free of complications. Hypertensive disorders are part of common pathologies during pregnancy. They can be classified into four categories: (i) pre-existing hypertension, characterized by being present before pregnancy or diagnosed before 20th week of gestation;(ii) pregnancy-associated hypertension as appearance of high blood pressure after 20th week of gestation, which in turn can be sub-classified according to the presence of proteinuria in preeclampsia, and gestational hypertension; (iii) superimposed preeclampsia; and (iv) eclampsia when convulsion is present in a pregnant woman with hypertension, or who later developes it.

Preeclampsia (PE) affects an estimated 2–10% of all pregnant women [1], and is the principal cause of maternal and foetal mortality [2, 3]. This systemic pregnancy disorder is characterized by high blood pressure (over 140/90 mmHg) and proteinuria (greater than 300 mg in a 24 hour urine collection), both of which disapear after delivery of the foetus [4].

Normal pregnancy is characterized by a fall in blood pressure due to peripheral vasodilatation during the second trimester, and increased cardiac output and blood volume by about 50%. By contrast, severe PE has usually been associated with low cardiac output and high peripheral resistance [5], decreasing in intravascular volume [6], low platelet count [6], fall in renal function [7, 8], liver damage and central nervous system dysfunction [6, 9]. There is no satisfactory treatment to prevent the development of the disease, except for measures to avoid or reduce complications [10, 11]. Indeed, early delivery is the only successful treatment. In about 20% of cases of early onset PE leads to delivery before 34 weeks. This pathology is more common in the following conditions: primagravid women, maternal age above 40 years and multiparous women with change of partner, increased body mass index and obesity, previous history of preeclampsia, antiphospholipid antibodies, pre-existing diabetes, and multiple pregnancies.

Preeclampsia as a syndrome, "the primary event" remains largely unknown, there are multiple mechanisms contributing to the pathophysiology of this complex obstetric condition. However, it is widely accepted that its origin is in the placenta [12-14]. This disease can be understood in two stages: a first stage "placental syndrome", and second the "maternal syndrome". A deficient invasion of the endometrium by extravillous trophoblast (EVT) cells during the first trimester of pregnancy is the most widely recognized predisposing factor for preeclampsia [15 16]. This failure in placental trophoblast invasion into the spiral arteries displays an abnormally high vascular resistance with reduced uteroplacental perfusion [17-18], giving rise to hypoxia–reoxygenation cycles. There are a series of intrinsic and extrinsic mechanisms that can alter the physiological process of placentation in the fetal-maternal interface. Among them, and related to hypoxia and reperfusion (or hypoxia by itself) is the increase of the EVT apoptosis. Also, the activation of apoptotic pathways could lead to increased deportation of syncytiotrophoblast microvesicles into the maternal circulation. These particles have been directly linked to activation of maternal neutrophils and the development of the maternal syndrome [19, 20]. Additionally, hypoxia generates an antiangiogenic state, mediated by a local and systemic increase of sFlt-1, the soluble receptor of the vascular endothelial growth factor (VEGF), which in turn, lowers the bioavailability of the latter and the placental growth factor (PlGF), thus resulting in an impaired angiogenesis and placentation.

Placental hemodynamics depends mainly on local factors, because it lacks autonomic innervations. Therefore, nitric oxide (NO) plays an important role in the maintenance of placental blood flow. In addition, NO regulates leukocyte adhesion to the endothelium, inhibits vascular smooth muscle cell proliferation and platelet aggregation. NO is synthesized by nitric oxide synthase (NOS). This is in fact a group of enzymes, but the most important in pregnancy is the endothelial isoform (eNOS). eNOS uses the amino acid L-arginine as substrate and tetrahydrobiopterin (BH_4) as a cofactor, producing NO. In pathological conditions, the bioavailability of NO is diminished due to the deficit of substrate (mediated by decreased substrate availability and especially an increased activity of arginase enzymes) and the increase of reactive oxygen species (ROS), which shifts the synthesis of NO by the eNOS to synthesis of peroxynitrite, a powerful oxidant. Moreover, the bioavailability of nitric oxide may be altered by higher levels of asymmetric dimetil-arginine (ADMA), a competitive inhibitor of eNOS. Accordingly, it is necessary an appropriate balance of local mediators and utero-placental perfusion without interruption for normal development of the placenta and fetus.

However, less than half of the pregnancies with PE have an altered placentation. There is growing doubt that failed transformation of the spiral arteries with subsequent placental ischemia is either sufficient or necessary to explain the pathogenesis of preeclampsia [21, 22]. Accordingly, new hypothesis have emerged to postulate that PE is a condition determined by an exacerbated systemic inflammatory response. This systemic inflammatory response is associated with an endothelial dysfunction.

The endothelial dysfunction plays a major role in the underlying pathophysiological mechanism of the disease. Most of the clinical attributes of PE, such as hypertension, proteinuria, and edema, are derived from pathological changes within the maternal vascular endothelium or involve endothelial dysfunction [23], but "the factors" that lead to this are not clear. The endothelium is a monolayer of polygonal flat cells that extend continuously over the luminal surface of the entire vasculature. It participates in the control of primary hemostasis, host defence and inflammation, transport of nutrients and other solutes [24], and its strategic location permits it to signal alterations in hemodynamics and humoral factors by synthesizing and releasing vasoactive substances. The terms "toxemia of pregnancy" were the earliest used to describe this clinical entity. The longest surviving theory held that the placenta produced toxins that were released into the maternal blood stream [25]. Observations that serum from patients with preeclampsia has mitogenic and cytotoxic effects on endothelial cells and fibroblasts, respectively, lend support to the theory of circulating toxins [26, 27]. Several placentally derived ''toxins'' were suggested as linkage between endothelial dysfunction and the maternal syndrome including cytokines [28], anti-angiogenic factors [29], syncytiotrophoblast microparticles [30] and formed blood products activated in the intervillus space [31]. This "toxemia" produced a shift of the endothelium's functions toward reduced vasodilation, a proinflammatory state, and prothrombic properties [32], which leads to hypertension and proteinuria. Alterations in the circulating levels of many markers of endothelial dysfunction have been reported in women that develop preeclampsia [33-37]. Also markers of endothelial dysfunction may serve as predictors of PE since many of them are often elevated weeks before observance of clinical manifestations.

The oxidative stress represents a point of convergence for several contributing factors potentially leading to endothelial cell dysfunction and eventually to the clinical manifestations of PE [38]. Pregnancy *per se* leads to oxidative stress [39], due to an increased mitochondrial activity, reduced antioxidant scavenging potential, and occurrence of ischemia–reperfusion events, in the placenta. The main source of ROS initiating the pathophysiological events appears to be the placenta [40]. Other mechanisms of ROS production in PE pregnancies should be the activation of maternal neutrophils by syncytiotrophoblast microvesicles following deportation due to increased aponecrotic mechanisms locally activated during the passage of maternal blood through the placenta [19]. Also ROS can activate monocytes and neutrophils, perpetuating the redox imbalance. In this context, oxidative stress is a consequence of an imbalance between excessive generation of ROS over the antioxidant defenses, causing placental damage, which in turn could account for the increased rates of infarction and syncytial necrosis observed in this condition. The most common ROS is the superoxide anion. Xanthine and NADPH oxidases have been identified as major vascular superoxide-forming enzyme systems, but the contribution of xanthine oxidase is generally minor [41]. NADPH oxidase activity, constitutively observed in the trophoblast of the human placenta, is highly stimulated in PE [42]. This enzyme consists mainly of 5 subunits and it has been observed that placentas from preeclamptic patients show increased expression of NADPH oxidase components p22, p47, and p67 [43]. Other forms of NADPH oxidase are also implicated in the pathophysiology of PE, such as those present in phagocytes (neutrophilic and eosinophilic granulocytes, monocytes, and macrophages) and vascular cells. NADPH oxidase mediates increased isolated neutrophils production of superoxide observed in women with PE [44]. It has been well established that vascular NADPH oxidase plays a major role in the development of hypertension [45] and is a target for a down-regulation exerted by antioxidant vitamins.

Despite the several studies and theories, it is still not possible to combine the knowledge of this pathology. In this chapter, we will to describe the recent findings about the pathophysiology of preeclampsia, and how these develop hypertension in the maternal syndrome.

2. Pathophysiology of Hypertension in Preeclampsia

Throughout gestation adaptive changes are produced in women to achieve a successful pregnancy. A normal pregnancy is characterized by vasodilation resulting in reduction of peripheral vascular resistance. Blood pressure begins to decrease early in the first trimester and nadirs are reached by 20 to 24 weeks' gestation, despite an increase in cardiac output [46]. The kidney is among the organs in the body most significantly affected by pregnancy. At the level of the kidney, these hormonal balance between vasodilatory and vasoconstricting hormones result in vasodilatation of the collecting system with a small increase in renal size, an increase in renal plasma flow, and thus the glomerular filtration rate. These renal physiologic changes appear critical for an optimal pregnancy outcome.

As previously mentioned, the key factor widely cited in preeclampsia is placental ischemia/hypoxia. This reduction in placental oxygenation is assumed to enhance the synthesis and release of vasoactive factors, which induce widespread injury of maternal vascular endothelium, and results in increased formation of endothelin, thromboxane, superoxide, increased vascular sensitivity to angiotensin II, and decreased formation of vasodilators such as NO and prostacyclin. These endothelial abnormalities, in turn, cause hypertension by impairing renal function and increasing total peripheral resistance [1, 47-50]. In preeclampsia, the glomerular endotelial cell has been established as the main site of renal injury, but recent data also emphasize the importance of the podocyte, manifesting as hypertension, depression of the glomerular filtration rate, and proteinuria.

The principal factors behind the development of hypertension in preeclampsia are analyzed in the following section.

2.1. Vasoconstrictor Factors

2.1.1. Angiogenic Imbalance

During the last years, the study of angiogenic/antiangiogenic imbalance in preeclampsia has become very important. One of the most studied pathways is that related to the vascular endothelial growth factor (VEGF) signalling. VEGF is an endothelial cell specific mitogen which promotes the placental vascularization. It regulates multiple endothelial cell functions including mitogenesis, permeability, vascular tone and vasoactive molecule production [51]. The biological effects of the VEGF are mediated by members of the class III subfamily of tyrosine kinase receptors: fms-like tyrosine kinase (Flt-1) and kinase insert domain-containing receptor [52]. VEGF is abundant in placental tissue and fetal membrane cells and its expression increases during gestation. Some studies have reported a decrease of this factor in PE [53], while in other studies report no change [54].

Also, VEGF is necessary for the maintenance of glomerular ultra-structure through the maintenance of glomerular fenestrated endothelium. It's highly expressed by glomerular podocytes, and VEGF receptors are present on glomerular endothelial cells [55]. Fenestrated endothelium is found in the renal glomerulus, choroid plexus, and the hepatic sinusoids, organs that are disproportionately affected in preeclampsia [56]. In humans, antiangiogenesis cancer trials with anti-VEGF therapies have led to proteinuria, hypertension, and glomerular endothelial damage [57, 58]. In addition, in the second trimester of PE pregnancies, decreased plasma levels of VEGF have been found to be associated with a diminution of NO. This has been suggested to represent an impaired stimulus to vascular formation and endothelial regulation that induces placental disease [59]. In addittion, placental growth factor (PlGF) has structural homology to VEGF-A and is also a potent angiogenic growth factor that is thought to amplify VEGF signaling by displacing VEGF from the Flt1 receptor [60] and allowing it to bind to the more active kinase insert domain (KDR) receptor (or VEGFR-2) instead [61]. PlGF appears to stimulate angiogenesis under conditions of ischemia, inflammation, and wound healing and may contribute to atherosclerosis [60, 62]. During pregnancy, inhibition of both PlGF and VEGF is necessary to produce a preeclampsia-like syndrome in pregnant rats [63]. Changes in PlGF are noted quite early in women destined to develop preeclampsia, suggesting that an abnormally low level of PlGF is an important risk factor [64]. It is clear then, that proper levels of VEGF are necessary for endothelial and vascular health.

To understand the changes in VEGF pathways, researches have focused on two circulating antiangiogenic proteins –soluble fms-like tyrosine kinase 1(sFlt1) [64], and its splicing form (sFlt1-14) [65]. sFlt1 is a truncated splice variant of the membrane-bound VEGF receptor Flt1. It consists of the extracelular ligand binding domain without the transmembrane and intracellular signaling domains; it captures free VEGF and PlGF, thus preventing these molecules from interacting with the respective endogenous receptor. An increased level of sFlt1 was suggested as a biomarker for the subsequent development of PE. Placental expression of sFlt1 is increased in preeclampsia and is associated with a marked increase in maternal circulating sFlt1 [63]. sFlt1 is released from placental villi and trophoblast cells in response to reduced oxygen tensions similar to that seen in an ischaemic placenta [36, 66, 67]. sFlt1 has also been found in monocytes [68]. Whilst sFlt-1 production appears to be regulated by the hypoxia inducible factor-1 (HIF-1), other factors such as tumour necrosis factor-α (TNF- α) and the agonistic auto-antibody to the angiotensin II type 1 receptor (AT1-AA) also appear to be involved. This last topic will be described later. On the other hand, sFlt1-14 (also referred to as sFlt1-e15a) is the predominant VEGF inhibitor produced by human nonendothelial cells. It accumulates in circulation throughout pregnancy and may induce endothelial damage in distant organs affected by preeclampsia [65, 69]. Chronic administration of sFlt-1 to pregnant rats, to mimic plasma concentrations observed in preeclamptic women, decreases free VEGF and PlGF and produces hypertension, proteinuria and glomerular endotheliosis [36, 37, 63]. Several investigators have confirmed that the increase in maternal circulating sFlt1 precedes the onset of clinical disease [69-71], including women with chronic hypertension, who developed subsequently superimposed preeclampsia [71, 72], and also is correlated with disease severity [64, 73-75]. Perni et al. examined angiogenic factors in patients who had preexisting hypertension with superimposed preeclampsia, and found higher circulating levels of sFlt-1 before the 20th week of gestation in patients with preeclampsia versus pregnant women who had preexisting hypertension but did not develop preeclampsia [76]. Murphy et al. showed that exogenous sFlt-1 administration into pregnant rats results in high arterial blood pressure and elevated renal preproendothelin mRNA expression [77]. The simultaneous administration of a selective endothelin type A receptor antagonist brought the blood pressure to normal-pregnant range, suggesting that endothelin-1, via endothelin type A receptor, is an important mediator of the hypertension secondary to excess sFlt-1 in pregnancy (the role of endothelin will be described later).

As we mentioned, NO may be an important downstream mediator of both VEGF and TGF-β and has been suggested to be involved in the pathogenesis of preeclampsia. More recently, impaired production of NO metabolites was observed in patients with preeclampsia, and the impairment correlated with circulating sFlt1 [78]. Li et al. also reported that reduced maternal endothelial NO synthase (eNOS) exacerbates the sFlt1 related preeclampsia-like phenotype through activation of the endothelin system [79]. According to this, increased endothelin-1 production and the decreased bioavailability of NO lead to the characteristic widespread vascular abnormalities in various organs, such as hypertension and proteinuria observed in this disorder.

Thus, VEGF deficiency, whether induced by anti-VEGF antibodies, gene deletion, or excess sFlt1, is probably responsible for hypertension, proteinuria and glomerular endotheliosis. A promising pilot study recently demonstrated that sFlt-1 could be removed from the maternal circulation of preeclamptic women by dextran sulfate apheresis safely and that this therapy reduced both blood pressure and proteinuria, with a trend towards increased gestational duration [80].

2.1.2. Renin Angiotensin System

This placental and systemic hemodynamic imbalance results in an activation of the renin angiotensin system.

The renin angiotensin system (RAS) is known to be an important regulator of blood pressure, sodium and fluid homeostasis. This system comprises the inactive peptide angiotensinogen (AGT), which is converted to angiotensin I and then the active peptide angiotensin II (Ang II) through the action of renin and angiotensin-converting enzyme (ACE), respectively [81]. There are two major angiotensin II receptors: AT1R and AT2R. Most of the actions of Ang II, including vasoconstriction and stimulation of aldosterone synthesis, angiogenesis and cell growth are mediated by the AT1R [82]. The AT2R is implicated in apoptosis, reduction in endothelial cell growth and migration, and vasodilation in the adult, and the reduction in neointima formation after vascular injury [83-87], although it is usually expressed at low density in adulthood. However, expression is much higher during fetal life, where it may counterbalance the effects of the AT1Rs during fetal development. It has been confirmed that the components of RAS are not unique to the kidney. There are synthesized in many tissues, among which one of the major local RAS during pregnancy is in the uteroplacental unit (placenta also named fetal origin and decidua named maternal origin) [88].

Hering et al. recently reported that local tissue Ang II stimulates trophoblast invasion *in vivo* in the rat and *in vitro* in human cells. The authors suggested that upregulation of tissue Ang II in the maternal part of the placenta represents an important growth factor for trophoblast migration and invasion, and abnormalities in this system may play a role in the pathophysiology of preeclampsia [89].

Several studies have suggested that RAS is implicated in the pathogenesis of preeclampsia [88, 90]. The plasma renin concentration and renin activity, angiotensin II levels are increased during normal pregnancy, but vascular responsiveness to Ang II is decreased. In contrast, preeclamptic patients are sensitive to Ang II, although the circulating Ang II concentrations are lower compared with control pregnancies [88]. In addittion, oxidative stress and increased pro renin receptor expression both enhance the cleavage of angiotensin I from AGT, potentially increasing circulating angiotensin II concentrations. AngII exerts part of its vasoconstrictor effect through the generation of ROS [82]. The absence of adequate antioxidant protection in preeclampsia might enhance the vasoconstrictor effect of locally-generated Ang II. The specific clustering (perivascular staining) of both the pro-renin receptor and AGT around some vessels, in conjunction with an elevated measure of oxidative stress, suggests that the RAS may be contributing to the heightened state of oxidative stress in placental tissue of preeclamptic pregnancies. Superoxide anion (O2_) has been implicated in Ang II-mediated hypertension [91] and experimental data in the non-pregnant state support the concept that Ang II mediated hypertension in pregnancy may also be due, in part, to effects on the oxidative state in vascular endothelial tissue [92].

Therefore, women with preeclampsia have increased vascular sensitivity to angiotensin II and other vasoconstrictive agents [93]. A further dysregulation of the RAS during preeclamptic disease is the presence of the activating autoantibodies to the AT1-AA in the circulation of preeclamptic patients.

2.1.3. Maternal Inflamatory Response

Maternal immune tolerance involves crucial interactions between regulatory CD4+ T cells and uterine natural killer cells recognizing and accepting the fetal antigens and facilitating placental growth. Abnormalities in this process have been proposed to lead to poor placentation, reduced placental perfusion and stress, and chronic immune activation. Next, will explain briefly how it would initiate the systemic inflammatory response, and how innate and adaptive immunity contribute in the development of hypertension in preeclampsia.

Apoptosis is a form of programmed cell death. Numerous stimuli, including oxidative stress, tumor necrosis factor-alfa (TNF-α) and high glucose are known to induce apoptosis in endothelial cells. Huppertz et al. have already characterized the role of apoptosis cascade in villous trophoblast turnover and syncytium formation of normal pregnancies [94]. It is well known that placentas from women complicated with PE show enhanced apoptosis as compared to placentas of normal pregnancies [95]. The increased apoptosis is mediated, partly, by a diminished bioavailability of NO and increased oxidative stress and pro-inflammatory factors. Apoptosis is one explanation for the derivation of serum toxins originating from placental tissue. Failed transformation of the uterine spiral arteries lead to release of ischemic placental factors into the maternal circulation. Trophoblastic debris (TD) are shed from the placenta and can be found in the maternal blood from as early as six weeks of pregnancy [96]. TD interact with the maternal immune and/or vascular systems leading to increased maternal blood pressure. Also cytokines/growth factors as IL-6 or TGF-β can induce excess trophoblast death and/or aberrant death (necrotic or aponecrotic), and alter the nature or the number of trophoblasts shed from preclamptic placenta. Maternal lung is the first capillary bed that circulating TD traverse. If TD are too large to pass through the capillaries of the maternal lungs and become trapped in the pulmonary capillaries where they may be phagocytosed by endothelial cells [97], and becoming activated and secreting increased amounts of IL-6, TGF-β and possibly other soluble factors. The IL-6 and TGF-β would lead to activation of additional maternal endothelial cells, and the increased IL-6 and TGF-β produced by the maternal endothelium and therefore raise blood pressure levels. Accordding to this, blocking calcium channels with nifedipine (or verapamil) reduces the adverse responses of endothelial cells following phagocytosis of necrotic trophoblast debris [98]. This beneficial effect of nifedipine may be mediated primarily by reducing the responsiveness of endothelial cells to IL-6/TGF-β1 which are produced by endothelial cells in response to phagocytosing [99]. Nifedipine may be acting in part by increasing the activity of endothelial *NO synthase (eNOS).* These actions of nifedipine may add to its direct vasodilatory actions on vascular smooth muscle to provide beneficial effects in women with preeclampsia.

Furthermore apoptosis will realese trophoblastic micro particles (MP). These phospholipid vesicles, are originated from different cell types including platelets, endothelial cells, leukocytes and red blood cells, besides several other cell types. Redman and Sargent [100] reviewed studies in normal pregnancies that detected the presence not only platelet, endothelium and leukocyte derived MP, but also syncytiotrophoblast derived. However, this increase is especially important in pregnant women with PE, which show an extensive activation on endothelial cells, leukocytes, and coagulation system [101,102]. MP have been proven to play key role in thrombosis, inflammation, and angiogenesis, as well as to mediate cell–cell communication by transferring mRNAs and microRNA from the cell of origin to target cells [103]. Microparticles from preeclamptic patients activate endothelial cells in the presence of monocytes [104]. And also, plasma from pregnant and preeclamptic women can activate monocytes *in vitro* [105]. Monocytes displayed an enhanced phagocytic rate with peak levels in the third trimester, a significantly higher baseline of reactive oxygen species, changes in the expression of the cell surface adhesion molecules, and an increased intracelular production of proinflammatory cytokines [22, 106-110]. Monocytes from preeclamptic patients demonstrated a further increase in basal intracellular ROS, a higher synthesis of interleukin 1b, 6 and 8 (IL-1b, IL-6, IL-8) and more pronounced changes in the expression profile of cell surface markers compared to monocytes from healthy pregnant women [109-112]. Activated monocytes play an important role in PE and that endothelial cell activation.

As mentioned, the productions of cytokines are exacerbated in PE. Interleukin-6 (IL-6) is a multifunctional cytokine with pivotal roles in the inflammatory response and in directing T cell differentiation in adaptive immunity. IL-6 is produced by placental trophoblasts and decidual cells, epithelial cells, and immune cells. Indeed, IL-6 is a reporter cytokine of obstetric stress conditions and endothelial dysfunction [113, 114]. Several studies have described an association between altered levels of IL-6 and PE. The majority of these report elevated serum IL-6 in the third trimester in patients with PE [115-117], although others report no change compared with normal pregnant women [118, 119]. IL-6 production in endothelial cells is elevated after endothelial cells phagocytose necrotic trophoblast debris, and is implicated in spreading the vascular activation response [120]. The elevated circulating IL-6 in preeclamptic women may exacerbate and amplify this response, by acting on trophoblasts to promote the excessive shedding of necrotic debris. Calcitriol plays an important role in limiting the inflammatory response, and suggests that it might also protect from endothelial damage that result from exacerbated Th1 cytokines. These suggest that calcitriol supplementation could balance the immunological milieu in PE women and, at the same time, point out the potential utility of vitamin D interventions for the treatment of other inflammatory pathologies [121].

Another component of the immune system that has been studied as part of the pathogenesis of PE is the complement system. This enzymatic amplification system is composed of endogenous plasma proteins that normally operate at a low steady state. The components are sequentially activated by any of three pathways (classical, mannose-binding lectin, and alternative) to function in host defense and inflammation and lead to pathogen opsonization and/or lysis. Regulation of this complement activation is important for a successful pregnancy. Though complement is necessary for a normal pregnancy, excessive activation of complement and generation of active fragments may be an important contributor to adverse pregnancy outcomes such as spontaneous miscarriage and PE. Inhibition of complement activation attenuates development of high blood pressure following placental ischemia in pregnancy, indicating that complement activation is a critical event leading to placental ischemia-induced hypertension. Complement activation occurs in concert with placental ischemia-induced hypertension important role for angiogenic imbalance in mediating the blood pressure increase [122]. During pregnancy, complement activation has been implicated in pathogenesis of hypertension in two different studies in mice; abnormal placental development (C1q deficiency) or infusion of AT1-AA. The C1q-deficient model investigates events leading to placental ischemia as well as resulting from placental ischemia. Mice deficient in C1q exhibit abnormal placental development during pregnancy resulting in preeclamptic symptoms including high blood pressure. In addittion, pregnant mice with the placenta already formed, adoptive transfer of human autoantibodies to the angiotensin II type I receptor (AT1-AA) results in symptoms resembling PE including increased blood pressure. A C3a antagonist prevents the AT1-AA-induced hypertension indicating that excessive complement activation during pregnancy mediates hypertension initiated by the immune complex formation of AT1- AA with its receptor [123, 124]. Clearly, inhibition of complement activation has the potential to increase susceptibility to infection and this limits its usefulness for long term therapy. A recent case report using eculizumab in a woman with PE/HELLP syndrome successfully normalized lab values and prolonged pregnancy by 17 days suggesting that therapeutic manipulation of the complement system during pregnancy may be feasible [125].

During last years, several studies have suggested that PE would be an autoimmune disease. There are characteristics shared between preeclamptic women with autoimmune patients. For example, T helper 17 lymphocyte has recently found to be elevated in the plasma of preeclamptic women [126]. Further evidence implicates an imbalance between regulatory (Treg) and effector T cells, subclasses of CD4+ T lymphocytes, in preeclamptic women [127]. Th17 secrete Interleukin 17, and play an important role in the development and progression of chronic inflammatory and autoimmune diseases such as lupus, allograft rejection, autoimmune arthritis, psoriasis, and multiple sclerosis. Inter-leukin 17 induces the synthesis of other cytokines such as IL-6, granulocyte colony stimulating factor, TNF alpha, IL-8, and macrophage colony stimulating factor, all of which are associated with PE and associated with hypertension in response to reductions in uterine placental perfusion in pregnant rats [128-130]. Continuing this autoimmune theory, recent studies have indicated that women with PE produce a novel agonistic autoantibody to the angiotensin II type I receptor (AT1-AA) [131-133], and also have demonstrated increased concentrations of AT1-AA in serum from women with PE compared to serum from women with normal pregnancies [134-136]. AT1-AA are not specific for PE, Walther et al. also described the AT1-AA in women with uneventful pregnancies and normotensive pregnant women with uterine growth-restricted fetuses [137]. Furthermore, AT1-AA were also detected outside of pregnancy, namely in kidney transplant recipients who had refractory vascular rejection, patients with systemic sclerosis, featuring autoimmunity, vasculopathy, and tissue fibrosis, and patients with malignant secondary hypertension, mainly attributable to renovascular diseases [138-140]

These autoantibodies start to increase at the time of development of the PE syndrome, and subside within 6 weeks after delivery. Hubel et al. could show that still 1 year after pregnancies, 17% of preeclamptic women showed circulating AT1-AA, whereas none in the control group [141]. In preeclamptic women, they may induce heterodimerization between the angiotensin I receptor for the vasopressor angiotensin II and the bradykinin 2 receptor for the vasodilator bradykinin. Expression of these heterodimers may result in the noted increased responsiveness to angiotensin II [142] AT1-AA signaling, via the AT1 receptor, results in a variety of physiological effects. AT1-AA induces signaling in vascular cells and trophoblasts including transcription factor activation. The signaling results in tumor necrosis factor alpha and ROSgeneration, both of which have been implicated in PE [43, 134-136]. Furthermore, maternal autoantibodies also may account for other features of PE such as increased plasminogen activator inhibitor 1 production, shallow trophoblast invasion, [132] and, finally, may also cause human trophoblasts and vascular smooth muscle cells to produce ROS [43]. Another important mechanism by which the AT1-AA exerted its hypertensive effects in pregnant rats was the increase of ROS in the placenta [144].

LaMarca et al. reported that hypertension in RUPP pregnant rats is associated with increased circulating levels of the AT1-AA [135]. Reduction in placental perfusion may be an important stimulus for AT1-AA production in PE. In addition, elevations of tumor necrosis factor-alpha (TNF-a) are also associated with increased production of the AT1-AA [145]. Furthermore, IL-6 is elevated in hypoxic pregnant rats, and, infusion of IL-6 into pregnant rats, increases arterial pressure and decreases renal hemodynamics [146]. The hypertension associated with IL-6 infusion in pregnant rats results in production of the AT1-AA.

A recent study also suggested that AT1-AA induced soluble fms like tyrosine kinase-1 (sFlt1) by angiotensin receptor activation and downstream calcineurin/nuclear factor of activated T-cell signaling may lead to inhibition of VEGF and its vasodilatory capacity [147]. According to this angiogenic hypothesis, circulating sFlt-1 and sEng to be significantly elevated in AT1-AA induced hypertensive pregnant rats. Both circulating anti-angio-genic factors, sFlt-1 and sEndoglin (sEng), are significantly elevated in AT1-AA-induced hypertensive pregnant rats [145]. Chronic immune activation in association with placental ischemia leads to sFlt 1 and sEng overexpression via stimulation of the AT1-receptor possibly by production of the AT1-AA. These demonstrate an important interaction between inflammatory and angiogenic markers found to be produced excessively in response to placental ischemia. VEGF is a potent angiogenic factor that plays a critical role in vascular development in health and neo-angiogenesis in disease states.

The administration of the AT1-AA to pregnant rats significantly increased endothelin-1 (ET-1) levels in renal cortices and placenta of pregnant rats. Increasing levels of AT1-AA to levels observed in preeclamptic women and in placental ischemic rats increases mean arterial pressure in pregnant rats by activation of the endothelin system. AT1-AA–induced hypertension in pregnant rats was attenuated by either oral administration of the AT1 receptor antagonist losartan or an ET type A receptor antagonist [136]. The majority of published studies indicate that there is a significant increase in the circulating levels of ET-1 in preeclamptic patients when compared to normal pregnant controls, and that these levels return to normal shortly after birth [148]. This is consistent with the resolution of preeclampsia-associated hypertension post-partum.

Recently the role of B cell depletion was determined, resulting AT1-AA suppression to mediate hypertension via activation of ET-1 in placental ischemic rat model of PE [149]. For B cell maturation and IgG production, several co-stimulatory signals must be occurring between the antibody producing B lymphocyte and CD4+T helper cells. One of these includes stimulation of the CD20 receptor on the surface of the B cell. This recognition stimulates the B cell to enter the circulation and mass produce specific immunoglobulin. In order to treat various autoimmune diseases, many therapeutic agents inhibiting specific interactions between immune molecules and cells have been developed. IL-6 serves as a stimulus of immune mechanisms leading to B cell production of AT1-AA. IL-6 is known to be a major stimulus for B-cell proliferation and is a regulator of various T cell signaling processes. Rituximab, a chemotherapeutic agent that has shown efficacy among autoimmune patients by blocking the CD20 co-stimulatory molecule and there by inhibiting B lymphocytes from entering the circulation and secreting antibody, a process coined as B cell depletion. Administration of Rituximab inhibits the release of B cells into circulation and subsequent secretion of antibody and therefore allows one to partially examine mechanisms of AT1-AA production in response to placental ischemia [149]. Via B cell depletion and AT1-AA suppression the proinflammatory cytokine, TNF alpha, was attenuated in the serum of placental ischemic rats. Furthermore, B cell depleted rats had lower ET-1 and blood pressure response to placental ischemia. The findings could have profound implications on our understanding and future therapies developed for treating women with PE. In hypertensive patients showing the AT1-AA, an AT1-receptor blocker-based therapy (candesartan) was able to lower blood pressure more efficiently than an ACE-inhibitor-based therapy (Imidapril) that was an adequate therapy in hypertensive patients without AT1-AA [150] However, an AT1-receptor blocker therapy is not appropriate in pregnant women as the treatment leads to severe maldevelopment of the kidney in the fetus [151, 152]

Hence, pregnancy is a state of controlled inflammation. Maternal mechanisms are evoked to prevent an immune response against the fetus and involve both innate and adaptive immunity. According to this, during PE, there is an exacerbated inflammatory response that triggers autoinmunity processes.

2.1.4. The Final Common Pathway: Endothelin-1

Endothelins are potent vasoconstrictor isopeptides that are produced in different vascular tissues, including the vascular endothelium, and endothelin-1 (ET-1) is the main ET generated by the endothelium and is the most important ET in the cardiovascular system, and given its increased concentrations in PE, there has been extensive research on the role of ET-1 in the induction of hypertension in the maternal syndrome. ET-1 is found to induce vasoconstriction via the ETA receptor. ET-1 mediates vasoconstriction via the activation of NADPH oxidase, xanthine oxidase, lipoxygenase (LOX), uncoupled eNOS, and mitochondrial respiratory chain enzymes. It has been reported that essential hypertension is characterized by increased ET-1 mediated vasoconstrictor tone, which is an effect that seems to be dependent on decreased endotelial mediated NO production that is attributable to the impaired NO bioavailability. ET-1 elicits inflammatory responses and contributes to the vascular remodeling and endotelial dysfunction found in hypertensive models that exhibit an ET-mediated component [153].

Antagonism of the ETA receptor has proved beneficial in numerous animal models of gestational hypertension and it remains an intriguing target for pharmacological intervention in PE [154, 155].

Fiore et al. has demonstrated that ET-1 plays a role in the induction of oxidative stress in PE. ET-1 treatment of human placental explants and JEG-3 cells (putative models of trophoblasts) was found to alter the balance between oxidant forces (increased malondialdehyde concentrations) and antioxidant forces (decreased glutathione and ascorbic acid) in favour of oxidation [156]. Recent evidence also implicates placental endoplasmic reticulum (ER) stress in the pathophysiology of PE [157], which together with oxidative stress can help explain a broader range of the symptoms in this disorder. The ER is a multifunctional organelle involved in the synthesis and packaging of membrane and secretory proteins, and also serves as a reservoir of calcium ions (Ca^{2+}) [158]. In the ER lumen, Ca^{2+} is buffered by calcium-binding proteins. Jain et al. showed taht ET-1 act through the ETB receptor to activate the PLC/IP3 pathway to induce Ca^{2+} reléase from the ER and thereby stimulate ER stress [159]. Furthermore, ROS are potent stimulators of ET-1 synthesis by endothelial cells and VSMCs [160]. According to this, increased production of ET-1 under oxidative stress can act in a positive feedback loop to generate more oxidative stress and thus more ET-1 production, and thus raise blood pressure.

An agent that has been used effectively for the prevention of recurrent preterm birth in singleton pregnancies is 17-alpha-hydroxyprogesterone caproate (17-OHPC) [161-164]. The mechanism of action pathway is thought to be based on its antiinflammatory properties, with some studies showing inhibition of basal and TNF-α-induced apoptosis in fetal membranes [165]. Progestin 17-hydroxyprogesterone caproate reduces the hypertensive response to placental ischemia in the RUPP rat model. Similar findings were demonstrated in pregnant human volunteers with PE. Progesterone was demonstrated to blunt ET-1 production by vascular endothelial cells whether stimulated by RUPP rat serum or serum from human subjects with PE [166]. This intervention has the potential to exert an antihypertensive effect through a decrease in the maternal intravascular inflammatory response and maternal vascular endothelial cell activation with secondary prolongation of pregnancy for maternal and fetal benefit.

In summary, anti-angiogenic protein soluble fms-like tyrosine kinase-1 (sFLT 1), inflammatory cytokines and agonistic AT1-AA induce hypertension experimentally through the production of ET-1 [154].

2.1.5. A New Factor: Urotensin II

Despite that endothelin is the point of convergence of the roads that would generate hypertension in PE; its vasoconstrictor power is not enough to explain the pathophysiological and clinical abnormalities that develop PE patients. According to this, several authors have recently tried to prove the role of urotensin in the development of hypertension in PE.

Urotensin is a peptide first biologically characterized by Bern and colleagues in 1967 and originally isolated from the urohypophysis of the goby (the urohypophysis being a neurosecretory organ found only in fishes) [167-169]. Urotensin II (UT-II) is a cyclic peptide of 11 aminoacids cleaved from a larger preprourotensin II (PP UT-II) precursor peptide of about 130 amino acids [168]. Messenger RNA encoding PP UT-II has been demonstrated to be present in various tissues such as brain, pituitary, heart, kidney, adrenal gland, placenta and colonic mucosa [170]. Urotensin-II is the most potent vasoconstrictor identified to date, nevertheless its activity is balanced most of the time for its indirect vasodilator effect by enhancing release of endothelium derived NO and prostacyclin [169, 171-175], in addition to its direct vasoconstrictor effect [167-170, 176]. That is why its net effect depends on the endothelium health. The particular interest of the UT-II system relies into its 'quasi-irreversible' binding to a G-protein-coupled receptor (GPCR), known as urotensin receptor (UTS2R) [177]. UTS2R is functionally linked to Gq and phospholipase C (PLC), and its activation promotes long-term effects such as vascular smooth muscle cells proliferation [177, 178].

It has been related to varied endothelium-impairing diseases. Several lines of evidence have demonstrated a major contribution of the UT-II system to cardiovascular diseases, metabolic syndrome, diabetes, or renal disease [179, 180]. UT-II and its receptor are known to be upregulated in atherosclerotic plaque from non-diabetic animals and human patients [170, 176, 181]. Recent studies have shown that UT-II may induce vascular remodeling in the adventitia by inducing the differentiation, migration and proliferation and collagen synthesis in adventitial fibroblasts [182, 183]. The above effects are mainly achieved through the binding of UT-II with their respective receptors to activate downstream pathways such as mitogen-activated protein kinase (MAPK), protein kinase C (PKC) and calcium channels [182].

Balat et al. were the first to establish a relationship between UT-II and PE, in which PE severity is correlated to UT-II plasma levels [184]. Months later, Cowley et al. found that UT-II levels from umbilical cord/vein in PE women were elevated compared to UT-II plasma concentration [185]. In turn, there was no significant difference in UT-II plasma levels in controls and PE patients. Besides, the study involved only 20 women in total, which could explain the lack of positive differences. Liu et al. further explored this line again finding an increase in plasma levels of UT-II in PE women [186], and Gould et al. showed that hypoxia augments levels of urotensin-II receptors in syncytiotrophoblasts, and the UT-II receptor expression is upregulated in preeclamptic placentas compared with controls [187]. Autocrine and paracrine effects of Urotensin-II, its reported high levels at circulation in cardiovascular disorders, and its interaction between vasoactive agents in the pathophysiology of PE like NO, prostaglandins, ET-1, and adrenomedullin may suggest a possible role of UT-II in the pathogenesis of PE. Moreover, UT-II is also reported to be a proangiogenic agent [187-189] and associated with increased sFlt-1 secretion from placental explants under hypoxic conditions. Hence, increased UT-II levels in the setting of endothelial dysfunction and increased UT-II receptors are likely to contribute to the pathophysiology of hypertension in PE.

2.1.6. An Unified Vision: Hypoxia Inducible Factor-1 in Preeclampsia

Finally, trying to unify the inflammatory and hypoxic theories, the hypoxia inducible factor-1 emerges as a new part in the pathogenesis of this syndrome.

Hypoxia inducible factor-1 has been mentioned as the master regulator of the cellular response to low oxygen tension and is central to maintenance of oxygen homeostasis. This heterodimeric transcription factor is formed by two subunits, α and β. While HIF-1β is constitutively active, HIF-1α is oxygensensitive, being rapidly inactivated and degraded in normoxia.

The first evidence establishing a role for HIF-1α in the pathogenesis of PE originated from the pioneering work of Caniggia et al., who demonstrated HIF-1α to be highly expressed in the low-oxygen environment of the placenta in early gestation, falling at around 9th week of gestation, when placental oxygen levels increase [190]. In a related work, these authors [191] showed that TGF-β3 placental expression parallels that of HIF-1α, with both being elevated in the low-oxygen environment of early gestation. In addition, they reported that TGF-β3 inhibits placental explant trophoblast differentiation and invasion, characteristic abnormalities of PE. In an elegant experiment [190], these same authors used antisense inhibition of HIF-1a in placental explant trophoblasts. This resulted in downregulation of TGF-β3, restoring trophoblast differentiation and invasive capabilities and suggesting a role for HIF-1α in inhibition of trophoblast invasion, an early key step in the pathogenesis of PE. Furthermore, this shallow trophoblast invasión and its consequent placental hypoxia could in turn promote continued HIF-1α production, potentially creating a vicious cycle.

The role of HIF-1 α in the development of hypertension in PE has been recently studied. ET-1 is a well-known transcriptional target of HIF-1α in response to hypoxia [192, 193]. Similarly, HIF-1α was shown to induce the antiangiogenic factor sFLT-1 in placental explants [194]. Administration of AT1-AA together with Ang II, but not separately, led to PE manifestations in pregnant rats along with increased placental expression of HIF-1α [195], suggesting that AT1-AA may affect HIF-1α indirectly by increasing tissue sensitivity to Ang II. In addition, UT-II has been reported to be upregulated via HIF-1α in response to hypoxia in a syncytiotrophoblast model [187]. Hypoxia might be an important stimulus for UT receptor expression. The hypoxic transcriptional regulator HIF-1 α appears to have a role in this induction, because antisense oligonucleotides that downregulate HIF-1α also downregulate UT receptor induction under hypoxic conditions. Analysis of the upstream sequence of the UT receptor revealed 4 putative hypoxia response elements. Hence UT receptor upregulation is mediated via HIF-1α, and also HIF-1α has a documented role in regulating sFlt1 release [194]. According to this, UT receptor stimulation might regulated sFlt1.

In summary, HIF-1 α suppression or antagonism of its downstream effectors may serve as targets for pharmacological intervention to prevent the development of PE, or its clinical features.

2.2. Vasodilator Factors

Vasodilation in response to increased flow is the correct function of normal endothelium [196]. The relaxation of smooth muscle cells within the vessel walls is mainly mediated through the secretion of three major endothelium-derived vasodilatory factors: NO [197-199], prostacyclin (PGI2) [200-203], and endothelial-derived hyperpolarizing factors (EDHFs) [204,205]. It has been proposed that a decreased bioavailability of any of them may result o contribute to the generation of hypertension [196]. Then, the contribution of of them is going to be review in the etiopathogenesis of the hypertension seen on PE.

2.2.1. Nitric Oxide Pathway

By definition NO is a free radical [206]. It is a small molecule that is generated in biological tissue by the three isoformsof NOS [207,208]. All isoforms of NOS utilize L-arginine as the substrate, and molecular oxygen and reduced nicotinamide-adenine-dinucleotide phosphate (NADPH) as co-substrates. Flavin adenine dinucleotide (FAD), flavin mononucleotide (FMN), and (6R-)5,6,7,8-tetrahydro- L-biopterin (BH4) are cofactors of all isozymes. All NOS proteins are homodimers. A functional NOS transfer electrons from NADPH, via the flavins FAD and FMN in the carboxyterminal reductase domain, to the haem in the amino-terminal oxygenase domain [209]. NO stability in a medium with a low oxygen concentration, its solubility in a lipid-rich environment plus a half-life of a few seconds in aqueous media, allow NO molecules to diffuse quickly within the cytoplasm and through plasma membranes [210, 211]. NO is a highly reactive molecule that performs an important oxidative biological signaling role in various processes: neurotransmission [212, 213] or vascular tone [214, 215], regulates gene transcription [216, 217] and mRNA translation [218, 219] and produces post-translational modifications of proteins [207, 220-222]. The major route for bioinactivation of NO in the tissues is by reaction with $O2^{\cdot}$ − forming the oxidative molecule, peroxynitrite (ONOO−) [223, 224]. NOS is also regarded as another major source of superoxide [225]. NOS generates superoxide when it undergoes a phenomenon called uncoupling. All isoforms of NOS can undergo uncoupling due to deficiency of either L-arginine, the substrate or co-factors such as BH_4 [226] which results in decreased NO formation and increased superoxide levels [227].

The NO generated by eNOS in response to shear stress [228] is one of the major endothelium-derives vasoactive mediators [229]. Is a potent endogenous vasodilator that plays an important role in the maintenance of endothelial function: regulation of blood flow, inhibition of platelet aggregation, leukocyte adhesion and vascular proliferation [229-231]. NO effects on vessels such as vasodilatation, decrease in vessel resistance, and an increase in blood flow, make NO a key factor on the pathophysiological genesis of hypertension [232]. Several studies have suggested an important role NO in modulating arterial pressure under various physiological and pathophysiological conditions [36]. During a normal pregnancy NO production is elevated [234, 235] Evidence from experimental and clinical studies strongly suggests it. This increment appears to play an important role in the physiological vascular adaptation that occurs in pregnancy: vasodilatation and the resulting decrease in vascular resistance [236, 237].

The pathophysiology of PE originates mainly from vasospasm and diffuse endothelial dysfunction [238]. NO bioavailability, as one of the most important factors in the development of vasospasm and endothelial dysfunction, was supported by investigations to be related to the etiopathogenesis of PE and its hypertension [235, 239-241]. Moreover different studies have support this hypothesis: Infusion of synthetic inhibitors of NOS causes pre-eclampsia-like symptoms in rodents, which can be reversed by infusion of L-arginine [36, 233, 242-245]. In knockout mice models, it has been shown that mice lacking endothelial nitric oxide (eNOS) have hypertension, insulin resistance, hyperlipidemia, and decreased NO production [246-249].

Nevertheless the results of the assessment of NO levels in preeclamptic women have been controversial. Some have shown increased levels of NO in maternal circulation [250, 251] and placenta [253], while others found decreased levels in maternal serum [230, 253-255] and placenta [256] or even normal levels [257]. A recently meta-analysis of 9 available studies indicates that maternal serum NO level was significantly decreased in PE [258]. Reduced bioavailability of NO in the vascular wall can be a result of diminished expression of eNOS, inadequate circulating L-arginine concentrations, absence of its substrates or cofactors, presence of inhibitors like ADMA, eNOS polymorphism or a change in cellular signaling. All of these may lead to improper inactivation of the enzyme and accelerated degradation of NO by ROS such as oxygen ions, free radicals and peroxides [239, 259].

L-arginine concentration has been asses. Lower than normal l-arginine concentrations have been found in preeclamptic women, in comparison to normotensive pregnant ones [260]. This reduction may be caused by arginase II over expression, an enzyme that competes with NOS for L-arginine [261,262] or an alteration in erythrocyte uptake of L-arginine [263]. Increased arginase II expression in the vasculature of women with PE could be enhanced by peroxynitrite via NFkB [262]. Furthermore, peroxynitrite formation is increased in the maternal vasculature of women with PE [264]. Finally, reduced levels of L-arginine can result in the uncoupling of eNOS with the subsequent formation of superoxide and peroxynitrite. The peroxynitrite formed could increase more the arginase II expression, enhancing this cycle and reducing NO bioavailability.

Despite the numerous studies addressed to examine NO production and eNOS expression [229]. Result has been controversial. No significant differences, decreased and increased expression and activity of eNOS have been found between preeclamptic and normotensive pregnant controls [265-269].

Activity is commonly assessed by monitoring plasma levels of the NO stable degradation products nitrites and nitrates (NOx) and its second messenger cGMP, in both normal pregnancy and PE. It is important to mention that the dietary intake of nitrate and the acute fluctuation in the renal tubular reabsortion can dramatically affect plasma levels and urinary excretion [270]. Conditions that can partly contribute to the differences observed in the studies.

eNOS expression is also been debated. Increased and decreased expression has been explained and linked with different hypothesis. A possible explication for the increased expression may be an adaptative response to the increased resistance and poor perfusion in the pathological pregnancies [229]. According to these authors, adaptative response fail in elevate NO levels due ADMA´s in vivo effects in these patients are not so much to inhibit NOS activity but to increase O_2^- production by NOS, leading to greater $ONOO^-$ and hence less available NO, even though NOS production of NO is increased [230]. Situations where endothelial dysfunction due to increased oxidative stress is encountered, the expression of the eNOS has been shown to be paradoxically increased rather than decreased. The mechanism underlying increased expression of eNOS is likely to be secondary to increased endothelial levels of H2O2 which increases the expression of eNOS at the transcriptional and translational level [271]. On the other hand, it was reported that decreased eNOS expression and activity may be associated with increased endothelial permeability in PE [272]. These authors suggested that IL-8, which is increased by oxidative stress [273], could be a candidate agent that mediates this effect. The inhibition of eNOS resulted in enhanced IL-8-induced endothelial monolayer permeability in preeclamptic endothelial cells compared with those from normal pregnancies. However this study didn't asses NO levels and the association could be more likely with NO bioavailability rather than with eNOS expression.

Recently, many studies have evaluated the rol of eNOS polymorphism and the risk of PE. G894T polymorphism has been largely studied, with different results. [274-277] A meta-analysis that review 22 publication of the risk of PE associated to this polymorphism, show that G894T do not contribute significantly to PE risk. The same study also review 11 studies about −786 T>C and 4b/a polymorphisms. The result was that −786 T>C polymorphism in the dominant model and 4b/a were related with increased PE risk and low NO levels, especially for Europeans [258].

In conclusion, the decrease of NO bioavailability is not exclusively due to a decrease in the activity or expression of eNOS, which could be even increased, but to a decrease of the activity or half-life of NO, measured by the concentration of cGMP [278, 279]. The more integrative explanation seems to be that the inadequate concentrations or absence of its substrates or cofactors, plus the presence of inhibitors, on a patient with susceptibilities, like a certain eNOS polymorphism, may lead to improper inactivation or even the uncoupling of the enzyme, accelerating the NO degradation. This process leads to the generation of ROS, such as oxygen ions, free radicals and peroxides, promoting and enhancing the cycle. Superoxide reacts with NO generating peroxynitrite, reducing NO bioavailability. Peroxynitrite also contribute diminishing NO bioavailability because it oxidises tetrahydrobiopterin, and reduce l-arginine concentration, by increasing arginase II expression. Thereby peroxynitrite leads to degradation and uncouple of the enzyme [280].

Finally, a recent study has demonstrated that testosterone plasma levels also participate in the reduction of NO bioavailability and PE´s hypertension [281]. Testosterone are increased ≈2- to 3-fold in pathological pregnancies, such as in PE [282–286] and androgen levels in preeclamptic women positively correlate with higher average systolic blood pressure. [286].This study mayor finding is that decreases in vascular mesenteric relaxations that are mediated by alterations in the endothelium dependent NO-pathway, but not EDHF- or PGI2-mediated pathways. Moreover, testosterone-induced reductions in endothelial NOS activity are associated with decreased phosphorylation of excitatory eNOS at Ser1177 and increased phosphorylation of inhibitory eNOS at Thr495 [281].

2.2.2. Asymmetric Dimethylarginine

Since Vallance and Leone [287] firstly described Asymmetric dimethylarginine (ADMA) as an endogenous inhibitor of the arginine-NO pathway and the subsequent description of ADMA elevated plasma concentration in preeclamptic pregnant women by Fickling et al. [288], ADMA has been postulated as an important and key factor in the development of PE and in the ethiopathogenesis of its hypertension [289], heightening investigators attention.

As mentioned, Asymmetric dimethylarginine (ADMA) is an endogenous inhibitor of the arginine-no-pathway. The antagonism of endothelium-dependent vasodilatation caused by ADMA, was first observed in chronic renal failure [290]. Since then several studies show a relation between ADMA levels and blood pressure [291]. Local intra-arterial infusion of ADMA can significantly reduce forearm blood flow [292]. Moreover, intravenous infusion of ADMA increased mean blood pressure by 6% and systemic vascular resistance by 24%, while reducing the effect of exercise on cardiac output (by ~15%), heart rate, and vascular responsiveness [293]. The administration of ADMA in rats causes an increase in the renal vascular resistance and blood pressure [294]. In human volunteers, infusion of ADMA has been shown to impair endothelium-dependent vasodilatation, increase systemic and renal vascular resistance, and decrease cardiac output [295].

ADMA is a naturally occurring amino acid that circulates in plasma [296]. At elevated concentrations is an endogenous inhibitor of the three types of NOS: endothelial NOS (eNOS), neuronal NOS (nNOS) and inducible NOS (iNOS). [297]. NOS inhibition works by competitive displacement of the physiological substrate, L-arginine [295]. The inhibition leads to decrease NO production in the endothelium of vessel walls and thus, when ADMA levels are elevated, endothelial dysfunction may result. ADMA is actually strongly linked to endothelial dysfunction [297-299].

ADMA have been found in multiple disorders where NOS dysfunction has been implicated [300] as atherosclerosis, hypertension, hypercholesterolemia, diabetes [295], insulin insensitivity, intermittent claudication, end-stage renal disease, congestive heart failure, thrombotic microangiopathy, diabetes and many vascular and endocrinologic disorders [297, 301-308]. In addition, elevated plasma ADMA concentration has been identified as an independent risk factor for progression of atherosclerosis, cardiovascular death and all-cause mortality [309-311]. Furthermore, several studies have shown that ADMA is increased in PE. [295, 297, 312-314].

ADMA is synthesized by post-translational modification, via methylation of arginine residues in proteins by protein argininemethyltransferases (PRMTs) [315]. There are two types of PRMT. Type 1 involved in the synthesis of ADMA, where two methyl groups are added to one of the guanidine nitrogens of arginina, which forms an asymmetrical molecule. Since ADMA contains two methyl groups, its synthesis is followed by the generation of two homocysteine equivalents. Explaining greatly the highly significant positive association that was identified between plasma ADMA and homocysteine in a large population study [295, 316]. Type 2 methylates both of the guanidine nitrogens and forms symmetrical molecule, symmetrical DMA (SDMA). Both types can also monomethylate, forming N(g)-monomethyl-l-arginine (L-NMMA) [296]. These methylated proteins are predominantly found in the nucleus and play a role in RNA processing and transcriptional control [317]. ADMA is released into the cytosol when these proteins are hydrolyzed, thereby being an obligatory product of protein turnover. Thus, the amount of ADMA generated depends on the extent of arginine methylation in proteins and on the rate of protein turnover [315]. Approximately 300 umol of ADMA is generated per day, while 10% of ADMA is extracted by kidneys [296], the rest is metabolized by dimethyl argininedimethyl aminohydrolase (DDAH), probably via a nucleophilic attack on the guanidine portion of the ADMA molecule by cysteine held in an activated state in the tertiary structure of the enzyme [296]. There are two isoforms of DDAH. DDAH 1 is mostly associated with nNOS and it weakly expressed in the blood vessels but strongly in the brain, pancreas, liver [296] and in the renal proximal tubules [318], while DDAH 2 is highly expressed in the endothelium, vascular smooth muscular cells and adventitia of blood vessels, macula densa cells, distal tubules and collecting ducts of kidney [319] and placenta [265], tissues that mostly co-express eNOS [296]. This different distribution may explain a distinct role of DDAH-1 and DDAH-2. Since the kidney is the major site for plasma ADMA clearance from the circulation in rats and humans [320-321]. Plasma levels of ADMA in non-pregnant patients would be dependent on DDAH- 1, while in pregnant patients, it can be supposed that the placenta contributes to the clearance of ADMA via degradation of ADMA by placental DDAH-2 [265]. Besides, endothelial function would be dependent on DDAH-2 [322]. Some studies assert this hypothesis. Over-expression of

DDAH-1 and DDAH- 2 appears to result in very similar phenotypic changes, [323] whereas only knockdown of DDAH-1 increased plasma ADMA. Only knockdown of DDAH-2 blunted the endothelial derived relaxing factor and NO responses of mesenteric resistance arterioles to acetylcholine. This is of high interest since prior studies had not found a significant role for DDAH-2 in metabolizing ADMA [324, 325].

The final result of the methylarginines-NOS pathway is the reduction in the NO bioavailability. Only ADMA and L-NMMA are inhibitors of NOS [326], with equal capacity of inhibition [327]. Although ADMA is present more than ten-fold higher concentrations than L-NMMA [296]. The three methylarginines interfere with the transport of L-arginine as mediated by the cationic amino acid carrier within the plasma membrane (y_+ channels), explaining the SDMA inhibitor effect in the context of NO generation [327]. Besides, the results of a study in eNOS knockout mice suggests that ADMA may also exert NO-independent effects via upregulation of ACE and augmentation of oxidative stress through angiotensin-1-dependent pathways [328]. And recently, it has been demonstrated that endothelial dysfunction caused by ADMA might be attributable to its inhibition of eNOS phosphorylation [329]. Finally ADMA can also uncouple NOS, generate superoxides, and it interfaces with other targets in the cell [330].

The regulation of this process is extremely complex, and multiples pathways related with ADMA formation or degradation have been described. ROS [296, 298], Estrogen [331], Homocysteine [332], tumor necrosis factor–alpha (TNF-alpha) [333], native or oxidized LDL [334], high levels of glucose [335] and the recently identify vaspin [336]; have demonstrated to participate in regulating ADMA levels.

It is well recognized that blood pressure falls in early normal pregnancy and rises again toward term [337-339]. ADMA concentration has a significant correlation with blood pressure at all stages of normal pregnancy [339]. Decrease in ADMA levels is at least partially responsible for the maternal vascular dilatation and blood pressure changes in normotensives pregnancies [296]. Holden et al. [339] showed that the lowered blood pressure in early pregnancy is accompanied by a significant decrease in the concentration of plasma ADMA and support a role for both ADMA and NO in the changes in blood pressure observed in both normal and preeclamptic pregnancy. Moreover even a slight increase in ADMA of 0.13–0.15 mmol/l was associated with an increase in adverse events of about 20–30% in previous, population based studies [340].

The mechanisms responsible for high plasma concentrations of ADMA in the second [341, 342] and third trimester [339, 343-345] in women who later develop PE is not completely known. The options are three; 1) increased production, 2) reduced degradation and 3) both options. Evidence shows that placental PRMT1 expression levels aren't significantly high in preeclamptic women [265]. Studies evaluating DDAH activity and expression are contradictory. Anderssohn et al. [290] found almost undetectable DDHA activity in PE, and it was significantly higher in controls. Furthermore, mRNA expression levels of DDAH 2 were significantly lower in pre-eclamptic women. Siroen et al. [346] didn't detect differences in DDAH activity between preeclamptic and healthy placental tissue. Discrepancy between these findings may be explained by the difference in the severity of PE in the groups investigated by the authors. Anderrssohn took more severe PEs. Severe or early onset PE had higher levels of ADMA in comparison with late onset PE [315, 346], indicating some ethiopathological difference between these two types of PE [347]. In conclusion, it seems that at list on some types of PE (early or severe) reduced degradation rather than an increased production causes the elevations in ADMA levels.

Additionally in the 3rd trimester, the impaired renal function due to established endothelial damages may represent an additional mechanism which also contributes to the elevated ADMA [346]. Also it has been proposed that accumulation of ADMA by reduced hepatic elimination due organ dysfunction plays a causal role in PE and HELLP syndrome [348].

2.2.3. Endothelium-Derived Hyperpolarizing Factor

Endothelial cells regulate vascular tone through the release of several soluble mediators [349-352]. They are released by a number of stimuli, including endothelial agonists such as bradykinin, acetylcholine and shear stress and mediate vasorelaxation. When NOS and cyclooxygenase (COX) are inhibited, the relaxations to acetylcholine decrease, but are not blocked, indicating that a component of the relaxations are mediated by another factor [353-355]. The residual vasodilatation to acetylcholine were inhibited by high extracellular K+ that blocks K+ channels and by mall-conductance Ca^{2+}-activated K+ channels (SKCa) and intermediate conductance Ca^{2+}- activated K+ channels (IKCa) inhibitors [356]. Additionally the persistent vasodilatation was associated with hyperpolarization of the smooth muscle cell membrane [350-352]. Thereby, this new factor was known as an endothelial derived hyperpolarizing factor (EDHF).

Studies have shown that EDHF is not just a single molecule but a family of compounds that mediate endothelium-dependent hyperpolarization and smooth muscle relaxation. These compounds include metabolites of arachidonic acid (AA) such as epoxyeicosatrienoic acids (EETs), 15-hydroxy-11,12-epoxyeicosatrienoic acids (15-H-11,12-EETA), and 11,12,15-trihydroxyeicosatrienoic acid (THETA), potassium (K) ion, hydrogen peroxide, C-type natriuretic peptide (CNP) [351-353, 357-361], carbon monoxide (CO) and hydrogen sulfide [362-363]. Despite differences in their chemical structure, all this molecules hyperpolarize by activating directly or indirectly different K+ channels [362]. Alternatively, endothelium dependent hyperpolarization may not require soluble mediators. Acetylcholine stimulates calcium influx into endothelial cells, activating KCa channels and causing the membrane of endothelial cells to hyperpolarize. The presence gap junctions between endothelial cells, smooth muscle cells, and between these two types, allow the transmission of the hyperpolarization along the vascular wall. Myoendothelial gap junctions transfer the endothelial hyperpolarization to the smooth muscle cells resulting in relaxation [352, 359, 364, 365]. Since a factor is not involved, this mechanism has been called just endothelium dependent hiperpolarization (EDH) [366]

Just as there are constitutively express and inducible forms of NOS, and COX, it has been proposed that some EDHFs may be constitutive of endothelium (cEDHF and cEDH) while others may be inducible forms (iEDHF) [366]. cEDHF and cEDH are released by endothelial agonists, and mediates a portion of endothelium dependent relaxation; however, the chemical or electrical nature may vary with vascular beds and with species. iEDHF is induced under various physiological and pathological conditions to participate in endothelium-dependent relaxation by endothelial agonists. Thus, the contribution of iEDHF to endothelium-dependent relaxation may be absent under basal conditions, but its contribution is enhanced when induced. Situation that could explain difference observed in normal pregnancy and PE.

In the normal physiological response to pregnancy, endothelial derived hyperpolarization has been shown to be a major contributor; along with NO, are predominantly involved in providing an increased vascular capacity for vasodilation [367]. Several studies have asses EDHFs and the EDH via myoendothelial gap junctions in PE and normal pregnancy. A significant loss of endothelium-dependent relaxation has been seen in myometrial resistance arteries in PE when compared to both non-pregnant and normotensive pregnant women. [368, 369]. Another study made in myometrial resistance arteries suggest that, in the absence of NO, an EDHF can mediate vasodilator responses to bradykinin during normal pregnancy, an effect not apparent in arteries from non-pregnant women or women with pre-eclampsia. The up-regulation of EDHF-type function may represent a vascular adaptation to normal pregnancy that is absent in PE [370, 371]. In comparison to myometrial arteries, the difference between PE and normal pregnancy in the endothelium-dependent relaxations of subcutaneous vessels was observed only after incubation with NOS and COX inhibitors [372]. Thus, it could be anticipated that myometrial arteries are particularly susceptible to the toxic environment that occurs in PE (e.g., pro-oxidative milieu and misbalance of pro- and antiangiogenic factors). The enhanced susceptibility for impairment in these vessels concurs with observations in which ex vivo incubation with PE plasma had an inhibitory effect on BK-induced dilatation in myometrial, but not omental, arteries from women with normal pregnancies [373] and with those studies of PE demonstrating severe reduction, or even total abolishment, of endothelium-dependent relaxation to ACh [374], BK [375-378], or flow [379] in this particular vascular bed. Recently, Mandala et al. [380] investigate the cellular mechanism involved in the potent vasodilatory action of PlGF on mesenteric resistance arteries from pregnant rats. Significant dilation remained, however, in the presence of NOS and cyclooxygenase inhibition. This study indicates part of the vasodilatory effect of PIGF is through EDHF, especially via SK Ca and BK Ca potassium channels.

Nowadays studies are trying to elucidate separately the contribution of every single EDHF and EHD via myoendothelial gap junctions. A few studies have assessed the particular contribution of EDH through myoendothelial gap junctions in normal pregnancy and in comparison to PE. [370, 381-383] demonstrated the important involvement of gap junctions in mediating EDH responses in myometrial, subcutaneous, and omental arteries and veins of pregnant women. In PE, bradykinin-induced relaxation was reduced via compromised EDHF-type responses, in which the contribution of myoendothelial gap junction's relaxation became negligible. The attenuated role of myoendothelial gap junctions to endothelium-dependent relaxation in PE was partly compensated through the contribution of an increase in hydrogen peroxide or other endothelium-derived relaxing factors [369].

Hydrogen peroxide (H2O2) is formed by hydration of superoxide by superoxide dismutase [384, 385]. It is constitutively present in some arteries and mediates a portion of the relaxation to endothelial agonists. Its mechanism of action has not been completely defined [386, 387]. Even though, it has been demonstrated that catalase, which dismutates hydrogen peroxide to form water and oxygen, significantly attenuated the response of myometrial arteries to bradykinin after NOS and COX inhibition in PE. Effect is not seen in arteries from women with normal pregnancy [369]. Several studies have shown elevate levels of H2O2 in PE [388-391]. Although the balance between beneficial and harmful roles of hydrogen peroxide in the pathogenesis of PE warrants more thorough research.

CNP is constitutively expressed in endothelial cells, is released by endothelial agonists, and relaxes smooth muscle by increasing cyclic guanosine monophosphate and membrane hyperpolarization. Its expression and secretion is increased by transforming growth factor-b, tumor necrosis factor-a, and interleukin-1 (IL-1). The role of platelet-derived growth factor (PDGF) and basic fibroblast growth factor is still being debated. [366]. CNP participation in PE has been poorly studied. In adult mice, the uterus and ovaries show the highest CNP expression [392] estradiol induces CNP gene expression at least in the mouse uterus [393] and CNP receptor are highly expressed in rat placenta. CNP mRNA was detected in human placenta and myometrium. In these tissues CNP expression levels did not differ between term and preterm pregnancies [392], and a recent study demonstrates that pro C-type natriuretic peptide remained constant during pregnancy [394]. Pregnancies with IUGR or pre-eclampsia show an opposite regulation of CNP with a decrease in the placenta and an increase in the myometrium compared with normal pregnancie. Interestingly, maternal CNP plasma levels are not significantly different in normal pregnancies and those complicated by gestational hypertension, PE or IUGR [392, 395]. Although different authors attribute these apparently contradictory facts to local functioning CNP, emphasizing that tissue CNP regulation does not reflect the circulating peptide [396,397].

CO is also described as an EDHF [362]. One key molecules implicated in PE pathogenesis is heme oxygenase-1 (HO-1), a rate-limiting enzyme that breaks down heme into carbon monoxide (CO), biliverdin and free iron [398]. Studies of HO-1 and HO-2 expression in mouse, rat and human placentas have been numerous [399-401] However, is still being quite controversial. Expression of HO-1 in pregnancy complications showed lower HO-1 protein expression in preeclamptic placentas [402]. Human *in vivo* studies demonstrate that while exhaled CO levels increase throughout gestation in healthy women, end-tidal CO measurements are lower in hypertensive pregnant women; especially those affected by sever PE, supporting the role of CO as a physiologic vasodilator implicated in gestational hemodynamic changes [403]. Assessment CO levels, by measuring carboxyhemoglobin (COHb) levels in the umbilical cord arterial blood of women with PE showed significantly lower COHb levels in the PE group compared with the normotensive [404]. Moreover, maternal exposure to moderate ambient CO is associated independently with a decreased risk of PE [405].

Hydrogen sulfide (H_2S) is a prominent EDHF [406], since mice lacking its biosynthetic enzyme, cystathionine γ-lyase (CSE), display pronounced hypertension with deficient vasorelaxant responses to acetylcholine [407-408]. The endothelial intermediate conductance (IK_{Ca}) and small conductance (SK_{Ca}) potassium channels mediate in part the effects of H_2S, as selective IK_{Ca} and SK_{Ca}channel inhibitors, charybdotoxin and apamin, inhibit glibenclamide-insensitive, H_2S-induced vasorelaxation. Two other enzymes have also been shown to generate H_2S in various tissues, namely cystathionine β-synthase (CBS) and 3-mercaptopyruvate sulfurtransferase (3-MST). In blood vessels however, CBS appears to play a negligible role in the production of H_2S [409] whereas the precise role of 3-MST has yet to have been defined despite its presence in vascular endothelium [410]. Studies show that plasma levels of H2S are significantly decreased in women with PE [411]. Moreover, perfusion of normal placentas with an H2S donor, after preconstriction with a thromboxane mimetic, resulted in dose-dependent vasorelaxation [412]. H2S producing enzymes expression has also been assessed. Reduced placental CSE expression has been found in PE [411]. Another investigation demonstrate that expression of CSE smooth muscle cells encircling arteries in stem villi is reduced in placentas associated with increased vascular resistance [412]. A recent study did not found difference in CSE expression, but was found that CBS mRNA expression was significantly down regulated in placental villous tissue derived from pregnancies complicated by early-onset PE when comparing to mode of delivery matched controls [413]. So far, in PE no CBS- and CSE-activity or H_2S-production is reported. Therefore, the exact role of endogenous H_2S in PE needs to be elucidated.

EETs are cytochrome P450 (CYP) metabolites of AA [414, 415] The EETs are synthesized by the endothelium and released by acetylcholine, bradykinin, and shear stress. [352, 357, 416]They hyperpolarize and relax vascular smooth muscle by activating large conductance KCa (BKCa) channels. [366]. There is not much work determination ETTs in PE, and result of ETTs levels are quite controversial. No difference between PE and normal pregnancies of levels of ETTs were found [417], while when the CYP subfamily 2J polypeptide 2 (CYP2J2) and the CYP2J2 metabolites, 5,6-epoxyeicosatrienoic acid, 14,15-EET, and the corresponding dihydroxyeicosatrienoic acids were measured, elevated levels of metabolites were found and CYP2J2was upregulated in preeclamptic placenta and decidua [418]. Besides, CYP2C9 products of arachidonic acid had no effect on EDHF-type relaxation in arteries of women with normal pregnancy or with PE [369].

15-H-11,12-EETA and 11,12,15-THETA are endothelial 15-lipoxygenase (15-LO) metabolites of AA [353, 354]. They mediate a portion of the relaxations to acetylcholine in several arteries by activating smooth muscle cell SKCa-like channels and causing hyperpolarization. The expression of 15-LO is increased in cultured smooth muscle cells or mesangial cells when compared with untreated cellsby angiotensin II, aldosterone, PDGF, transforming growth factor-b, IL-8, growth hormone–releasing peptide-2, peroxisome proliferator–activated receptor-g agonist, and high glucose [419-425]. Also cytokines, estrogen, hypoxia, and hypercholesterolemia, increase 15-Lo expression resulting in enhanced production of hydroxyepoxyeicosatrienoic acid [HEETA)/THETAs and enhanced relaxations to acetylcholine [426-428]. The 15-LO/HEETA/THETA pathway is an iEDHF [366]. 15-LO expression is increased in human umbilical arteries from patients with PE compared with normal patients [429]. More work is needed to elucidate the mechanism exact mechanism.

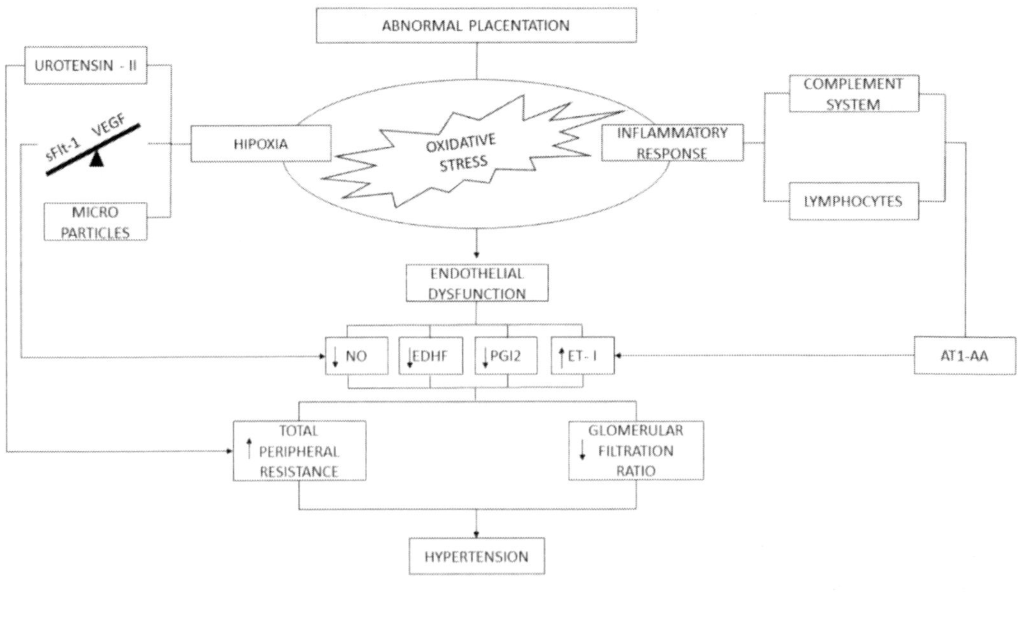

Figure 3-1. Hypertension in preeclampsia. Both placental hypoxia as the exacerbated inflammatory state is a continuous process in the pathogenesis of preeclampsia, which would lead to the endothelial dysfunction. The endothelial dysfunction plays a major role in the underlying pathophysiological mechanism of the disease.

Is it Possible to Prescribe an Appropriate Treatment against this Disease?

As mentioned, there is no satisfactory treatment to prevent the development of PE, except for measures to avoid or reduce complications [10, 11]. Although some traditional antihypertensive drugs that may be given in severe cases are often ineffective, and rarely achieve normal pressure. Consequently, management of PE focuses on prolonging pregnancy as long as possible and without risk to the mother through a combination of bed rest and anticonvulsant therapy. Indeed, early delivery is the only successful treatment. In about 20% of cases of early onset PE leads to delivery before 34 weeks. Clinical features can start manifesting from the 20th week, but damage to the placenta occurs before, the question is when. If there is no probable starting time it is very difficult to raise the idea of a preventive treatment to apply.

Analyzing the inflammatory state in PE; calcitriol plays an important role in limiting the inflammatory response, and suggests that it might also protect from endothelial damage that result from exacerbated Th1 cytokines (IL-6) [121]. Control of the complement system by eculizumab in a woman with PE syndrome / HELLP successfully normalized laboratory values and prolong the pregnancy by 17 days suggesting that therapeutic manipulation of the during pregnancy may be feasible [125]. Furthermore, a chemotherapeutic agent, Rituximab, has shown efficacy among autoimmune patients by blocking the CD20 co-stimulatory molecule and there by inhibiting B lymphocytes from entering the circulation and subsequent secretion of antibody and therefore allows one to partially examine mechanisms of AT1-AA production in response to placental ischemia [149]. Clearly, inhibition of complement activation as B cell depletion has the potential to increase susceptibility to infection and this limits its usefulness for long term therapy, but the findings could have profound implications on our understanding and future therapies developed for treating women with PE.

Moreover, in hypertensive patients showing the AT1-AA, an AT1-receptor blocker-based therapy (candesartan) was able to lower blood pressure more efficiently than an ACE-inhibitor-based therapy (Imidapril) that was an adequate therapy in hypertensive patients without AT1-AA [150] However, an AT1-receptor blocker therapy is not appropriate in pregnant women as the treatment leads to severe maldevelopment of the kidney in the fetus [151, 152].

Recently, studies have shown encouraging results to antagonize the effects of urotensin in diabetes [430] and pulmonary hypertension [431], as also was tested statin use against myocardial dysfunction by blocking the effects of HIF-1α [432]. These therapeutic targets should be considered as a possible treatment in PE.

An agent that has been used effectively for the prevention of recurrent preterm birth in singleton pregnancies is 17-α-hydroxyprogesterone caproate (17-OHPC) [161-164]. The mechanism of action pathway is thought to be based on its antiinflammatory properties that can reduce the hypertensive response to placental ischemia blunting ET-1 production by vascular endothelial cells [166]. This intervention has the potential to exert an antihypertensive effect through a decrease in the maternal intravascular inflammatory response and maternal vascular endothelial cell activation with secondary prolongation of pregnancy for maternal and fetal benefit. More research is needed to achieve general acceptance.

In relation to enhancing vasodilator factors; several studies have postulated increase NO levels in pregnant women through the supply of the amino acid L-arginine, but the results have been mixed, without achieving universal acceptance. To maintain adequate levels of NO, there have been studies with Phosphodiesterase 5 (PDE5) inhibitors such as Sildenafil. Besides there are phase 2 clinical trials of sildenafil administration with no apparent adverse effects on the mother or offspring, there was also no concurrent benefit to sildenafil treatment in the preeclamptic patients [433]. In addition, carbon monoxide (CO) has beneficial properties for the body, one of which is its vasodilator effect. A source of carbon monoxide is the free hem metabolism by hem oxygenase 1 (HO-1). CO functions in a manner quite similar to NO. It has recently been shown that at least in an in vitro context, HO-1 or CO alone can down regulate sFlt-1expression [434]. Therefore, increased HO-1 activity might be one way to decrease vascular oxidative stress and improve endotelial function. Indeed, HO-1 has been shown to have beneficial effects in diverse models of hypertension which share several common pathways with PE [435]. These suggest that manipulation of the HO-1 pathway might prove an efficacious approach to the treatment of PE.

According to this, more research is needed to find appropriate preventive treatments and better management of its symptoms and complications.

Conclusion and Perspectives

As mentioned, it is necessary an appropriate balance of local mediators and utero placental perfusion without interruption for normal development of the placenta and fetus. Even less than half of the pregnancies with PE have an altered placentation; placental ischemia/hipoxia is the most widely recognized factor in PE. This reduction in placental oxygenation is assumed to enhance the synthesis and release of vasoactive factors, which induce widespread injury of maternal vascular endothelium and also activates the maternal inflammatory response. Both placental hypoxia as the exacerbated inflammatory state is a continuous process in the pathogenesis of PE, which would lead to the endothelial dysfunction.

Increased formation of endothelin, urotensin thromboxane, superoxide, increased vascular sensitivity to angiotensin II, chronic immune activation, angiogenic imbalance and decreased formation of vasodilators such as NO, prostacyclin and endothelial derived hyperpolarizing factor are some of the mediators involved in the development of hypertension in PE.

More research is needed to explain the pathogenesis of this disease, as also find appropriate preventive treatments and better management of its symptoms and complications.

Acknowledgment

Supported by FONDECYT, grant 1120594

References

[1] American College of Obstetricians and Gynecologists. *Diagnosis and management of preeclampsia and eclampsia.* 2002; 99: 159–167.

[2] Roberts JM, Cooper DW. Pathogenesis and genetics of preeclampsia. *Lancet* 2001; 357, 53–56.

[3] Davison JM, Homuth V, Jeyabalan A, Conrad KP, Karumanchi SA, Quaggin S, Dechend R, Luft FC. New aspects in the pathophysiology of preeclampsia. *J Am Soc Nephrol* 2004; 15: 2440–2448.

[4] Davey DA, MacGillivray I. The classification and definition of hypertensive disorders of pregnancy. *Am J Obstet Gynecol* 1988:892-898.

[5] Walker J.J. Severe pre-eclampsia and eclampsia. *Baillieres Best Pract Res Clin Obstet Gynaecol.* 2000; 14:57-71.

[6] Brown MA. Pregnancy-induced hypertension: current concepts. *Anaesth Intensive Care* 1989; 17:185–197.

[7] Martin Jr. JN, May WL, Magann EF, Terrone DA, Rinehart BK, Blake PG. The spectrum of severe preeclampsia: comparative analysis by HELLP (hemolysis, elevated liver enzyme levels, and low platelet count) syndrome classification. *Am J Obstet Gynecol* 1999; 180:1373-1384.

[8] Saphier CJ, Repke JT. Hemolysis, elevated liver enzymes, and low platelets (HELLP) syndrome: a review of diagnosis and management. *Semin Perinatol* 1998; 22:118-133.

[9] Leitch CR, Cameron AD, Walker JJ. The changing pattern of eclampsia over a 60 year period. *Br J Obstet Gynaecol* 1997; 104: 917-922.

[10] Afifi Y, Churchill D. Pharmacological treatment of hypertension in pregnancy. *Curr Pharm Des 2003*; 9:1745-1753.

[11] Meher S, Duley L. Interventions for preventing pre-eclampsia and its consequences: generic protocol. *Cochrane Database Syst Rev* 2005; 2:CD005301.

[12] Redman CW. Current topic: pre-eclampsia and the placenta. *Placenta* 1991; 12:301-308.

[13] Scott JS. Pregnancy toxaemia associated with hydrops foetalis, hydatidiform mole and hydramnios. *J Obstet Gynaecol Br Emp* 1958; 65:689-701.

[14] Hou HL, Wan XR, Xiang Y, Qi QW, Yang XY. Changes of clinical features in hydatidiform mole: analysis of 113 cases. *J Reprod Med* 2008; 53:629-633.

[15] Khong TY, De Wolf F. Inadequate maternal vascular response to placentation in pregnancies complicated by preeclampsia and by small-for-gestational age infants. *Br J Obstet Gynaecol* 1986, 93:1049-1059.

[16] Hubel CA. Oxidative stress in the pathogenesis of preeclampsia. *Proc Soc Exp Biol Med* 1999; 222: 222–235.

[17] Aquilina J, Harrington K. Pregnancy hypertension and uterine artery Doppler ultrasound. *Curr Opin Obstet Gynecol* 1996; 8:435–440.

[18] Merviel P, Carbillon L, Challier JC, Rabreau M, Beaufils M, & Uzan S. Pathophysiology of preeclampsia: links with implantation disorders. *Eur J Obstet Gynecol Reprod Biol* 2004; 115, 134– 147.
[19] Raijmakers MT, Dechend R, Poston L. Oxidative stress and preeclampsia: rationale for antioxidant clinical trials. *Hypertension*. 2004; 44:374–380.
[20] Holthe MR, Staff AC, Berge LN, Lyberg T. Leukocyte adhesion molecules and reactive oxygen species in preeclampsia. *Obstet Gynecol*. 2004; 103:913-922.
[21] Huppertz B. Placental origins of preeclampsia: challenging the current hypothesis. *Hypertension* 2008; 51:970–975.
[22] Roberts JM, Hubel CA. The two stage model of preeclampsia: variations on the theme. Placenta 2009; 30:S32–37.
[23] Luscher TF, Barton M. Biology of the endothelium. *Clin Cardiology* 1997; 20:11:II3–II10.
[24] Endemann, DH, Schiffrin EL. Endothelial dysfunction. *J Am Soc Nephrol* 2004; 15:1983–1992.
[25] Roberts, J. M. Endothelial dysfunction in preeclampsia. *Semin Reprod Endocrinol* 1998; 16:5 – 15.
[26] DeLee, J. B. Theories of Eclampsia. *Am J Obstet Gynecol*. 1905; 51:325–330.
[27] Rodgers, G. M.; Taylor, R. N.; Roberts, J. M. Preeclampsia is Associated with a Serum Factor Cytotoxic to Human Endothelial Cells. *Am J Obstet Gynecol*. 1988; 159:908–914.
[28] Taylor RN, Heilbron DC, Roberts JM. Growth Factor Activity in the blood of Women in Whom Preeclampsia Develops is Elevated from Early Pregnancy. *Am J Obstet Gynecol*. 1990; 163, 1839–1844.
[29] Schipper EJI, Bolte AC, Schalkwijk CG, Van Geijn HP, Dekker GA. Tnf-receptor levels in preeclampsia – results of a longitudinal study in high-risk women. *J Matern Fetal Neonatal* 2005; 18:283–287.
[30] Maynard SE, Venkatesha S, Thadhani R, Karumanchi SA. Soluble fms-like tyrosine kinase 1 and endothelial dysfunction in the pathogenesis of preeclampsia. *Pediatr Res* 2005; 57:1R–7R.
[31] Redman CW, Sargent IL. Latest advances in understanding preeclampsia. *Science* 2005; 308:1592–1594.
[32] Mellembakken JR, Aukrust P, Olafsen MK, Ueland T, Hestdal K, Videm V. Activation of leukocytes during the uteroplacental passage in preeclampsia. *Hypertension* 2002; 39:155–160.
[33] Roberts JM, Taylor RN, Goldfien A. Clinical and biochemical evidence of endothelial cell dysfunction in the pregnancy syndrome preeclampsia. *Am J Hypertens* 1991; 4:700–708.
[34] Krauss T, Kuhn W, Lakoma C, Augustin HG. Circulating endothelial cell adhesion molecules as diagnostic markers for the early identification of pregnant women at risk for development of preeclampsia. *Am J Obstet Gynecol* 1997; 177:443–449.
[35] Roberts JM, Gammill HS. Preeclampsia: recent insights. *Hypertension* 2005; 46: 1243–1249.
[36] Gilbert JS, Ryan MJ, LaMarca BB, Sedeek M, Murphy SR, Granger JP. Pathophysiology of hypertension during preeclampsia: linking placental ischemia with endothelial dysfunction. *Am J Physiol Lung Cell Mol Physiol* 2008; 294:H541–H550.

[37] LaMarca BD, Gilbert J, Granger JP. Recent progress toward the understanding of the pathophysiology of hypertension during preeclampsia. *Hypertension.* 2008; 51:982–988.

[38] Roberts JM, Hubel CA. Is oxidative stress the link in the two-stage model of pre-eclampsia? *Lancet* 1999; 354: 788–789.

[39] Wisdom SJ, Wilson R, McKillop JH, Walker JJ. Antioxidant systems in normal pregnancy and in pregnancy-induced hypertension. *Am J Obstet Gynecol* 1991; 165:701– 1704.

[40] Serdar Z, Gur E, Develioglu O, Colakogullari M, Dirican M. Placental and decidual lipid peroxidation and antioxidant defenses in preeclampsia. Lipid peroxidation in preeclampsia. *Pathophysiology.* 2002; 9:21.

[41] Poston L, Raijmakers MT. Trophoblast oxidative stress, antioxidants and pregnancy outcome--a review. *Placenta.* 2004; 25:S72-S78.

[42] Matsubara S, Takizawa T, Takayama T, Izumi A, Watanabe T, Sato I. Immuno-electron microscopic localization of endothelial nitric oxide synthase in human placental terminal villous trophoblasts-normal and pre-eclamptic pregnancy. *Placenta.* 2001; 22:782-786.

[43] Dechend R, Viedt C, Müller DN, Ugele B, Brandes RP, Wallukat G, Park JK, Janke J, Barta P, Theuer J, Fiebeler A, Homuth V, Dietz R, Haller H, Kreuzer J, Luft FC. AT1 receptor agonistic antibodies from preeclamptic patients stimulate NADPH oxidase. *Circulation.* 2003; 107:1632-1639.

[44] Lee VM, Halligan AW, Ng LL. Neutrophil intracellular pH and Na+/H+ exchanger activity in pre-eclampsia. *Metabolism.* 2003;52:87-93.

[45] Touyz RM, Yao G, Quinn MT, Pagano PJ, Schiffrin EL. p47phox associates with the cytoskeleton through cortactin in human vascular smooth muscle cells: role in NAD(P)H oxidase regulation by angiotensin II. *Arterioscler Thromb Vasc Biol* 2005; 25:512-518.

[46] Chapman AB, Abraham, Zamudio S, Coffin C, Merouani A, Young D, Johnson A, Osorio F, Goldberg C, Moore LG, Dahms T, Schrier RW. Temporal relationships between hormonal and hemodynamic changes in early human pregnancy. *Kidney Int.* 1998; 54:2056-2063.

[47] Cunningham FG, Gant NF, Leveno KJ, Gilftrap III LC, Hauth JC, Wenstrom KD, editors. Hypertensive Disorders of Pregnancy. 21th ed. McGraw-Hill: Williams *Obstetrics*; 2001: 567–618.

[48] Creasy RK, Resnik R, editors. *Preeclampsia–Eclampsia. Maternal-Fetal Medicine. 4th ed. Philadelphia,* WB Saunders; 1999: 833–872.

[49] Report of The National High Blood Pressure Education Program Working Group on High Blood Pressure in Pregnancy. *Am J Obstet Gynecol* 2000; 183:1–22.

[50] Granger JP, Alexander BT, Llinas MT, Bennett WA, Khalil RA. Pathophysiology of preeclampsia: Linking placental ischemia/hipoxia with microvascular dysfunction *Microcirculation* 2002; 9:147–160.

[51] Zachary I. Vascular endothelial growth factor. *Int J Biochem Cell Biol.* 1998;30:1169-1174.

[52] Zachary I, Gliki G. Signaling transduction mechanisms mediating biological actions of the vascular endothelial growth factor family. *Cardiovasc Res.* 2001; 49:568-571.

[53] Lyall F, Yong A, Boswell F, Kingdom JCP, Greer IA. Placental expression of vascular endothelial growth factors in placenta from pregnancies complicated by pre-eclampsia and intrauterine growth restriction does not support placental hypoxia at delivery. *Placenta*. 1997; 18:269-276.

[54] Oh MJ, Lee JK, Lee NW, Shin JH, Yeo MK, Kim A, Kim IS, Kim HJ. Vascular endothelial growth factor expression is unaltered in placentae and myometrial resistance arteries from preeclampsia patients. *Acta Obstet Gynecol Scand.* 2006; 85:545-550.

[55] Maharaj AS, Saint-Geniez M, Maldonado AE, D'Amore PA. Vascular endothelial growth factor localization in the adult. *Am J Pathol* 2006;168:639–648.

[56] Esser S, Wolburg K,Wolburg H, Breier G, Kurzchalia T, Risau W. Vascular endothelial growth factor induces endothelial fenestrations in vitro. *J Cell Biol* 1998; 140:947–959.

[57] Eremina V, Jefferson JA, Kowalewska J, Hochster H, Haas M, Weisstuch J, Richardson C, Kopp JB, Kabir MG, Backx PH, Gerber HP, Ferrara N, Barisoni L,Alpers CE, Quaggin SE.VEGF inhibition and renal thrombotic microangiopathy. *N Engl J Med* 2008;358:1129–1136.

[58] Patel TV, Morgan, Demetri GD, George S, Maki RG, Quigley M, Humphreys BD. A preeclampsia-like síndrome characterized by reversible hypertension and proteinuria induced by the multitargeted kinase inhibitors sunitinib and sorafenib. *J Natl Cancer Inst* 2008; 100:282–284.

[59] Sugimoto H, Hamano Y, Charytan D, Cosgrove D, Kieran M, Sudhakar A, Kalluri R. Neutralization of circulating vascular endothelial growth factor (VEGF) by anti-VEGF antibodies and soluble VEGF receptor 1 (sFlt-1) induces proteinuria. *J Biol Chem.* 2003;278:12605–12608.

[60] Autiero M, Luttun A, Tjwa M, Carmeliet P. Placental growth factor and its receptor, vascular endothelial growth factor receptor-1: novel targets for stimulation of ischemic tissue revascularization and inhibition of angiogenic and inflammatory disorders. *J Thromb Haemost.* 2003;1:1356–1370.

[61] Kendall RL, Wang G, Thomas KA. Identification of a natural soluble form of the vascular endotelial growth factor receptor, FLT-1, and its heterodimerization with KDR. *Biochem Biophys Res Commun* 1996; 226:324–328.

[62] Carmeliet P, Moons L, Luttun A, Vincenti V, Compernolle V, De Mol M, Wu Y, Bono F, Devy L, Beck H, Scholz D, Acker T, DiPalma T, Dewerchin M, Noel A,Stalmans I, Barra A, Blacher S, VandenDriessche T, Ponten A, Eriksson U, Plate KH, Foidart JM, Schaper W, Charnock-Jones DS, Hicklin DJ, Herbert JM,Collen D, Persico MG. Synergism between vascular endothelial growth factor and placental growth factor contributes to angiogenesis and plasma extravasation in pathological conditions. *Nat Med:* 2001;7:575–583.

[63] Maynard SE, Min JY, Merchan J, Lim KH, Li J, Mondal S, Libermann TA, Morgan, Sellke FW, Stillman IE, Epstein FH, Sukhatme VP, Karumanchi SA. Excess placental soluble fms-like tyrosine kinase 1 (sFlt1) may contribute to endothelial dysfunction, hypertension, and proteinuria in preeclampsia. *J Clin Invest* 2003;111:649–658.

[64] Levine RJ, Maynard SE, Qian C, Lim KH, England, Yu KF, Schisterman EF, Thadhani R, Sachs BP, Epstein FH, Sibai BM, Sukhatme VP, Karumanchi SA. Circulating angiogenic factors and the risk of preeclampsia. *N Engl J Med* 2004;350:672–683.

[65] Sela S, Itin A, Natanson-Yaron S, Greenfield C, Goldman-Wohl D. A novel human specific soluble vascular endothelial growth factor receptor 1. Circ Res. 2008;102:1566-1584.

[66] Mutter, W.P. & Karumanchi, S.A. Molecular mechanisms of preeclampsia. *Microvasc Res* 2008;75, 1–8.

[67] Wang A, Rana S & Karumanchi SA. Preeclampsia: the role of angiogenic factors in its pathogenesis. *Physiology* (Bethesda) 2009;24, 147–158.

[68] Rajakumar A, Michael HM, Rajakumar PA, Shibata E, Hubel CA, Karumanchi SA, Thadhani R, Wolf M, Harger G, Markovic N. Extra-placental expression of vascular endothelial growth factor receptor-1 (Flt-1), and soluble Flt-1 (sFlt-1), by peripheral blood mononuclear cells (PBMCs) in normotensive and preeclamptic pregnant women. *Placenta* 2005;26:563–573.

[69] Thomas CP, Andrews JI, Liu KZ. Intronic polyadenylation signal sequences and alternate splicing generate human soluble Flt1 variants and regulate the abundance of soluble Flt1 in the placenta. *FASEB J*. 2007;21:3885–3895.

[70] Ohkuchi A, Hirashima C, Matsubara S, Takahashi K, Matsuda Y, Suzuki M. Threshold of soluble fms-like tyrosine kinase 1/placental growth factor ratio for the imminent onset of preeclampsia. *Hypertension*. 2011;58:859–866.

[71] Rana S, Powe CE, Salahuddin S, Verlohren S, Perschel FH, Levine RJ, Lim KH, Wenger JB, Thadhani R, Karumanchi SA. Angiogenic factors and the risk of adverse outcomes in women with suspected preeclampsia. *Circulation*. 2012;125:911–919.

[72] Garovic VD. The role of angiogenic factors in the prediction and diagnosis of preeclampsia superimposed on chronic hypertension. *Hypertension*. 2012;59:555–557.

[73] Wathén KA, Tuutti E, Stenman UH, Alfthan H, Halmesmäki E, Finne P, Ylikorkala O, Vuorela P. Maternal serum-soluble vascular endothelial growth factor receptor-1 in early pregnancy ending in preeclampsia or intrauterine growth retardation. *J Clin Endocrinol Metab* 2006;91:180–184.

[74] McKeeman GC, Ardill JE, Caldwell CM, Hunter AJ, McClure N. Soluble vascular endotelial growth factor receptor-1 (sFlt-1) is increased throughout gestation in patients who have preeclampsia develop. *Am J Obstet Gynecol* 2004;191:1240–1246.

[75] Hertig A, Berkane N, Lefevre G, Toumi K, Marti HP, Capeau J, Uzan S, Rondeau E. Maternal serum sFlt1 concentration is an early and reliable predictive marker of preeclampsia. *Clin Chem* 2004;50:1702–1703.

[76] Perni U, Sison C, Sharma V, Helseth G, Hawfield A, Suthanthiran M, August P. Angiogenic factors in superimposed preeclampsia: a longitudinal study of women with chronic hypertension during pregnancy. *Hypertension*. 2012;59:740–746.

[77] Murphy SR, LaMarca BB, Cockrell K, Granger JP. Role of endothelin in mediating soluble fms-like tyrosine kinase 1-induced hypertension in pregnant rats. *Hypertension*. 2010;55:394–398.

[78] Sandrim VC, Palei AC, Metzger IF, Gomes VA, Cavalli RC, Tanus-Santos JE. Nitric oxide formation is inversely related to serum levels of antiangiogenic factors soluble fms-like tyrosine kinase-1 and soluble endogline in preeclampsia. *Hypertension* 2008;52:402–407.

[79] Li F, Hagaman JR, Kim HS, Maeda N, Jennette JC, Faber JE, Karumanchi SA, Smithies O, Takahashi N. eNOS deficiency acts through endothelin to aggravate sFlt-1-induced pre-eclampsia-like phenotype. *J Am Soc Nephrol* 2012;23:652–660.

[80] Thadhani R, Kisner T, Hagmann H, Bossung V, Noack S, Schaarschmidt W, Jank A, Kribs A, Cornely OA, Kreyssig C, Hemphill L, Rigby AC, Khedkar S, Lindner TH, Mallmann P, Stepan H, Karumanchi SA, Benzing T. Pilot study of extracorporeal removal of soluble fms-like tyrosine kinase 1 in preeclampsia. *Circulation* 2011; 124: 940–950.
[81] Welches WR., Brosnihan KB., and Ferrario CM. A comparison of the properties and enzymatic activities of three angiotensin processing enzymes: angiotensin converting enzyme, prolyl endopeptidase and neutral endopeptidase 24.11. *Life Sci* 1993; 52: 1461–1480.
[82] Higuchi S, Ohtsu H, Suzuki H, Shirai H, Frank GD, Eguchi S. Angiotensin II signal transduction through the AT1 receptor: novel insights into mechanisms and pathophysiology. *Clin Sci* 2007;112:417-428.
[83] Nguyen Dinh Cat A, Touyz RM. A new look at the renin-angiotensin systeme focusing on the vascular system. *Peptides* 2011;32:2141-2150.
[84] Csikos T, Chung O, Unger T. Receptors and their classification: focus on angiotensin II and the AT2 receptor. *J Hum Hypertens* 1998;12:311-318.
[85] Arima S, Endo Y, Yaoita H, Omata K, Ogawa S, Tsunoda K, Abe M, Takeuchi K, Abe K, Ito S.Possible role of P-450 metabolite of arachidonic acid in vasodilator mechanism of angiotensin II type 2 receptor in the isolated microperfused rabbit afferent arteriole. *J Clin Invest* 1997;100:2816-2823.
[86] Janiak P, Pillon A, Prost JF, Vilaine JP. Role of angiotensin subtype 2 receptor in neointima formation after vascular injury. *Hypertension* 1992;20:737-745.
[87] Haberl RL, Anneser F, Villringer A, Einhaupl KM. Angiotensin II induces endothelium-dependent vasodilation of rat cerebral arterioles. *Am J Physiol* 1990;258:H1840-1846.
[88] Shah DM. The role of RAS in the pathogenesis of preeclampsia. *Curr Hypertens Rep* 2006;8:144–152.
[89] Hering L, Herse F, Geusens N, Verlohren S, Wenzel K, Staff AC, Brosnihan KB, Huppertz B, Luft FC, Muller DN, Pijnenborg R, Cartwright JE, Dechend R. Effects of circulating and local uteroplacental angiotensin II in rat pregnancy. *Hypertension.* 2010;56:311–318.
[90] Li C, Ansari R, Yu Z, Shah D: Definitive molecular evidence of renin-angiotensin system in human uterine decidual cells. *Hypertension* 2000; 36:159–164.
[91] McIntyre M, Bohr DF, Dominiczak AF. Endothelial function in hypertension: the role of superoxide anion. *Hypertension* 1999;34:539-545.
[92] Shah DM. Role of the renineangiotensin system in the pathogenesis of preeclampsia. *Am J Physiol Renal Physiol* 2005;288:F614-625.
[93] Anguiano-Robledo L, Reyes-Melchor PA, Bobadilla-Lugo RA, Perez-Alvarez VM, Lopez-Sanchez P. Renal angiotensin-II receptors expression changes in a model of preeclampsia. *Hypertens Pregnancy* 2007;26:151–161.
[94] Huppertz B, Tews DS, Kaufmann P. Apoptosis and syncytial fusion in human placental trophoblast and skeletal muscle. *Int Rev Cytol*, 2001;205:215–253.
[95] Ishihara N, Matsuo H, Murakoshi H, Laoag-Fernandez JB, Samoto T, Maruo T. Increased apoptosis in the syncytiotrophoblast in human term placentas complicated by either preeclampsia or intrauterine growth retardation. *Am J Obstet Gynecol* 2002;186:158-166.

[96] Covone AE, Mutton D, Johnson PM, Adinolfi M. Trophoblast cells in peripheral blood from pregnant women. *Lancet* 1984;2:841–843.

[97] Chen Q, Stone PR, McCowan LM, Chamley LW. Phagocytosis of necrotic but not apoptotic trophoblasts induces endothelial cell activation. *Hypertension* 2006; 47:116–121.

[98] Chen Q, Guo F, Liu S, Xiao J, Wang C, Snowise S, Stone PR, Chamley LW. Calcium channel blockers prevent endothelial cell activation in response to necrotic trophoblast debris: possible relevance to pre-eclampsia. *Cardiovasc Reserch.* 2012;96:484-493.

[99] Chen Q, Chen L, Liu B, Vialli C, Stone P, Ching LM, Chamley LThe role of autocrine TGFbeta1 in endothelial cell activation induced by phagocytosis of necrotic trophoblasts: a possible role in the pathogenesis of preeclampsia. *J Pathol* 2010;221:87 – 95.

[100] Redman CW, Sargent IL. Circulating microparticles in normal pregnancy and pre-eclampsia. *Placenta* 2008;29:73–77.

[101] Han KH, Hong KH, Park JH, Ko J, Kang DH, Choi KJ, Hong MK, Park SW, Park SJ. C-reactive protein promotes monocyte chemoattractant protein-1-mediated chemotaxis through upregulating CC chemokine receptor 2 expression in human monocytes. *Circulation* 2004;109:2566–2569.

[102] Meziani F, Tesse A, David E, Martinez MC, Wangesteen R, Schneider F, Andriantsitohaina R. Shed membrane particles from preeclamptic women generate vascular wall inflammation and blunt vascular contractility. *Am J Pathol* 2006;169:1473–1483.

[103] Freyssinet JM, Toti F. Formation of procoagulant microparticles and properties. *Thromb Res* 2010;125:S46-48.

[104] Lok CA, Snijder KS, Nieuwland R, Van Der Post JA, de Vos P, Faas MM. Microparticles of pregnant women and preeclamptic patients activate endothelial cells in the presence of monocytes. *Am J Reprod Immunol.* 2012;67:206-215.

[105] Donker RB, Asgeirsdottir SA, Gerbens F, Van Pampus MG, Kallenberg CG, Te Meerman GJ, Aarnoudse JG, Molema G. Plasma factors in severe early-onset preeclampsia do not substantially alter endothelial gene expression in vitro. *J Soc Gynecol Investig.* 2005;12, 98–106.

[106] Sacks GP, Studena K, Sargent K, Redman CW. Normal pregnancy and preeclampsia both produce inflammatory changes in peripheral blood leukocytes akin to those of sepsis. *American Journal of Obstetrics & Gynecology* 1998; 179:80 86.

[107] Koumandakis E, Koumandaki I, Kaklamani E, Sparos L, Aravantinos D, Trichopoulos D. Enhanced phagocytosis of mononuclear phagocytes in pregnancy. *Br J Obstet Gynaecol* 1986;93:1150–1154.

[108] Shibuya T, Izuchi K, Kuroiwa A, Okabe N, Shirakawa K. Study on nonspecific immunity in pregnant women: increased chemiluminescence response of peripheral blood phagocytes. *Am J Reprod Immunol Microbiol* 1987;15:19–23

[109] Luppi P, Haluszczak C, Betters D, Richard CA, Trucco M, DeLoia JA. Monocytes are progressively activated in the circulation of pregnant women. *J Leukoc Biol* 2002;72:874–884.

[110] Sacks GP, Redman CW, Sargent IL. Monocytes are primed to produce the Th1 type cytokine IL-12 in normal human pregnancy: an intracellular flow cytometric analysis of peripheral blood mononuclear cells. *Clin Exp Immunol* 2003;131:490–497.

[111] Gervasi MT, Chaiworapongsa T, Naccasha N, Blackwell S, Yoon BH, Maymon E, Romero R. Phenotypic and metabolic characteristics of maternal monocytes and granulocytes in preterm labor with intact membranes. *Am J Obstet Gynecol* 2001;185:1124–1129.

[112] Luppi P, Deloia JA. Monocytes of preeclamptic women spontaneously synthesize pro-inflammatory cytokines. *Clin Immunol* 2006;118:268–75.

[113] Santhanam U, Avila C, Romero R, Viguet H, Ida N, Sakurai S, Sehgal PB. Cytokines in normal and abnormal parturition: elevated amniotic fluid interleukin-6 levels in women with premature rupture of membranes associated with intrauterine infection. *Cytokine* 1991;3:155–163.

[114] Erzen B, Sabovic M, Sebestjen M, Keber I, Poredos P. Interleukin-6 correlates with endothelial dysfunction in young post-myocardial infarction patients. *Cardiology* 2007;107:111–116.

[115] Greer IA, Lyall F, Perera T, Boswell F, Macara LM. Increased concentrations of cytokines interleukin-6 and interleukin-1 receptor antagonist in plasma of women with preeclampsia: a mechanism for endothelial dysfunction? *Obstet Gynecol.* 1994;84:937–940.

[116] Vince GS, Starkey PM, Austgulen R, Kwiatkowski D, Redman CW. Interleukin-6, tumour necrosis factor and soluble tumour necrosis factor receptors in women with pre-eclampsia. *Br J Obstet Gynaecol* 1995;102:20–25.

[117] Kupferminc MJ, Peaceman AM, Aderka D, Wallach D, Socol ML. Soluble tumor necrosis factor receptors and interleukin-6 levels in patients with severe preeclampsia. *Obstet Gynecol.* 1996;88:420–427.

[118] Al-Othman S, Omu AE, Diejomaoh FM, Al-Yatama M, Al-Qattan F. Differential levels of interleukin 6 in maternal and cord sera and placenta in women with pre-eclampsia. *Gynecol Obstet Invest.* 2001;52:60–65.

[119] Borekci B, Aksoy H, Al RA, Demircan B, Kadanali S. Maternal serum interleukin-10, interleukin-2 and interleukin-6 in pre-eclampsia and eclampsia. *Am J Reprod Immunol* 2007;58:56–64.

[120] Chen Q, Stone P, Ching LM, Chamley L. A role for interleukin-6 in spreading endothelial cell activation after phagocytosis of necrotic trophoblastic mate-rial: implications for the pathogenesis of pre-eclampsia. *J Pathol* 2009;217:122–130.

[121] Noyola-Martínez N, Díaz L, Avila E, Halhali A, Larrea F, Barrera D. Calcitriol downregulates TNF-α and IL-6 expression in cultured placental cells from preeclamptic women. *Cytokine* 2013;61:245-250.

[122] Gilbert JS, Verzwyvelt J, Colson D, Arany M, Karumanchi SA, Granger JP. Recombinant vascular endothelial growth factor 121 infusion lowers blood pressure and improves renal function in rats with placentalischemia-induced hypertension. *Hypertension* 2010;55:380–385.

[123] Wang W, Irani RA, Zhang Y, Ramin SM, Blackwell SC, Tao L, Kellems RE, Xia Y. Autoantibody-mediated complement C3a receptor activation contributes to the pathogenesis of preeclampsia. *Hypertension* 2012;60, 712–721.

[124] Zhou CC, Zhang Y, Irani RA, Zhang H, Mi T, Popek EJ, Hicks MJ, Ramin SM, Kellems RE, Xia Y. Angiotensin receptor agonistic autoantibodies induce pre-eclampsia in pregnant mice. *Nat Med* 2008;14:855–862.

[125] Burwick RM, Feinberg BB. Eculizumab for the treatment of preeclampsia/HELLP syndrome. *Placenta* 2013;34:201–203.

[126] Santner-Nanan B, Peek MJ, Khanam R, Richarts L, Zhu E, Fazekas de St GB, Nanan R. Systemic increase in the ratio between Foxp3+ and IL-17-producing CD4+ T cells in healthy pregnancy but not in preeclampsia. *J Immunol.* 2009; 183:7023–7030.

[127] Prins JR, Boelens HM, Heimweg J, Van der Heide S, Dubois AE, Van Oosterhout AJ, Erwich JJ. Preeclampsia is associated with lower percentages of regulatory T cells in maternal blood. *Hypertens Pregnancy* 2009,28:300-311.

[128] Alexander BT, Kassab SE, Miller MT, Abram SR, Reckeihoff JF, Bennett WA, Granger JP. Reduced uterine perfusion pressure during pregnancy in the rat is associated with increases in arterial pressure and changes in renal nitric oxide. *Hypertension* 2001,37:1191-1195.

[129] Granger JP, LaMarca BB, Cockrell K, Sedeek M, Baizi C, Chandler D, Bennett W. Reduced uterine perfusion pressure (RUPP) model for studying cardiovascular-renal dysfunction in response to placental ischemia. *Methods Mol Med* 2006;122:383-392.

[130] LaMarca B. The role of immune activation in contributing to vascular dysfunction and the pathophysiology of hypertension during preeclampsia. *Minerva Ginecol* 2010,62:105-120.

[131] Wallukat G, Homuth V, Fischer T, Lindschau C, Horstkamp B, Jüpner A, Baur F, Nissen E, Vetter K, Neichel D, Dudenhausen JW, Haller H, Luft FC. Patients with preeclampsia develop agonistic autoantibodies against the angiotensin AT1 receptor. *J Clin Invest*1999,103:945-952.

[132] Xia Y, Wen H, Bobst S, Day MC, Kellems RE. Maternal autoantibodies from preeclamptic patients activate angiotensin receptors on human trophoblast cells. *J Soc Gynecol Investig.* 2003;10:82-93.

[133] Xia Y, Ramin SM, Kellems RE: Potential roles of angiotensin receptor-activating autoantibody in the pathophysiology of preeclampsia. *Hypertension* 2007,50:269-275.

[134] LaMarca B, Bennett W, Alexander B, Cockrell K, Granger J: Hypertension produced by reductions in uterine perfusion in the pregnant rat: role of tumor necrosis factor-alpha. *Hypertension* 2005,46:1022-1025.

[135] LaMarca B, Wallukat G, Llinas M, Herse F, Dechend R, Granger JP: Autoantibodies to the angiotensin type I receptor in response to placental ischemia and tumor necrosis factor alpha in pregnant rats. *Hypertension* 2008,52:1168-1172.

[136] LaMarca B, Parrish M, Ray LF, Murphy SR, Roberts L, Glover P, Wallukat G, Wenzel K, Cockrell K, Martin JN Jr, Ryan MJ, Dechend R. Hypertension in response to autoantibodies to the angiotensin II type I receptor (AT1-AA) in pregnant rats: a role of endothelin-1. *Hypertension* 2009,54:905-909.

[137] Walther T, Wallukat G, Jank A, Bartel S, Schultheiss HP, Faber R, Stepan H: Angiotensin II type 1 receptor agonistic antibodies reflect fundamental alterations in the uteroplacental vasculature. *Hypertension* 2005; 46:1275–1279.

[138] Fu ML, Herlitz H, Schulze W, Wallukat G, Micke P, Eftekhari P, Sjogren KG, Hjalmarson A, Muller-Esterl W, Hoebeke J: Autoantibodies against the angiotensin receptor (AT1) in patients with hypertension. *J Hypertens* 2000; 18:945–953.

[139] Dragun D, Muller DN, Brasen JH, Fritsche L, Nieminen-Kelha M, Dechend R, Kintscher U, Rudolph B, Hoebeke J, Eckert D, Mazak I, Plehm R, Schonemann C,

Unger T, Budde K, Neumayer HH, Luft FC, Wallukat G: Angiotensin II type 1-receptor activating antibodies in renal-allograft rejection. *N Engl J Med* 2005; 352:558–569.

[140] Riemekasten G, Philippe A, Nather M, Slowinski T, Muller DN, Heidecke H, Matucci-Cerinic M, Czirjak L, Lukitsch I, Becker M, Kill A, van Laar JM, Catar R, Luft FC, Burmester GR, Hegner B, Dragun D: Involvement of functional autoantibodies against vascular receptors in systemic sclerosis. *Ann Rheum Dis* 2011; 70:530–536.

[141] Hubel CA, Wallukat G, Wolf M, Herse F, Rajakumar A, Roberts JM, Markovic N, Thadhani R, Luft FC, Dechend R: Agonistic angiotensin II type 1 receptor autoantibodies in postpartum women with a history of preeclampsia. *Hypertension* 2007; 49:612–617.

[142] AbdAlla S, Lother H, el Massiery A, Quitterer U. In-creased AT(1) receptor heterodimers in preeclampsia mediate enhanced angiotensin II responsiveness. *Nat Med.* 2001;7:1003-1009.

[143] Xia Y, Wen H, Bobst S, Day MC, Kellems RE. Maternal autoantibodies from preeclamptic patients activate angiotensin receptors on human trophoblast cells. *J Soc Gynecol Investig*. 2003;10:82-93.

[144] Parrish MR, Wallace K, Tam Tam KB, Herse F, Weimer A, Wenzel K, Wallukat G, Ray LF, Arany M, Cockrell K, Martin JN, Dechend R, LaMarca B. Hypertension in response to AT1-AA: role of reactive oxygen species in pregnancy induced hypertension. *Am J Hypertens*. 2011;24:835– 840.

[145] Parrish MR, Murphy SR, Rutland S, Wallace K, Wenzel K, Wallukat G, Keiser S, Ray LF, Dechend R, Martin JN, Granger JP, LaMarca B.The effect of immune factors, tumor necrosis factor-alpha, and agonistic autoantibodies to the angiotensin II Type I receptor on soluble fms-like tyrosine-1 and soluble endoglin production in response to hypertension during pregnancy. *Am J Hypertens* 2010;23:911-916.

[146] LaMarca B, Speed J, Ray LF, Cockrell K, Wallukat G, Dechend R, Granger J. Hypertension in response to IL-6 during pregnancy: role of AT1-receptor activation. International Journal of Iinterferon, *Int J Infereron Cytokine Mediator Res*. 2011;3:65–70.

[147] Zhou CC, Ahmad S, Mi T, Abbasi S, Xia L, Day MC, Ramin SM, Ahmed A, Kellems RE, Xia Y. Autoantibody from women with preeclampsia induces soluble Fms-like tyrosine kinase-1 production via angiotensin type 1 receptor and calcineurin/nuclear factor of activated T-cells signaling. *Hypertension*. 2008;51:1010-1019.

[148] Taylor RN, Varma M, Teng NN, Roberts JM. Women with pre-eclampsia have higher plasma endothelin levels than women with normal pregnancies. *J Clin Endocrinol Metab* 1990;71:1675-1677.

[149] LaMarca B, Wallace K, Herse F, Wallukat G, Martin Jr JN, Weimer A, Dechend R. Hypertension in response to placental ischemia during pregnancy: role of B lymphocytes. *Hypertension* 2011; 57:865–871.

[150] Wei F, Jia XJ, Yu SQ, Gu Y, Wang L, Guo XM, Wang M, Zhu F, Cheng X, Wei YM, Zhou ZH, Fu M, Liao YH: Candesartan versus imidapril in hypertension: a randomised study to assess effects of anti-AT1 receptor autoantibodies. *Heart* 2011;97:479–484.

[151] Daikha-Dahmane F, Levy-Beff E, Jugie M, Lenclen R. Foetal kidney maldevelopment in maternal use of angiotensin II type I receptor antagonists. *Pediatr Nephrol* 2006; 21:729–732.

[152] Vendemmia M, Garcia-Meric P, Rizzotti A, Boubred F, Lacroze V, Liprandi A, Simeoni U: Fetal and neonatal consequences of antenatal exposure to type 1 angiotensin II receptor-antagonists. *J Matern Fetal Neonatal Med* 2005; 18:137–140.

[153] Schiffrin EL. Vascular endothelin in hypertension. *Vascul Pharmacol.* 2005;43:19-29.

[154] George EM, Granger JP. Endothelin: key mediator of hypertension in preeclampsia. *Am J Hypertens* 2011;24, 964–969.

[155] Tam Tam KB, George E, Cockrell K, Arany M, Speed J, Martin Jr JN, Lamarca B, Granger JP. Endothelin type A receptor antagonist attenuates placental ischemia-induced hypertension and uterine vascular resistance. *Am J Obstet Gynecol* 2011;204,331–334.

[156] Fiore, G., Florio, P., Micheli, L., Nencini, C., Rossi, M., Cerretani, D., Ambrosini, G., Giorgi, G., Petraglia, F., Endothelin-1 triggers placental oxidative stress pathways: putative role in preeclampsia. *J Clin Endocrinol Metab.* 2005;90: 4205–4210.

[157] Yung, H.W., Calabrese, S., Hynx, D., Hemmings, B.A., Cetin, I., Charnock-Jones, D.S., Burton, G.J., Evidence of placental translation inhibition and endoplasmic reticulum stress in the etiology of human intrauterine growth restriction. *Am J Pathol.* 2008;173:451–462.

[158] Zhang K, Kaufman RJ. From endoplasmic-reticulum stress to the inflammatory response. *Nat Med* 2008; 454: 455–462.

[159] Jain A. Olovsson M, Burton GJ, Yung HW. Endothelin- 1 induces endoplasmic reticulum stress by activating the PLC-IP(3) pathway: implications for placental pathophysiology in preeclampsia. *Am J Pathol* 2012;180;2309–2320.

[160] Kähler, Jan; Ewert, Anne; Weckmüller, Jörn; Stobbe, Silvia; Mittmann, Clemens*; Köster, Ralf; Paul, Martin†; Meinertz, Thomas; Münzel, Thomas. Oxidative Stress Increases Endothelin-1 Synthesis in Human Coronary Artery Smooth Muscle Cells. *J Cardiovasc Pharmacol* 2001;38 :49–57.

[161] Sfakianaki A, Norwitz E. Mechanisms of progesterone action in inhibiting prematurity. *J Matern Fetal Neonatal Med* 2006;19:763-772.

[162] Saghafi N, Khadem N, Mohajeri T, Shakeri M. Efficacy of 17-alpha-hydroxyprogesterone caproate in prevention of preterm delivery. *J Obstet Gynaecol Res* 2011;37: 1342-1345.

[163] Merlob P, Stahl B, Klinger G. 17-alpha- Hydroxyprogesterone caproate for prevention of recurrent spontaneous preterm birth. *Reprod Toxicol* 2012;33:15-19.

[164] Society for Maternal-Fetal Medicine Publications Committee; Berghella V. Progesterone and preterm birth prevention: translating clinical trials data into clinical practice. *Am J Obstet Gynecol* 2012;5:376-386.

[165] Luo, Abrahams VM, Tadesse S, Funai EF, Hodgson EJ, Gao J, Norwitz ER. Progesterone inhibits basal and TNF-alpha-induced apoptosis in fetal membranes: a novel mechanisms to explain progesterone-mediated prevention of preterm birth. *Reprod Sci* 2010;17: 532-539.

[166] Kiprono LV, Wallace K, Moseley J, Martin J Jr, Lamarca B. Progesterone blunts vascular endothelial cell secretion of endothelin-1 in response to placental ischemia. *Am J Obstet Gynecol* 2013;209:44-46.

[167] Maguire JJ, Kuc RE, Davenport AP. Orphan receptor ligand human urotensin II: receptor localization in human tissues and comparison of vasocontrictor responses with endothelin 1. *Br J Pharmacol* 2000;13: 441–446.

[168] Affolter J, Webb DJ. Urotensin II: a new mediator in cardiopulmonary regulation? *Lancet* 2001;358:774–775.

[169] Maguire JJ, Davenport AP. Is urotensin II the new endothelin? *Br J Pharmacol* 2002;137:579–88.

[170] Totsune K, Takahashi K, Arihata Z. Role of urotensin II in patients on dialysis. *Lancet* 2001;358:810–811.

[171] Gray AG, Jones MR, Sharif I. Human urotensin II increases coronary perfusion pressure in the isolated rat heart potentiation by nitric oxide synthase and cyclooxygenase inhibition. *Life Sci* 2001;69:175–180.

[172] MacLean MR, Alexander D, Stirrat A, Gallagher M, Douglas SA, Ohlstein EH, Morecroft I, Polland K. Contractile responses to human urotensin-II in rat and human pulmonary arteries: effect of endothelial factors and chronic hypoxia in the rat. *Br J Pharmacol* 2000;130:201–204.

[173] Krum H, Gilbert RE. Urothensin: a new player in vascular and myocardial disease. *Clin Sci* 2003;104:65–67.

[174] Bottril FE, Douglas SA, Hiley CR, White R. Human urotensin II is an endothelium dependent vasodilator in rat small arteries. *Br J Pharmacol* 2000;130:1865–70.

[175] Affolter JT, Newby DE, Wilkinson IB,Winter MJ, Balment RJ,Webb DJ. No effect on central or peripheral blood pressure of systemic urotensin II infusion in humans. *Br J Clin Pharmacol* 2002;54:617–621.

[176] Matsushita M, Shichiri M, Imai T, Iwashina M, Tanaka H, Takasu N, Hirata Y. Co-expression of urotensin II and its receptor (GPR14) in human cardiovascular and renal tissues. *J Hypertens* 2001;19:2185–2190.

[177] Douglas SA, Sulpizio AC, Piercy V, Sarau HM, Ames RS, Aiyar NV, Ohlstein EH, Willette RN. Differential vasoconstrictor activity of human urotensin-II in vascular tissue isolated from the rat, mouse, dog, pig, marmoset and cynomolgus monkey. *Br J Pharmacol* 2000;131:1262–1274.

[178] Song W, McDonald J, Camarda V, Calo G, Guerrini R, Marzola E, Thompson JP, Rowbotham DJ, Lambert DG. Cell and tissue responses of a range of urotensin II analogs at cloned and native urotensin II receptors: evidence for coupling promiscuity. *Naunyn Schmiedebergs Arch Pharmacol* 2006;373:148–157.

[179] Ross B, McKendy K, Giaid A. Role of urotensin II in health and disease. *Am J Physiol Regul Integr Comp Physiol* 2010;298:R1156–R1172.

[180] Tsoukas P, Kane E, Giaid A. Potential clinical implications of the urotensin ii receptor antagonists. *Front Pharmacol* 2011;2:38.

[181] Douglas SA, Ohlstein EH. Human urotensin II, the most potent mammalian vasoconstrictor identified to date, as a therapeutic target for the management of cardiovascular disease. *Trends Cardiovasc Med* 2000;10:229–237.

[182] Zhang YG, Li J, Li YG, Wei RH. Urotensin II induces phenotypic differentiation, migration and collagen synthesis of adventitial fibroblasts from rat aorta. *J Hypertens* 2008; 26: 1119 – 1126.

[183] Pan P, Fu H, Zhang L, Huang H, Luo, Wu W, Guo Y, Liu X.Angiotensin II upregulates the expression of placental growth factor in human vascular endothelial cells and smooth muscle cells. *BMC Cell Biol* 2010; 26: 36.

[184] Balat O, Aksoy F, Kutlar I, Ugur MG, Iyikosker H, Balat A, Anarat R. Increased plasma levels of Urotensin-II in preeclampsia-eclampsia: a new mediator in pathogenesis? *Eur J Obstet Gynecol Reprod Biol.*2005;120:33-38.

[185] Cowley E, Thompson JP, Sharpe P, Waugh J, Ali N, Lambert DG. Effects of pre-eclampsia on maternal plasma, cerebrospinal fluid, and umbilical cord urotensin II concentrations: a pilot study. *Br J Anaesth.* 2005;95:495-499.

[186] Liu Y, Li Y, Xu X, Chen X, Chen H. Neurokinin B and urotensin II levels in preeclampsia. *J Matern Fetal Neonatal Med.* 2010;23:869-873.

[187] Gould PS, Gu M, Liao J, Ahmad S, Cudmore MJ, Ahmed A, Vatish M. Upregulation of urotensin II receptor in preeclampsia causes in vitro placental release of soluble vascular endothelial growth factor receptor 1 in hypoxia. *Hypertension.* 2010;56:172–178.

[188] Spinazzi R, Albertin G, Nico B, Guidolin D, Di Liddo R, Rossi GP, Ribatti D, Nussdorfer GG. Urotensin-II and its receptor (ut-r) are expressed in rat brain endothelial cells, and urotensin-II via ut-r stimulates angiogenesis in vivo and in vitro. *Int J Mol Med.* 2006;18:1107–1112.

[189] Albertin G, Guidolin D, Sorato E, Spinazzi R, Mascarin A, Oselladore B, Montopoli M, Antonello M, Ribatti D. Pro-angiogenic activity of urotensin-ii on different human vascular endothelial cell populations. *Regul Pept.* 2009;157:64 –71.

[190] Caniggia I, Mostachfi H, Winter J, Gassmann M, Lye SJ, Kuliszewski M, Post M. Hypoxia-inducible factor-1 mediates the biological effects of oxygen on human trophoblast differentiation through TGFbeta(3). *J Clin Invest* 2000; 105:577–587.

[191] Caniggia I, Grisaru-Gravnosky S, Kuliszewsky M, Post M, Lye SJ. Inhibition of TGF-beta 3 restores the invasive capability of extravillous trophoblasts in preeclamptic pregnancies. *J Clin Invest* 1999; 103: 1641–1650.

[192] Yamashita K, Discher DJ, Hu J, Bishopric NH, Webster KA. Molecular regulation of the endothelin-1 gene by hypoxia. Contributions of hypoxia-inducible factor-1, activator protein-1, GATA-2, and p300/ CBP. *J Biol Chem* 2001; 276:12645–12653.

[193] Minchenko A, Caro J. Regulation of endothelin-1 gene expression in human microvascular endothelial cells by hypoxia and cobalt: role of hypoxia responsive element. *Molecular and Cellular Biochemistry* 2000; 208:53–62.

[194] Nevo O, Soleymanlou N, Wu Y, Xu J, Kingdom J, Many A, Zamudio S, Caniggia I. Increased expression of sFlt-1 in in vivo and in vitro models of human placental hypoxia is mediated by HIF-1. *Am J Physiol Regul Integr Comp Physiol* 2006; 291:R1085–R1093.

[195] Wenzel K, Rajakumar A, Haase H, Geusens N, Hubner N, Schulz H, Brewer J, Roberts L, Hubel CA, Herse F, Hering L, Qadri F, Lindschau C, Wallukat G,Pijnenborg R, Heidecke H, Riemekasten G, Luft FC, Muller DN, Lamarca B, Dechend R. Angiotensin II type 1 receptor antibodies and increased angiotensin II sensitivity in pregnant rats. *Hypertension* 2011; 58:77–84.

[196] Giles TD, Sander GE, Nossaman BD, Kadowitz PJ. Impaired vasodilation in the pathogenesis of hypertension: focus on nitric oxide, endothelial-derivedhyperpolarizing factors, and prostaglandins. *J Clin Hypertens.* 2012:4:198-205.

[197] Conrad KP, Joffe GM, Kruszyna H, Kruszyna R, Rochelle LG, Smith RP, Chavez JE, Mosher MD. Identification of increased nitric oxide biosynthesis during pregnancy in rats. *FASEB J.* 1993;7:566–571.

[198] Williams DJ, Vallance PJ, Neild GH, Spencer JA, Imms FJ. Nitric oxidemediated vasodilation in human pregnancy. *Am J Physiol*. 1997;27:748–752.

[199] Sladek SM, Magness RR, Conrad KP. Nitric oxide and pregnancy. *Am J Physiol* 1997;272:441–463.

[200] Kawano M, Mori N. Prostacyclin producing activity of human umbilical, placental and uterine vessels. *Prostaglandins*. 1983;26:645–662.

[201] Magness RR, Shideman CR, Habermehl DA, Sullivan JA, Bird IM. Endothelial vasodilator production by uterine and systemic arteries. V. Effects of ovariectomy, the ovarian cycle, and pregnancy on prostacyclin synthase expression. *Prostaglandins Other Lipid Mediat*. 2000;60:103–118.

[202] Magness RR, Rosenfeld CR, Hassan A, Shaul PW. Endothelial vasodilator production by uterine and systemic arteries. I. Effects of ANG II on PGI2 and NO in pregnancy. *Am J Physiol*. 1996;270:1914–1923.

[203] Magness RR, Mitchell MD, Rosenfeld CR. Uteroplacental production of eicosanoids in ovine pregnancy. *Prostaglandins*. 1990;39:75–88.

[204] Gillham JC, Kenny LC, Baker PN. An overview of endothelium-derived hyperpolarising factor (EDHF) in normal and compromised pregnancies. *Eur J Obstet Gynecol Reprod Biol*. 2003;109:2–7.

[205] Gokina NI, Kuzina OY, Vance AM. Augmented EDHF signaling in rat uteroplacental vasculature during late pregnancy. *Am J Physiol Heart Circ Physiol*. 2010;299:1642–1652.

[206] Hogg N, Kalyanaraman B, Joseph J, Struck A, Parthasarathy S. Inhibition of low-density lipoprotein oxidation by nitric oxide. Potential role in atherogenesis. *FEBS Lett;* 1993: 334: 170-174.

[207] Forstermann U, Sessa W. Nitric oxide synthases: regulation and function. *Eur Hear J;* 2012; 33, 829–837

[208] Tsao PS, Buitrago R, Chan JR, Cooke JP. Fluid flow inhibits endothelial adhesiveness. Nitric oxide and transcriptional regulation of VCAM-1. *Circulation* 1996; 94: 1682-1689.

[209] Boger RH, Bode-Boger SM, Szuba A, Tsao PS, Chan JR, Tangphao O, Blaschke TF, Cooke JP Asymmetric dimethylarginine (ADMA): a novel risk factor for endothelial dysfunction: its role in hypercholesterolemia. *Circulation* 1998; 98: 1842-1847.

[210] Heitzer T, Schlinzig T, Krohn K, Meinertz T, Munzel T. Endothelial dysfunction, oxidative stress, and risk of cardiovascular events in patients with coronary artery disease. *Circulation* 2001; 104: 2673-2678.

[211] Vallance P, Leone A, Calver A, Collier J, Moncada S. Accumulation of an endogenous inhibitor of nitric oxide synthesis in chronic renal failure. *Lancet* 1992; 339: 572-575.

[212] Schachinger V, Britten MB, Zeiher AM. Prognostic impact of coronary vasodilator dysfunction on adverse long-term outcome of coronary heart disease. *Circulation* 2000; 101: 1899-1906.

[213] O'Dell TJ, Hawkins RD, Kandel ER, Arancio O. Tests of the roles of two diffusible substances in long-term potentiation: evidence for nitric oxide as a possible early retrograde messenger. *Proc Natl Acad Sci USA* 1991;88:11285–11289.

[214] Schuman EM, Madison DV. A requirement for the intercellular messenger nitric oxide in long-term potentiation. *Science* 1991;254:1503–1506.

[215] Rapoport RM, Draznin MB, Murad F. Endothelium-dependent relaxation in rat aorta may be mediated through cyclic GMP-dependent protein phosphorylation. *Nature* 1983;306:174–176.

[216] Forstermann U, Mulsch A, Bohme E, Busse R. Stimulation of soluble guanylate cyclase by an acetylcholine-induced endothelium-derived factor from rabbit and canine arteries. *Circ Res* 1986;58:531–538.

[217] Khan BV, Harrison DG, Olbrych MT, Alexander RW, Medford RM. Nitric oxide regulates vascular cell adhesion molecule 1 gene expression and redox-sensitive transcriptional events in human vascular endothelial cells. *Proc Natl Acad Sci USA* 1996;93:9114–9119.

[218] Gudi T, Hong GK, Vaandrager AB, Lohmann SM, Pilz RB. Nitric oxide and cGMP regulate gene expression in neuronal and glial cells by activating type II cGMP-dependent protein kinase. *FASEB J* 1999;13:2143–2152.

[219] Pantopoulos K, Hentze MW. Nitric oxide signaling to iron-regulatory protein: direct control of ferritin mRNA translation and transferrin receptor mRNA stability in transfected fibroblasts. *Proc Natl Acad Sci USA* 1995;92:1267–1271.

[220] Liu XB, Hill P, Haile DJ. Role of the ferroportin iron-responsive element in iron and nitric oxide dependent gene regulation. *Blood Cells Mol Dis* 2002;29: 315–326.

[221] Pozdnyakov N, Lloyd A, Reddy VN, Sitaramayya A. Nitric oxide-regulated endogenous ADP-ribosylation of rod outer segment proteins. *Biochem Biophys Res Commun* 1993;192:610–615.

[222] Brune B, Dimmeler S, Molina y Vedia L, Lapetina EG. Nitric oxide: a signal for ADP-ribosylation of proteins. *Life Sci* 1994;54:61–70.

[223] Rubanyi GM, Vanhoutte PM. Superoxide anion and hyperoxia inactivate endothelium-derived relaxing factor. *Am J Physiol*. 1986; 250:H822–H827.

[224] Wilcox CS; Asymmetric dimethylarginine and reactive oxygen species: unwelcome twin visitors to the cardiovascular and kidney disease tables. *Hypertension*. 2012;59:375–381.

[225] Feletou M, Vanhoutte PM; Endothelial dysfunction: a multifaceted disorder (The Wiggers Award Lecture). Am J Physiol Heart Circ Physiol 2006;291:H985-H1002.

[226] Alp NJ, Channon KM. Regulation of endothelial nitric oxide synthase by tetrahydrobiopterin in vascular disease. Arterioscler Thromb Vasc Biol 2004;24:413-420.

[227] VasquezVivar J, Kalyanaraman B, Martasek P, Hogg N, Masters BS, Karoui H. Supero xide generation by endothelial nitric oxide synthase: the influence of cofactors. Proc Natl Acad Sci USA 1998;95:9220-9225.

[228] Cooke JP, Rossitch E, Jr., Andon NA, Loscalzo J, Dzau VJ. Flow activates an endothelial potassium channel to release an endogenous nitrovasodilator. *J Clin Invest* 1991; 88: 1663-1671.

[229] Slaghekke F, Dekker G, Jefries B; Endogenous inhibitors of nitric oxide and preeclampsia: A Review. *J Matern Fetal Neonatal Med cine*. 2006; 19: 447-452.

[230] Demir B, Demir S, Pasa S, Guven S, Atamer Y, Atamer A, Kocyigit Y.; The role of homocysteine, asymmetric dimethylarginine and nitric oxide in pre-eclampsia.; *J Obstet Gynaecol*; 2012:32:525-528.

[231] Mao D, Che J, Li K, Han S, Yue Q, Zhu L, Zhang W, Li L. Association of homocysteine, asymmetric dimethylarginine, and nitric oxide with preeclampsia. *Arch Gynecol Obstet,* 2010;282:371–375.

[232] Alacam H, Dikmen ZG, Yaman H, Cakir E, Deren O, Akgul EO, Aydin I, Kurt YG, Keskin U, Akalin S, Polat B, Danisman N, Dogan P; The Role of Asymmetric Dimethyl Arginine and Oxidant/Antioxidant System in Preeclampsia.*; Fetal Pediatr Patho*2011; 30:387–393.

[233] LaMarca BD, Gilbert J, Granger JP. Recent progress toward the understanding of the pathophysiology of hypertension during preeclampsia. *Hypertension* 2008; 51, 982–988.

[234] Palei AC, Spradley FT, Warrington JP, George EM, Granger JP. Pathophysiology of hypertension in pre-eclampsia: a lesson in integrative physiology; *Acta Physiol* 2013, 208, 224–233.

[235] Rytlewski K, Olszanecki R, Korbut R, Zdebski Z. Effects of prolonged oral supplementation with L-arginine on blood pressure and nitric oxide synthesis in preeclampsia. *Eur J Clin Invest* 2005; 35: 32–37.

[236] Davidge ST, Stranko CP, Roberts JM. Urine but not plasma nitric oxide metabolites are decreased in women with preeclampsia. *Am J Obstet Gynecol* 1996; 174, 1008–1013.

[237] Conrad KP, Kerchner LJ, Mosher MD. Plasma and 24-h NO(x) and cGMP during normal pregnancy and preeclampsia in women on a reduced NO(x) diet. *Am J Physiol* 1999:277: 48–57.

[238] Altun ZS, Uysal S, Guner G, Yilmaz O, Posaci,C. Effects of oral L-arginine supplementation on blood pressure and *asymmetric dimethylarginine in stress-induced preeclamptic rats. Cell* Biochemistry And Function; 2008:5, 648-653.

[239] Staff AC, Berge L, Haugen G, Lorentzen B, Mikkelsen B, Henriksen T. Dietary supplementation with L-arginine or placebo in women with pre-eclampsia. *Acta Obstet Gynecol Scand* 2004; 83: 103–107.

[240] Garcia RG, Celedón J, Sierra-Laguado J, Alarcón MA, Luengas C, Silva F, Arenas-Mantilla M, López-Jaramillo P. Raised C-reactive protein and impaired flow-mediated vasodilation precede the development of preeclampsia. *Am. J. Hypertens*. 2007.20, 98–103.

[241] Savvidou MD, Hingorani AD, Tsikas D, Frolich JC., Vallance P, Nicolaides KH. Endothelial dysfunction and raised plasma concentrations of asymmetric dimethylarginine in pregnant women who subsequently develop pre-eclampsia. *Lancet* 2003. 361, 1511–1517.

[242] Buhimschi I, Yallampalli C, Chwalisz K, Garfield RE. Pre-eclampsia-like conditions produced by nitric oxide inhibition: effects of L-arginine, D-arginine and steroid hormones. *Hum Reprod* 1995;10:2723–2730.

[243] Bahtiyar MO, Buhimschi C, Ravishankar V, Copel J, Norwitz E, Julien S, Guller S, Buhimschi IA. Contrasting effects of chronic hypoxia and nitric oxide synthase inhibition on circulating angiogenic factors in a rat model of growth restriction. *Am J Obstet Gynecol* 2007;196: e1–e6.

[244] Yallampalli C, Garfield RE. Inhibition of nitric oxide synthesis in rats during pregnancy produces signs similar to those of preeclampsia. *Am J Obstet Gynecol* 1993;169:1316–1320.

[245] Deng A, Engels K, Baylis, C. Impact of nitric oxide deficiency on blood pressure and glomerular hemodynamic adaptations to pregnancy in the rat. *Kidney Int*; 1996:50: 1132–1138.

[246] Duplain H, Burcelin R, Sartori C, Cook S, Egli M, Lepori M, Vollenweider P, Pedrazzini T, Nicod P, Thorens B, Scherrer U;Insulin resistance, hyperlipidemia, and hypertension in mice lacking endothelial nitric oxide synthase. *Circulation*; 2001:104:342–345.

[247] W. Niu and Y. Qi,. An updated meta-analysis of endothelial nitric oxide synthase gene: three well-characterized polymorphisms with hypertension,. *PLoS ONE,* 2011:6:9:e24266.

[248] Serrano NC, Casas JP, Díaz LA, Páez C, Mesa CM, Cifuentes R, Monterrosa A, Bautista A, Hawe E, Hingorani AD, Vallance P, López-Jaramillo P;Endothelial NO synthase genotype and risk of preeclampsia: a multicenter case-control study. *Hypertension* 2004; 44:702–707.

[249] Fatini C, Sticchi E, Gensini F, Genuardi M, Tondi F, Gensini GF, Riviello C, Parretti E, Mello G, Abbate R. Endothelial nitric oxide synthase gene influences the risk of pre-eclampsia, the recurrence of negative pregnancy events, and the maternalfetal flow. *J Hypertens* 2006:24:1823– 1829.

[250] Bhatnagar S, Bhattacharjee J, Vaid M, Madan T, Trivedi SS, Sarma PU. Inducible nitric oxide synthase (iNOS) gene polymorphism in preeclampsia: a pilot study in North India. Australian and New Zealand. *Journal of Obstetrics and Gynaecology* 2007.47:477 – 482.

[251] Vural P. Nitric oxide/endothelin-1 in pre-eclampsia. *Clinica Chimica Acta* 2002. 317:65–70.

[252] Shaamash AH, Elsnosy ED, Makhlouf AM, Zakhari MM, Ibrahim OA, EL-dien HM. Maternal and fetal serum nitric oxide (NO) concentrations in normal pregnancy, pre-eclampsia and eclampsia. *International Journal of Gynaecology and Obstetrics* 2000. 68:207 – 214.

[253] Sandrim VC, Palei AC, Metzger IF, Gomes VA, Cavalli RC, Tanus-Santos JE. Nitric oxide formation is inversely related to serum levels of antiangiogenic factors soluble fms-like tyrosine kinase-1 and soluble endogline in preeclampsia. *Hypertension* 2008. 52:402 – 407.

[254] Aris A, Benali S, Ouellet A, Moutquin JM, Leblanc S. Potential biomarkers of preeclampsia: inverse correlation between hydrogen peroxide and nitric oxide early in maternal circulation and at term in placenta of women with preeclampsia. *Placenta* 2009. 30, 342–347.

[255] Bernardi F, Constantino L, Machado R, Petronilho F, Dal-Pizzol F. Plasma nitric oxide, endothelin-1, arginase and superoxide dismutase in pre-eclamptic women. *J. Obstet. Gynaecol. Res*. 2008. 34, 957–963.

[256] Schonfelder G, Fuhr N, Hadzidiakos D, John M, Hopp H, Paul M. Pre eclampsia is associated with loss of neuronal nitric oxide synthase expression in vascular smooth muscle cells of the human umbilical cord. *Histopathology* 2004. 44:116– 128.

[257] Orange SJ, Painter D, Horvath J, Yu B, Trent R, Hennessy A. Placental endothelial nitric oxide synthase localization and expression in normal human pregnancy and pre-eclampsia. *Clinl Exp Pharmacol Physiol*. 2003. 30:376– 381.

[258] Dai B, Liu T, Zhang B, Zhang X, Wang Z. The polymorphism for endothelial nitric oxide synthase gene, the level of nitric oxide and the risk for pre-eclampsia: A meta-analysis. *Gene* 519. 2013. 187–193.

[259] Landim M, Casella Filho A, Chagas A. Asymmetric dimethylarginine (ADMA) and endothelial dysfunction: implications for atherogenesis. *Clinics*. 2009;64:471.

[260] Tamás P, Bódis J, Sulyok E, Kovács GL, Hantosi E, Molnár G, Martens-Lobenhoffer J, Bode-Böger SM. L-arginine metabolism in early-onset and late-onset pre-eclamptic pregnancies. *Scand J Clin Lab Invest.* 2013;73:436-443.

[261] Noris M, Todeschini M, Cassis P, Pasta F, Cappellini A, Bonazzola S, Macconi D, Maucci R, Porrati F, Benigni A, Picciolo C, Remuzzi G. L-Arginine depletion in preeclampsia orients nitric oxide synthase toward oxidant species. *Hypertension.* 2004;43:614–622.

[262] Sankaralingam S, Xu H, Davidge ST. Arginase contributes to endothelial cell oxidative stress in response to plasma from women with preeclampsia. *Cardiovasc Res*; 2010:85: 194–203.

[263] da Costa BP, Steibel JP, Antonello IC, Guimaraes JA, Poli de Figueiredo C E. l-Arginine erythrocyte transport in normal pregnant and preeclamptic women. *Am J Obstet Gynecol.* 2004;190:468–71.

[264] Poston L, Chappell LC; Is oxidative stress involved in the aetiology of pre-eclampsia? *Acta Paediatr Suppl* 2001;90:3-5.

[265] Anderssohn M, Maass LM, Diemert A, Lüneburg N, Atzler D, Hecher K, Böger RH; Severely decreased activity of placental dimethylarginine dimethylaminohydrolase in pre-eclampsia.; *Eur J Obstet Gynecol Reprod Biol*; 2012:161:152–156.

[266] Myatt L., Eis A.L., Brockman D.E., Kossenjans W., Greer I.A., Lyall F. Endothelial nitric oxide in placental villous tissue from normal, pre-eclamptic and intrauterine restricted pregnancies. *Hum. Reprod.* 1997;12:714–718.

[267] Nobunaga T, Tokugawa Y, Hashimoto K, Kimura T, Matsuzaki N, Nitta Y, Fujita T, Kidoguchi KI, Azuma C, Saji F. Plasma nitric oxide levels in pregnant patients with preeclampsia and essential hypertension. *Gynecol Obstet Invest.* 1996;41:189–193.

[268] Choi JW, Im MW, Pai SH. Nitric oxide production increases during normal pregnancy and decreases in preeclampsia. *Ann Clin Lab Sci.* 2002;32:257–263.

[269] Diejomaoh FM, Omu AE, Al-Busiri N, Taher S, Al-Othman S, Fatinikun T, *Fernandes S.. Nitric oxide production is not altered in preeclampsia.* Arch Gynecol Obstet. 2004;269:237–243.

[270] Conrad KP, Kerchner L J, Mosher MD. Plasma and 24-h NO(x) and cGMP during normal pregnancy and preeclampsia in women on a reduced NO(x) diet. *Am J Physiol.* 1999;277:F48– F57.

[271] Drummond GR, Cai H, Davis ME, Ramasamy S, and Harrison DG. Transcriptional and posttranscriptional regulation of endothelial nitric oxide synthase expression by hydrogen peroxide. *Circ. Res.* 2000;86:347–354.

[272] Wang Y, Gu Y, Zhang Y, Lewis DF. Evidence of endothelial dysfunction in preeclampsia: decreased endothelial nitric oxide synthase expression is associated with increased cell permeability in endothelial cells from preeclampsia. *Am J Obstet Gynecol.* 2004;190:817-824.

[273] Scholz H, Yndestad A, Damås JK, Waehre T, Tonstad S, Aukrust P, Halvorsen B. 8-Isoprostane increases expression of interleukin-8 in human macrophages through activation of mitogenactivated protein kinases. *Cardiovasc Res.* 2003;59:945–954.

[274] Qi HP, Fraser WD, Luo, Julien P, Audibert F, Wei SQ. Endothelial Nitric Oxide Synthase Gene Polymorphisms and Risk of Preeclampsia. *Am J Perinatol.* 2013 [in press].

[275] Singh A, Sharma D, Raghunandan C, Bhattacharjee J. Role of inflammatory cytokines and eNOS gene polymorphism in pathophysiology of pre-eclampsia. *Am J Reprod Immunol.* 2010 1;63:244–251.

[276] Sharma D, Trivedi SS, Bhattacharjee J. Oxidative stress and eNOS (Glu298Asp) gene polymorphism in preeclampsia in Indian population. *Mol Cell Biochem*; 2011:353:189-193.

[277] Turan F, Ilhan N, Kaman D, Ate? K, Kafkasli A. Glu298Asp polymorphism of the endothelial nitric oxide synthase gene and plasma concentrations of asymmetric dimethylarginine in Turkish pre-eclamptic women without fetal growth retardation. *J Obstet Gynaecol Res.* 2010;36:495-501.

[278] Aydin S, Benian A, Madazli R, Uludag S, Uzun H, Kaya S. Plasma malondialdehyde, superoxide dismutase, sE-selectin, fibronectin, endothelin-1 and nitric oxide levels in women with preeclampsia. *Eur J Obstet Gynecol Reprod Biol.* 2004;113:21–25.

[279] Var A, Yildirim Y, Onur E, Kuscu NK, Uyanik BS, Goktalay K, Guvenc Y. Endothelial dysfunction in preeclampsia. Increased homocysteine and decreased nitric oxide levels. *Gynecol Obstet Invest.* 2003;56:221–224.

[280] Szabo I, Vizer M, Ertl T. Fetal betamethasone treatment and neonatal outcome in preeclampsia and intrauterine growth restriction. *Am J Obstet Gynecol.* 2003;189:1812–1813.

[281] Chinnathambi V, Balakrishnan M, Ramadoss J, Yallampalli C, Sathishkumar K. Testosterone alters maternal vascular adaptations: role of the endothelial NO system. *Hypertension.* 2013:61:647-654.

[282] Salamalekis E, Bakas P, Vitoratos N, Eleptheriadis M, Creatsas G. Androgen levels in the third trimester of pregnancy in patients with preeclampsia. *Eur J Obstet Gynecol Reprod Biol.* 2006;126:16–19.

[283] Acromite MT, Mantzoros CS, Leach RE, Hurwitz J, Dorey LG. Androgens in preeclampsia. *Am J Obstet Gynecol.* 1999;180:60–63.

[284] Ghorashi V, Sheikhvatan M. The relationship between serum concentration of free testosterone and pre-eclampsia. *Endokrynol Pol.* 2008;59:390–392.

[285] Carlsen SM, Romundstad P, Jacobsen G. Early second-trimester maternal hyperandrogenemia and subsequent preeclampsia: a prospective study. *Acta Obstet Gynecol Scand.* 2005;84:117–121.

[286] Troisi R, Potischman N, Roberts JM, Ness R, Crombleholme W, Lykins D, Siiteri P, Hoover RN. Maternal serum oestrogen and androgen concentrations in preeclamptic and uncomplicated pregnancies. *Int J Epidemiol.* 2003;32:455–460.

[287] Vallance P, Leone A, Calver A, Collier J, Moncada S. Accumulation of an endogenous inhibitor of nitric oxide synthesis in chronic renal failure. *Lancet.* 1992;10:572–575.

[288] Fickling SA, Leone AM, Moncada S, Nussey SS, Vallance P, Whitley GS. Synthesis of NG,NG dimethylarginine by human endothelial cells. *Endothelium* 1993;1:137-140.

[289] Anderssohn M, Maass LM, Diemert A, Lüneburg N, Atzler D, Hecher K, Böger RH; Severely decreased activity of placental dimethylarginine dimethylaminohydrolase in pre-eclampsia.; *Eur J Obstet Gynecol Reprod Biol* 2012; 161: 152–156.

[290] Vallance P, Leone A, Calver A, Collier J, Moncada S. Accumulation of an endogenous inhibitor of nitric oxide synthesis in chronic renal failure. *Lancet.* 1992;10:572–575.

[291] Slaghekke F, Dekker G, Jefries B; Endogenous inhibitors of nitric oxide and preeclampsia: A Review. *J Matern Fetal Neonatal Med* 2006; 19:447-452.

[292] Calver A, Collier J, Leone A, Moncada S, Vallance P. Effect of local intra-arterial asymmetric dimethylarginine (ADMA) on the forearm arteriolar bed of healthy volunteers. *J Hum Hypertension* 1993; 7: 193-194.

[293] Achan V, Broadhead M, Malaki M, Whitley G, Leiper J, MacAllister R, Vallance P. Asymmetric dimethylarginine causes hypertension and cardiac dysfunction in humans and is actively metabolized by dimethylarginine dimethylaminohydrolase. *Arterioscler Thromb Vasc Biol* 2003; 23: 1455-1459.

[294] Gardiner SM, Kemp PA, Bennett T, Palmer RM, Moncada S. Regional and cardiac haemodynamic effects of NG, NG, dimethyl-L-arginine and their reversibility by vasodilators in conscious rats. *Br J Pharmacol.* 1993;110:1457-1464.

[295] Mao D, Che J, Li K, Han S, Yue Q, Zhu L, Zhang W, Li L. Association of homocysteine, asymmetric dimethylarginine, and nitric oxide with preeclampsia. *Arch Gynecol Obstet,* 2010;282:371–375.

[296] Slaghekke F, Dekker G, Jefries B; Endogenous inhibitors of nitric oxide and preeclampsia: A Review. *J Matern Fetal Neonatal Med*; 2006; 19: 447-452.

[297] Demir B, Demir S, Pasa S, Guven S, Atamer Y, Atamer A, Kocyigit Y.; The role of homocysteine, asymmetric dimethylarginine and nitric oxide in pre-eclampsia.; *J Obstet Gynaecol.* 2012; 32:525-528.

[298] Alacam H, Dikmen ZG, Yaman H, Cakir E, Deren O, Akgul EO, Aydin I, Kurt YG, Keskin U, Akalin S, Polat B, Danisman N, Dogan P; The Role of Asymmetric Dimethyl Arginine and Oxidant/Antioxidant System in Preeclampsia.; *Fetal and Pediatric Pathology*, 2011. 30:387–393.

[299] Rizos D, Eleftheriades M, Batakis E, Rizou M, Haliassos A, Hassiakos D, Botsis D. Levels of asymmetric dimethylarginine throughout normal pregnancy and in pregnancies complicated with preeclampsia or had a small for gestational age baby. *J Matern Fetal Neonatal Med.* 2012;25:1311–1315.

[300] Kielstein JT, Impraim B, Simmel S, Bode-Böger SM, Tsikas D, Frölich JC, Hoeper MM, Haller H, Fliser D. Cardio vascular eVects of systemic nitric oxide synthase inhibition with asymmetrical dimethylarginine in humans. *Circulation* 2004. 109:172–177

[301] Böger RH, Bode-Böger SM, Szuba A, Tsao PS, Chan JR, Tangphao O, Blaschke TF, Cooke JP.. Asymmetric dimethylarginine (ADMA): a novel risk factor for endothelial dysfunction: its role in hypercholesterolemia. *Circulation* 1998; 98: 1842-1847.

[302] Miyazaki H, Matsuoka H, Cooke JP, Usui M, Ueda S, Okuda S, Imaizumi T. Endogenous nitric oxide synthase inhibitor: a novel marker of atherosclerosis. *Circulation* 1999; 99: 1141-1146.

[303] Surdacki A, Nowicki M, Sandmann J, Tsikas D, Boeger RH, Bode-Boeger SM, Kruszelnicka-Kwiatkowska O, Kokot F, Dubiel JS, Froelich JC. Reduced urinary

excretion of nitric oxide metabolites and increased plasma levels of asymmetric dimethylarginine in men with essential hypertension. *J Cardiovasc Pharmacol* 1999; 33: 652-658.

[304] Abbasi F, Asagmi T, Cooke JP, Lamendola C, McLaughlin T, Reaven GM, Stuehlinger M, Tsao PS. Plasma concentrations of asymmetric dimethylarginine are increased in patients with type 2 diabetes mellitus. *Am J Cardiol* 2001; 88: 1201-1203.

[305] Lundman P, Eriksson MJ, Stuhlinger M, Cooke JP, Hamsten A, Tornvall P. Mild-to-moderate hypertriglyceridemia in young men is associated with endothelial dysfunction and increased plasma concentrations of asymmetric dimethylarginine. *J Am Coll Cardiol* 2001; 38: 111-116.

[306] Stühlinger MC, Abbasi F, Chu JW, Lamendola C, McLaughlin TL, Cooke JP, Reaven GM, Tsao PS. Relationship between insulin resistance and an endogenous nitric oxide synthase inhibitor. *JAMA* 2002; 287: 1420-1426.

[307] Stühlinger MC, Oka RK, Graf EE, Schmölzer I, Upson BM, Kapoor O, Szuba A, Malinow MR, Wascher TC, Pachinger O, Cooke JP. Endothelial dysfunction induced by hyperhomocyst(e)inemia: role of asymmetric dimethylarginine. *Circulation* 2003; 108: 933-938.

[308] Boger RH, Zoccali C. ADMA: a novel risk factor that explains excess cardiovascular event rate in patients with end-stage renal disease. *Atheroscler Suppl* 2003; 4: 23-28.

[309] Moncada S, Higgs A. The L-argininc-nitric oxide pathway. *N Engl J Med* 1993. 329:2002–2012.

[310] Cayatte AJ, Palacino JJ, Horten K, Cohen RA. Chronic inhibition of nitric oxide production accelerates neointima formation and impairs endothelial function in hypercholesterolemic rabbits. *Arterioscler Thromb* 1994. 14:753–759.

[311] MacAllister RJ, Parry H, Kimoto M, Ogawa T, Russell RJ, Hodson H, Whitley GS, Vallance P. Regulation of nitric oxide synthesis by dimethylarginine dimethylaminohydrolase. *Br J Pharmacol* 1996: 119:1533–1540.

[312] Sandvik MK, Leirgul E, Nygård O, Ueland PM, Berg A, Svarstad E, Vikse BE; Preeclampsia in healthy women and endothelial dysfunction 10 years later. *Am J Obstet Gynecol.* 2013 [in press].

[313] Laskowska M, Laskowska K, Leszczyńska-Gorzelak B, Oleszczuk J. Asymmetric dimethylarginine in normotensive pregnant women with isolated fetal intrauterine growth restriction: a comparison with preeclamptic women with and without intrauterine growth restriction; *J Matern Fetal Neonatal Med* 2011;24:936-942.

[314] Speer PD, Powers RW, Frank MP, Harger G, Markovic N, Roberts JM. Elevated asymmetric dimethylarginine concentrations precede clinical preeclampsia, but not pregnancies with small-for-gestational-age infants. *Am J Obstet Gynecol.* 2008;198:e1–7

[315] Alpoim PN, Godoi LC, Freitas LG, Gomes KB, Dusse LM. Assessment of l-arginine asymmetric 1 dimethyl (ADMA) in early-onset and late-onset (severe) preeclampsia. *Nitric Oxide.* 2013 [in press]

[316] Teerlink T. Measurement of asymmetric dimethylarginine in plasma: methodological considerations and clinical relevance. *Clin. Chem. Lab. Med.* 2005;43:1130-1138.

[317] Siroen MP, Teerlink T, Nijveldt RJ, Prins HA, Richir MC, Van Leeuwen PA. The clinical significance of asymmetric dimethylarginine, *Annu. Rev. Nutr..* 2006; 26 162: 203–228.

[318] Onozato ML, Tojo A, Leiper J, Fujita T, Palm F, Wilcox CS. Expression of DDAH and PRMT isoforms in the diabetic rat kidney; effects of angiotensin II receptor blockers. *Diabetes*. 2008; 57:172–180.

[319] Tojo A, Kimoto M, Wilcox CS. Renal expression of constitutive NOS and DDAH: separate effects of salt intake and angiotensin. *Kidney Int*. 2000; 58:2075–2083.

[320] Nijveldt RJ, van Leeuwen PAM, van Guldener C, Stehouwer CDA, Rauwerda JA, Teerlink T. Net renal extraction of asymmetrical (ADMA) and symmetrical (SMDA) dimethylarginine in fasting humans. *Nephrol Dial Tranplant*. 2002; 17:1999–2002.

[321] Nijveldt RJ, Teerlink T, van Guldener C, Prins HA, van Lambalgen AA, Stehouwer CDA, Rauwerda JA, van Leeuwen PAM. Handling of asymmetrical dimethylarginine and symmetrical dimethylarginine by the rat kidney under basal conditions and during endotoxaemia. *Nephrol Dial Tranplant*. 2003; 18:2542–2550.

[322] Wilcox CS; Asymmetric dimethylarginine and reactive oxygen species: unwelcome twin visitors to the cardiovascular and kidney disease tables.*Hypertension*. 2012;59:375–381.

[323] Sibal L, Agarwal SC, Home PD, Boger RH. The role of asymmetric dimethylarginine (ADMA) in endothelial dysfunction and cardiovascular disease. *Curr Cardiol Rev*. 2010;6:82–90.

[324] Hu X, Atzler D, Xu X, Zhang P, Guo H, Lu Z, Fassett J, Schwedhelm E, Boger RH, Bache RJ, Chen Y. Dimethylarginine dimethylaminohydrolase-1 is the critical enzyme for degrading the cardiovascular risk factor asymmetrical dimethylarginine. *Arterioscler Thromb Vasc Biol*. 2011; 31:1540–1546.

[325] Pope AJ, Karrupiah K, Kearns PN, Xia Y, Cardounel AJ. Role of dimethylarginine dimethylaminohydrolases in the regulation of endothelial nitric oxide production. *J Biol Chem*. 2009; 284:35338–35347.

[326] Wada K, Inoue K, Hagiwara M. Identification of methylated proteins by protein arginine N-methyltransferase 1, PRMT 1, with a new expression cloning strategy. *Biochim Biophys Acta*. 2002;1591:1-10.

[327] Landim M, Casella Filho A, Chagas A. Asymmetric dimethylarginine (ADMA) and endothelial dysfunction: implications for atherogenesis. *Clinics*. 2009;64:471.

[328] Suda O, Tsutsui M, Morishita T, Tasaki H, Ueno S, Nakata S, Tsujimoto T, Toyohira Y, Hayashida Y, Sasaguri Y, Ueta Y, Nakashima Y, Yanagihara N. Asymmetric dimethylarginine produces vascular lesions in endothelial nitric oxide synthase-deficient mice: involvement of renin-angiotensin system and oxidative stress. *Arterioscler Thromb Vasc Biol* 2004; 24: 1682-1688.

[329] Kajimoto H, Kai H, Aoki H, Yasuoka S, Anegawa T, Aoki Y, Ueda S, Okuda S, Imaizumi T. Inhibition of eNOS phosphorylation mediates endothelial dysfunction in renal failure: new effect of asymmetric dimethylarginine. *Kidney Int*. 2012. 81: 762–768.

[330] Pou S, Keaton L, Surichamom W, Rosen GM. Mechanism of superoxide generation by neuronal nitric oxide synthase. *J Biol Chem*. 1999;274:9573-9580.

[331] Holden DP, Cartwright JE, Nussey SS, Whitley GS. Estrogen stimulates dimethylarginine dimethylaminohydrolase activity and the metabolism of asymmetric dimethylarginine. *Circulation*.2003;108:1575–1580.

[332] Stühlinger MC, Tsao PS, Her JH, Kimoto M, Balint RF, Cooke JP. Homocysteine impairs the nitric oxide synthase pathway: role of asymmetric dimethylarginine. *Circulation*. 2001;104:2569-2575.

[333] Ito A, Tsao PS, Adimoolam S, Kimoto M, Ogawa T, Cooke JP. Novel mechanism for endothelial dysfunction: dysregulation of dimethylarginine dimethylaminohydrolase. *Circulation*. 1999;99:3092-3095.

[334] Leiper JM, Santa Maria J, Chubb A, MacAllister RJ, Charles IG, Whitley GS, Vallance P. Identification of two human dimethylarginine dimethylaminohydrolases with distinct tissue distributions and homology to microbial arginine deiminases. *Biochem J*. 1999;343:209-214.

[335] Lin KY, Ito A, Asagami T, Tsao PS, Adimoolam S, Kimoto M, Tsuji H, Reaven GM, Cooke JP. Impaired nitric oxide synthase pathway in diabetes mellitus: role of asymmetric dimethylarginine and dimethylarginine dimethylaminohydrolase. *Circulation*. 2002;106;987-992.

[336] Jung CH, Lee WJ, Hwang JY, Lee MJ, Seol SM, Kim YM, Lee YL, Kim HS, Kim MS, Park JY; Vaspin increases nitric oxide bioavailability through the reduction of asymmetric dimethylarginine in vascular endothelial cells; *PLoS One* 2012;7:e52346.

[337] MacGillivray I, Rose GA, Rowe B. Blood pressure survey in pregnancy. *Clin Sci* 1969;37:395-407.

[338] Gant NF, Daley GL, Chand S, Whalley PJ, MacDonald PC. A study of angiotensin II pressor response throughout primigravid pregnancy. *J Clin Invest* 1973;52:2682-2689.

[339] Holden DP, Fickling SA, Whitley GS, Nussey SS. Plasma concentrations of asymmetric dimethylarginine, a natural inhibitor of nitric oxide synthase, in normal pregnancy and preeclampsia. *American Journal of Obstetrics and Gynecology* 1998; 178:551-556.

[340] Boger RH, Maas R, Schulze F, Schwedhelm E. Asymmetric dimethylarginine (ADMA) as a prospective marker of cardiovascular disease and mortality—an update on patient populations with a wide range of cardiovascular risk. *Pharmacol Res* 2009;60:481–487.

[341] Savvidou MD, Hingorani AD, Tsikas D, Frölich JC, Vallance P, Nicolaides KH. Endothelial dysfunction and raised plasma concentrations of asymmetric dimethylarginine in pregnant women who subsequently develop pre-eclampsia. *Lancet* 2003;361:1511–1517.

[342] Speer PD, Powers RW, Frank MP, Harger G, Markovic N, Roberts JM. Elevated asymmetric dimethylarginine concentrations precede clinical preeclampsia, but not pregnancies with small-for-gestational-age infants. *Am J Obstet Gynecol* 2008;198:112–117.

[343] Pettersson A, Hedner T, Milsom I. Increased circulating concentrations of asymmetric dimethyl arginine (ADMA), an endogenous inhibitor of nitric oxide synthesis, in preeclampsia. *Acta Obstet Gynecol Scand* 1998;77:808–813.

[344] Ellis J, Wennerholm UB, Bengtsson A, Lilja H, Pettersson A, Sultan B, Wennergren M, Hagberg H. Levels of dimethylarginines and cytokines in mild and severe preeclampsia. *Acta Obstet Gynecol Scand* 2001;80:602–608.

[345] Fickling SA, Williams D, Vallance P, Nussey SS, Whitley GS. Plasma concentrations of endogenous inhibitor of nitric oxide synthesis in normal pregnancy and pre-eclampsia. *Lancet* 1993;342:242–243.

[346] Siroen MP, Teerlink T, Bolte AC, van Elburg RM, Richir MC, Nijveldt RJ, van der Hoven B, van Leeuwen PA. No compensatory upregulation of placental dimethylarginine dimethylaminohydrolase activity in preeclampsia. *Gynecol Obstet Invest* 2006;62:7–13.

[347] Roberts JM, Hubel CA. The two stage model of preeclampsia: variations on the theme. *Placenta* 2009; 30: 32–37.

[348] Nijveldt RJ, Teerlink T, Van Leeuwen PAM. The asymmetrical dimethylarginine (ADMA) – multiple organ failure hypothesis. *Clin Nutr* 2003;22:99–104.

[349] Furchgott RF. Role of endothelium in responses of vascular smooth muscle. *Circ Res.* 1983;53:557–573.

[350] Cohen RA, Vanhoutte PM. Endothelium-dependent hyperpolarization: beyond nitric oxide and cyclic GMP. *Circulation*. 1995;92:3337–3349.

[351] Feletou M, Vanhoutte PM. Endothelium-derived hyperpolarizing factor. Where are we now? *Arterioscler Thromb Vasc Biol*. 2006;26:1215–1225.

[352] Campbell WB, Fleming I. Epoxyeicosatrienoic acids and endothelium dependent responses. *Pflugers Arch.* 2010;459:881–895.

[353] Chawengsub Y, Gauthier KM, Campbell WB. Role of arachidonic acid lipoxygenase metabolites in the regulation of vascular tone. *Am J Physiol.* 2009;297:H495–H507.

[354] Campbell WB, Spitzbarth N, Gauthier KM, Pfister SL. 11,12,15-Trihydroxyeicosatrienoic acid mediates acetylcholine-induced relaxations in the rabbit aorta. *Am J Physiol.* 2003;285:H2648–H2656.

[355] Gauthier KM, Goldman DH, Aggarwal NT, Chawengsub Y, Falck JR. Role of arachidonic acid lipoxygenase metabolites in acetylcholine-induced relaxations in mouse arteries. *Am J Physiol.* 2010;300:H725–H735.

[356] Gillham JC, Myers JE, Baker PN, Taggart MJ.Regulation of endothelial-dependent relaxation in human systemic arteries by SKCa and IKCa channels. *Reprod Sci.* 2007;14:43-50.

[357] Campbell WB, Falck JR. Arachidonic acid metabolites as endotheliumderived hyperpolarizing factors. *Hypertension*. 2007;49:590–596.

[358] Matoba T, Shimokawa H, Nakashima M, Hirakawa Y, Mukai Y, Hirano K, Kanaide H, Takeshita A.. Hydrogen peroxide is an endothelium-derived hyperpolarizing factor in mice. *J Clin Invest*. 2000;106:1521–1530.

[359] Griffith TM. Endothelium-dependent smooth muscle hyperpolarization: do gap unctions provide a unifying hypothesis? *Br J Pharmacol*. 2004;141:881–903.

[360] Chauhan SD, Nilsson H, Ahluwalia A, Hobbs AJ.Release of c-type natriuretic peptide accounts for the biological activity of endothelium-derived hyperpolarizing factor. *Proc Natl Acad Sci U S A*. 2003;100:1426–1431.

[361] Edwards G, Dora KA, Gardener MJ, Garland CJ, Weston AH. K is an endothelium-derived hyperpolarizing factor in rat arteries. *Nature*. 1998;396:269–272.

[362] Giles TD, Sander GE, Nossaman BD, Kadowitz PJ. Impaired vasodilation in the pathogenesis of hypertension: focus on nitric oxide, endothelial-derived hyperpolarizing factors, and prostaglandins. *J Clin Hypertens.* 2012:4:198-205

[363] Mustafa AK, Sikka G, Gazi SK, Steppan J, Jung SM, Bhunia AK, Barodka VM, Gazi FK, Barrow RK, Wang R, Amzel LM, Berkowitz DE, Snyder SH. Hydrogen sulfide as endothelium-derived hyperpolarizing factor sulfhydrates potassium channels. *Circ Res*; 201;109:1259-1268.

[364] Edwards G, Félétou M, Gardener MJ, Thollon C, Vanhoutte PM, Weston AH. Role of gap junctions in the responses to EDHF in rat and guinea-pig small arteries. *Br J Pharmacol.* 1999;128:1788–1794.

[365] Edwards G, Feletou M, Weston AH. Endothelium-derived hyperpolarizing factors and associated pathways: a synopsis. *Pflugers Arch.* 2010; 459:863–879.

[366] Campbell WB, Gauthier KM. Inducible endothelium – derived hyperpolarizing factor: role of the 15-lipoxygenase-EDHF pathway. *J Cardiovasc Pharmacol.* 2013;61:3:176-187.

[367] Morton JS, Davidge STJ Arterial endothelium 2013; 61:197-203.

[368] Ashworth JR, Warren AY, Baker PN, Johnson IR. Loss of endothelium-dependent relaxation in myometrial resistance arteries in preeclampsia. *Br J Obstet Gynaecol.* 1997;104:1152–1158.

[369] Luksha L, Luksha N, Kublickas M, Nisell H, Kublickiene K. Diverse mechanisms of endothelium-derived hyperpolarizing factor-mediated dilatation in small myometrial arteries in normal human pregnancy and preeclampsia. Biol Reprod. 2010;83:728-735.

[370] Kenny LC, Baker PN, Kendall DA, Randall MD, Dunn WR. Differential mechanisms of endothelium-dependent vasodilator responses in human myometrial small arteries in normal pregnancy and pre-eclampsia.*Clin Sci.* 2002;103:67-73.

[371] Mateev S, Sillau AH, Mouser R, McCullough RE, White MM, Young DA, Moore LG. Chronic hypoxia opposes pregnancy-induced increase in uterine artery vasodilator response to flow. *Am J Physiol Heart Circ Physiol.* 2003;284:H820-829.

[372] Luksha L, Nisell H, Luksha N, Kublickas M, Hultenby K, Kublickiene K. Endothelium-derived hyperpolarizing factor in preeclampsia: heterogeneous contribution, mechanisms, and morphological prerequisites. *Am Physiol Regul Integr Comp Physiol* 2008; 294:R510–R519.

[373] Hayman R, Warren A, Johnson I, Baker P. Inducible change in the behavior of resistance arteries from circulating factor in preeclampsia: an effect specific to myometrial vessels from pregnant women. *Am J Obstet Gynecol* 2001; 184:420–426.

[374] Wimalasundera RC, Thom SAM, Regan L, Hughes AD. Effects of vasoactive agents on intracellular calcium and force in myometrial and subcutaneous resistance arteries isolated from preeclamptic, pregnant, and nonpregnant woman. *Am J Obstet Gynecol* 2005; 192:625–632.

[375] Ashworth JR, Warren AY, Baker PN, Johnson IR. Loss of endotheliumdependent relaxation in myometrial resistance arteries in pre-eclampsia. *BJOG* 1997; 104:1152–1158.

[376] Ashworth JR, Baker PN, Warren AY, Phil M, Johnson IR. Mechanisms of endothelium-dependent relaxation in myometrial resistance vessels and their alteration in preeclampsia. *Hypertens Pregnancy* 1999; 18:57–71.

[377] Wareing M, Myers JE, O'Hara M, Kenny LC, Warren AY, Taggart MJ, Skillern L, Machin I, Baker PN. Effects of a phosphodiesterase-5 (PDE5) inhibitor on endothelium-dependent relaxation of myometrial small arteries. *Am J Obstet Gynecol* 2004; 190:1283–1290.

[378] Ong SS, Moore RJ, Warren AY, Crocker IP, Fulford J, Tyler DJ, Gowland PA, Baker PN. Myometrial and placental artery reactivity alone cannot explain reduced placental perfusion in pre-eclampsia and intrauterine growth restriction. *BJOG* 2003; 110:909–915.

[379] Svedas E, Nisell H, VanWijk MJ, Nikas Y, Kublickiene KR. Endothelial dysfunction in uterine circulation in preeclampsia: can estrogens improve it? *Am J Obstet Gynecol* 2002; 187:1608–1616.

[380] Mandalà M, Gokina N, Barron C, Osol G.Endothelial-derived hyperpolarization factor (EDHF) contributes to PlGF-induced dilation of mesenteric resistance arteries from pregnant rats. *J Vasc Res.* 2012;49:43-49.

[381] Lang NN, Luksha L, Newby DE, Kublickiene K. Connexin 43 mediates endothelium-derived hyperpolarising factor-induced vasodilatation in subcutaneous resistance arteries from healthy pregnant women *Am. J. Physiol*;2007:292:1026–1032.

[382] Luksha L, Nisell H, Kublickiene K. The mechanism of EDHF-mediated responses in subcutaneous small arteries from healthy pregnant women. *Am. J. Physiol.* 2004:286:1102–1109.

[383] Hammond S, Mathewson AM, Baker PN, Mayhew TM, Dunn WR. Gap junctions and hydrogen peroxide are involved in endothelium-derived hyperpolarising responses to bradykinin in omental arteries and veins isolated from pregnant women. *Eur J Pharmacol.* 2011:668:225-232.

[384] Faraci FM, Didion SP. Vascular protection: superoxide dismutase isoforms in the vessel wall. *Arterioscler Thromb Vasc Biol.* 2004;24:1367–1373.

[385] Shimokawa H. Hydrogen peroxide as an endothelium-derived hyperpolarizing factor. *Pflugers Arch.* 2010;459:915–922.

[386] Edwards DH, Li Y, Griffith TM. Hydrogen peroxide potentiates the EDHF phenomenon by promoting endothelial Ca2þ mobilization. *Arterioscle Thromb Vasc Biol* 2008; 28:1774–1781.

[387] Drouin A, Thorin-Trescases N, Hamel E, Falck JR, Thorin E. Endothelial nitric oxide synthase activation leads to dilatory H2O2 production in mouse cerebral arteries. *Cardiovasc Res* 2007; 73:73–81.

[388] Zhou X, Zhang GY, Wang J, Lu SL, Cao J, Sun LZ.A novel bridge between oxidative stress and immunity: the interaction between hydrogen peroxide and human leukocyte antigen G in placental trophoblasts during preeclampsia. *Am J Obstet Gynecol;* 2012:206:e7-16.

[389] Leblanc S, Ouellet A, Giguère Y, Forest JC, Moutquin JM, Aris A..A positive correlation between hydrogen peroxide and soluble TNF-alpha receptor 2 early in maternal blood and at term in placenta of pregnant women with preeclampsia. *Hypertens Pregnancy.* 2012;31:357-366.

[390] Kharfi, Y. Giguère, P. De Grandpré, J.M. Moutquin, J.C. Forest Human chorionic gonadotropin (hCG) may be a marker of systemic oxidative stress in normotensive and preeclamptic term pregnancies *Clin Biochem*, 2005; 38: 717–721.

[391] Aris A, Benali S, Ouellet A, Moutquin JM, Leblanc s. Potential biomarkers of preeclampsia: inverse correlation between hydrogen peroxide and nitric oxide early in maternal circulation and at term in placenta of women with preeclampsia. *Placenta.* 2009:30:342-347.

[392] Stepan H, Leitner E, Bader M, Walther T: Organ-specific mRNA distribution of C-type natriuretic peptide in neonatal and adult mice. *Regul Pept*; 2000:95:81–85.

[393] Acuff CG, Huang H, Steinhelper ME. Estradiol induces C-type natriuretic peptide gene expression in mouse uterus. *Am J Physiol* 1997; 273: H2672–H2677.

[394] Bayoğlu Tekin Y, Güvendağ Güven ES, Cobanoğlu U, Colak S, Doğan OD, Kir Şahin F. Alterations of Natriuretic Peptides Amino-Terminal Pro B-Type Natriuretic Peptide and Amino-Terminal Pro C-Type Natriuretic Peptide During the Pregnancy. *J Matern Fetal Neonatal Med.* 2013 [In press].

[395] Walther T, Stepan H.C-type natriuretic peptide in reproduction, pregnancy and fetal development. *J Endocrinol.* 2004:180:17-22.

[396] Itoh H, Sagawa N, Hasegawa M, Nanno H, Kobayashi F, Ihara Y, Mori T, Komatsu Y, Suga S, Yoshimasa T, Itoh H, Nakao K Expression of biologically active receptors for natriuretic peptides in the human uterus during pregnancy. *Biochem Biophys Res Commun;* 1994:203:602–607.

[397] Hatjis CG, Grogan DM. Atrial natriuretic peptide receptors in normal human placentas. *Am J Obstet Gynecol*;1988:159 587–591.

[398] Levytska K, Kingdom J, Baczyk D, Drewlo S. Heme oxygenase-1 in placental development and pathology. *Placenta*;2013:34:291-298.

[399] Kreiser D, Kelly DK, Seidman DS, Stevenson DK, Baum M, Dennery PA. Gestational pattern of heme oxygenase expression in the rat. *Pediatr Res*; 2003: 54:172–178

[400] Watanabe S, Akagi R, Mori M, Tsuchiya T, Sassa S. Marked developmental changes in heme oxygenase-1 (HO-1) expression in the mouse placenta: correlation between HO-1 expression and placental development *Placenta*; 2004:25:387–395.

[401] Zhao H, Wong RJ, Doyle TC, Nayak N, Vreman HJ, Contag CH, Stevenson DK. Regulation of maternal and fetal hemodynamics by heme oxygenase in *mice Biol Reprod;* 2008:78:744–751

[402] Ehsanipoor RM, Fortson W, Fitzmaurice LE, Liao WX, Wing DA, Chen DB, Chan K. Nitric oxide and carbon monoxide production and metabolism in preeclampsia. *Reprod Sci.* 2013:20:542-548.

[403] Baum M, Schiff E, Kreiser D, Dennery PA, Stevenson DK, Rosenthal T, Seidman DS. End-tidal carbon monoxide measurements in women with pregnancy-induced hypertension and preeclampsia *Am J Obstet Gynecol*; 2000:183: 900–903

[404] Yusuf K, Kamaluddeen M, Wilson RD, Akierman A. Carboxyhemoglobin levels in umbilical cord blood of women with pre-eclampsia and intrauterine growth restriction. *J Perinat Med.* 2012 [In press]

[405] Zhai D, Guo Y, Smith G, Krewski D, Walker M, Wen SW. Maternal exposure to moderate ambient carbon monoxide is associated with decreased risk of preeclampsia. *Am J Obstet Gynecol.* 2012:207:e1-9.

[406] Mustafa AK, Sikka G, Gazi SK, Steppan J, Jung SM, Bhunia AK, Barodka VM, Gazi FK, Barrow RK, Wang R, Amzel LM, Berkowitz DE, Snyder SH.Hydrogen sulfide as endothelium-derived hyperpolarizing factor sulfhydrates potassium channels. *Circ Res.* 2011;109:1259-1268

[407] Yang G, Wu L, Jiang B, Yang W, Qi J, Cao K, Meng Q, Mustafa AK, Mu W, ZhangS, Snyder SH, Wang R. H2S as a physiologic vasorelaxant: hypertension in mice with deletion of cystathionine gamma-lyase. Science.2008;322:587–590.

[408] Huang PL, Huang Z, Mashimo H, Bloch KD, Moskowitz MA, Bevan JA, Fishman MC. Hypertension in mice lacking the gene for endothelial nitric oxide synthase. *Nature.*1995;377:239–242.

[409] Zhao W, Zhang J, Lu Y, Wang R. The vasorelaxant effect of H(2)S as a novel endogenous gaseous K(ATP) channel opener. *EMBO J.*2001;20:6008–6016.

[410] Shibuya N, Mikami Y, Kimura Y, Nagahara N, Kimura H. Vascular endothelium expresses 3-mercaptopyruvate sulfurtransferase and produces hydrogen sulfide. *J Biochem.* Nov. 2009;146:623–626.

[411] Wang K, Ahmad S, Cai M, Rennie J, Fujisawa T, Crispi F, Baily J, Miller MR, Cudmore M, Hadoke PW, Wang R, Gratacós E, Buhimschi IA, Buhimschi CS,Ahmed A. Dysregulation of hydrogen sulfide producing enzyme cystathionine γ-lyase contributes to maternal hypertension and placental abnormalities in preeclampsia. *Circulation.* 2013;127:2514-2522.

[412] Cindrova-Davies T, Herrera EA, Niu Y, Kingdom J, Giussani DA, Burton GJ. Reduced cystathionine γ-lyase and increased miR-21 expression are associated with increased vascular resistance in growth-restricted pregnancies: hydrogen sulfide as a placental vasodilator. *Am J Pathol.* 2013:182:1448-1458.

[413] Holwerda KM, Bos EM, Rajakumar A, Ris-Stalpers C, van Pampus MG, Timmer A, Erwich JJ, Faas MM, van Goor H, Lely AT..Hydrogen sulfide producing enzymes in pregnancy and preeclampsia. *Placenta.* 2012:33:518-521.

[414] Capdevila J, Chacos N, Werringloer J, Prough RA, Estabrook RW. Liver microsomal cytochrome P450 and the oxidative metabolism of archidonic acid. *Proc Natl Acad Sci U S A.* 1981;78:5362–5366.

[415] Zeldin DC. Epoxygenase pathways of arachidonic acid metabolism. *J Biol Chem.* 2001;276:36059–36062

[416] Campbell WB, Gebremedhin D, Pratt PF, Harder DR.. Identification of epoxyeicosatrienoic acids as endothelium-derived hyperpolarizing factors. *Circ Res.* 1996;78:415–423.

[417] Jiang H, McGiff JC, Fava C, Amen G, Nesta E, Zanconato G, Quilley J, Minuz P.Maternal and fetal epoxyeicosatrienoic acids in normotensive and preeclamptic pregnancies. *Am J Hypertens.* 2013:26:271-278.

[418] Herse F, Lamarca B, Hubel CA, Kaartokallio T, Lokki AI, Ekholm E, Laivuori H, Gauster M, Huppertz B, Sugulle M, Ryan MJ, Novotny S, Brewer J, Park JK, Kacik M, Hoyer J, Verlohren S, Wallukat G, Rothe M, Luft FC, Muller DN, Schunck WH, Staff AC, Dechend R.Cytochrome P450 subfamily 2J polypeptide 2 expression and circulating epoxyeicosatrienoic metabolites inpreeclampsia. *Circulation*; 2012;126:2990-2999.

[419] Natarajan R, Gu JL, Rossi J, Gonzales N, Lanting L, Xu L, Nadler J. Elevated glucose and angiotensin II increase 12-lipoxygenase activity and expression in porcine aortic smooth muscle cells. *Proc Natl Acad Sci U S A.* 1993;90:4947–4951.

[420] Natarajan R, Bai W, Rangarajan V, Gonzales N, Gu JL, Lanting L, Nadler JL. Platelet-derived growth factor BB mediated regulation of 12-lipoxygenase in porcine aortic smooth muscle cells. *J Cell Physiol.* 1996;169:391–400.

[421] Limor R, Kaplan M, Sharon O, Knoll E, Naidich M, Weisinger G, Keidar S, Stern N. Aldosterone up-regulates 12- and 15-lipoxygenase expression and LDL oxidation in human vascular smooth muscle cells. *J Cell Biochem.* 2009;108: 1203–1210.

[422] Kim YS, Xu ZG, Reddy MA, Li SL, Lanting L, Sharma K, Adler SG, Natarajan R. Novel interactions between TGFbeta1 actions and the 12/15-lipoxygenase pathway in mesangial cells. *J Am Soc Nephrol.* 2005;16:352–362.

[423] Kim JH, Kang YJ, Kim HS. IL-8/CXCL8 upregulates 12-lipoxygenase expression in vascular smooth muscle cells from spontaneously hypertensive rats. *Immune Netw.* 2009;9:106–113.

[424] Titterington JS, Sukhanov S, Higashi Y, Vaughn C, Bowers C, Delafontaine P. Growth hormone-releasing peptide-2 suppresses vascular oxidative stress in ApoE2/2 mice but does not reduce atherosclerosis. *Endocrinology*. 2009;150:5478–5487.

[425] Limor R, Sharon O, Knoll E, Many A, Weisinger G, Stern N. Lipoxygenase-derived metabolites are regulators of peroxisome proliferator-activated receptor gamma-2 expression in human vascular smooth muscle cells. *Am J Hypertens*. 2008;21:219–223.

[426] de Wit C, Boettcher M, Schmidt VJ. Signaling across myoendothelial gap junctions: fact or fiction? Cell Commun Adhes 2008; 15:231–245. Hayman R, Warren A, Johnson I, Baker P. Inducible change in the behavior of resistance arteries from circulating factor in preeclampsia: an effect specific to myometrial vessels from pregnant women. *Am J Obstet Gynecol* 2001; 184:420–426.

[427] Kublickiene KR, Lindblom B, Kru¨ger K, Nisell H. Preeclampsia: evidence for impaired shear stress-mediated nitric oxide release in uterine circulation. *Am J Obstet Gynecol* 2000; 183:160–166.

[428] Pascoal IF, Lindheimer MD, Nalbantian-Brandt C, Umans JG. Preeclampsia selectively impairs endothelium-dependent relaxation and leads to oscillatory activity in small omental arteries. *J Clin Invest* 1998; 101:464– 470.

[429] Wang Y, Zhu D, An Y, Sun J, Cai L, Zheng J. Preeclampsia activates 15-lipoxygenase and its metabolite 15-hydroxyeicosatetraenoic acid enhances constriction in umbilical arteries. *Prostaglandins Leukot Essent Fatty Acids.* 2012;86:79–84.

[430] Watson AM, Olukman M, Koulis C, Tu Y, Samijono D, Yuen D, Lee C, Behm DJ, Cooper ME, Jandeleit-Dahm KA, Calkin AC, Allen TJ. Urotensin II receptor antagonism confers vasoprotective effects in diabetes associated atherosclerosis: studies in humans and in a mouse model of diabetes. *Diabetologia* 2013;56:1155-1165.

[431] Onat AM, Pehlivan Y, Turkbeyler IH, Demir T, Kaplan DS, Ceribasi AO, Orkmez M, Tutar E, Taysi S, Sayarlioglu M, Kisacik B. *Urotensin Inhibition with Palosuran Could Be a Promising Alternative in Pulmonary Arterial Hypertension. Inflammation* 2013; 36;405-412.

[432] Thirunavukkarasu M, Selvaraju V, Dunna NR, Foye JL, Joshi M, Otani H, Maulik N. Simvastatin treatment inhibits hypoxia inducible factor 1-alpha (HIF-1alpha)-prolyl-4-hydroxylase 3 (PHD 3) and increases angiogenesis after myocardial infarction in streptozotocin-induced diabetic rat. *Int J Cardiol* 2013;168:2474–2480.

[433] Samangaya RA, Mires G, Shennan A, Skillern L, Howe D, McLeod A, Baker PN. A randomised, doublé blinded, placebo controlled study of the phosphodiesterase type 5 inhibitor sildenafil for the treatment of preeclampsia. *Hypertens Pregnancy* 2009;28:369-382.

[434] Cudmore M, Ahmad S, Al-Ani B, Fujisawa T, Coxall H, Chudasama K, Devey LR, Wigmore SJ, Abbas A, Hewett PW, Ahmed A.Negative regulation of soluble Flt-1 and soluble endoglin reléase by hemeoxygenase-1. *Circulation* 2007;115:1789-1797.

[435] Cao J, Inoue K, Li X, Drummond G, Abraham NG. Physiological significance of hemeoxygenase in hypertension. *Int J Biochem Cell Biol* 2009;41:1025-1033.

In: Advances in Hypertension Research
Editor: Ramón Rodrigo

ISBN: 978-1-62948-857-8

Chapter 4

Renovascular Hypertension*

***Matías Libuy*† *and Andrés Carreño*††**
Molecular and Clinical Pharmacology Program, Institute of Biomedical Sciences, Faculty of Medicine, University of Chile, Chile

Abstract

Renovascular hypertension is among the most common causes of secondary hypertension worldwide. In fact, renal artery stenosis, especially the one due to atherosclerotic peripheral vascular disease, is increasing among the population. The pathophysiology of renovascular hypertension is complex and involves multiple mechanisms. Synthesis and secretion of renin and angiotensin II, stimulation of sympathetic nervous system, endothelial dysfunction, increased aldosterone synthesis, oxidative stress and increased proinflammatory cytokine release, constitute major pathways in the pathophysiology of renovascular hypertension. This chapter is an updated mechanistic approach to the molecular basis of pathophysiology of renovascular hypertension. Moreover, it presents a structured perspective for diagnoses and therapy in this pathology.

Keywords: Renovascular hypertension, oxidative stress, renin, angiotensin II, sympathetic nervous system

Abbreviations

ACEI	angiotensin converting enzyme inhibitor
ARAS	atherosclerotic renal artery stenosis

* Supported by FONDECYT, grant 1120594

† Corresponding author: Lic. Matías Libuy Ríos, Molecular and Clinical Pharmacology Program Institute of Biomedical Sciences, Faculty of Medicine, University of Chile, 1027 Independencia Avenue, P.O Box 70058, Santiago 7, Chile. Telephone: 56-2-29786126 Fax: 56-2-29786126, E-mail: mlibuy@med.uchile.cl.

†† MSc in Surgical Sciences (c) University of Edinburgh, UK.

Ang II	angiotensin II
ARB's	angiotensin-receptor blocking agents
ARNA	afferent renal nerve activity
AT-1	angiotensin II type I receptor
AVP	arginine vasopressin hormone
BP	blood pressure
eNOS	endothelial nitric oxide synthase
ET-1	endothelin - 1
FMD	fibromuscular dysplasia
GFR	glomerular filtration rate
MCP-1	monocyte chemoattractant protein -1
MMPs	matrix metalloproteinases
NO	nitric oxide
NADPH	reduced nicotinamide adenine dinucleotide phosphate-oxidase
PRA	plasma renin activity
RAAS	renin angiotensin aldosterone system
RAS	renal artery stenosis
ROS	reactive oxygen species
RSNA	renal sympathetic nerve activity
RVH	renovascular hypertension
SHR	spontaneously hypertensive rat
SHRSP	stroke-prone spontaneously hypertensive rat
SNS	sympathetic nervous system
TGF	tubuloglomerular feedback
TGF- β1	transforming growth factor- β1
1K1C	one kidney- one clip
2K1C	two kidney-one clip
2K2C	two kidney-two clip

1. Introduction

Renovascular hypertension (RVH) syndrome was proposed after the classic animal model experiments carried out by Goldblatt, who clipped the renal arteries in two different settings (two kidneys, one clip, and one kidney, one clip), producing systemic hypertension in both of them [1]. These experiments, among others, finally led to its definition as a rise in blood pressure (BP) induced by reduced renal perfusion. RVH is the most common 'correctable' cause of secondary hypertension [2]. It comprises several types of disorders; most of them listed in Table 4-1, which share the common feature of constantly decreased renal blood flow.

The influence of the kidney function and their vasoactive mediators started to be described in the beginning of the 20th century, progressively giving way to a solid body of knowledge known as the renin-angiotensin-aldosterone system, reviewed elsewhere [3]. Currently, several further mediators and mechanisms have been described or proposed as part of this complex system, which will be discussed along this chapter.

Table 4-1. Etiologies of renovascular hypertension

Atherosclerotic renal artery stenosis (ARAS)	
	Unilateral ARAS
	Bilateral ARAS
	Unilateral ARAS in a Solitary functioning kidney
Fibromuscular dysplasia	
	Medial fibroplasia
	Intimal fibroplasia
	Perimedial fibroplasia
	Medial fibroplasia
Renal artery aneurism	
Arterial embolus	
Arteriovenous fistula	
Segmental arterial occlusion (postraumatic)	
Extrinsec compression of the renal artery	
Renal compression	
Aortic coarction	
Systemic vasculitis	
Atheroembolic disease	
Vascular occlusion due to endovascular aortic stent graft	

Epidemiological studies show that among patients with mild to moderate hypertension the prevalence of RVH is low, ranging from 0,6 to 3% [4]. However, in treating resistant hypertension, it could rise up to 20% [5]. The two most frequent lesions producing RVH are fibromuscular dysplasia (FMD) and atherosclerotic renal artery stenosis (ARAS), each of them usually having characteristic features.

FMD is a non-inflammatory, nonatherosclerotic vascular disorder that produces arterial stenosis, occlusion, aneurysm, and dissection. It has been described in nearly every arterial bed, but most commonly it affects renal and internal carotid arteries, and less often vertebral, iliac, subclavian, and other visceral arteries [6]. It usually affects women, producing an early onset hypertension (between 30 and 50 years old) with unusual severity. These lesions rarely lead to major renal function loss, although progression may be seen, particularly in smokers [7]. Among patients with RVH, FMD accounts for 35 to 50 percent of cases in children, and 5 to 10 percent of cases in adults under the age of 50 years [8-10]. It can also occur in older patients either in isolation or in combination with atherosclerosis, but the prevalence is not well described. FMD of the renal arteries is bilateral in 35 to 50 percent [11, 12] and approximately 65 percent of patients with renal artery FMD also have other vascular beds involvement, usually carotid or vertebral FMD. Similarly, patients with carotid or vertebral FMD are likely to have renal involvement. FMD of the renal arteries can be an incidental finding in asymptomatic patients. Neymark et al. reported a 7 per cent of renal arteries FMD in healthy potential kidney donors using catheter-based renal angiograms [13]. Lorenz et al. reported 2.8% of renal arteries FMD in a similar setting using computed tomography angiograms [14].

On the other hand, ARAS usually affects older patients, with concomitant atherosclerotic involvement in coronary, carotid and peripheral arteries. The narrowing of the artery lumen is clinically significant when it goes beyond 70%, creating a pressure gradient big enough to compromise renal perfusion [15]. It usually leads to glomerular filtration rate (GFR) reduction, as the renal adaptation mechanisms to ischemia, which will be discussed below, produce kidney structural changes and ultimately medullary fibrosis [16].

As stated by most important medical and research institutions, the emphasis of treatment of atherosclerotic disease is nowadays put on the reduction of exposure to major risk factors, and there is an open discussion about who would benefit from a more aggressive approach when there is renovascular involvement. Several prospective studies have addressed these questions, but most of them have received criticism and the results have not given concluding evidence to support a single recommendation. The last available data will be presented and discussed in this chapter focusing on future perspectives in terms of basic science research, new pathophysiological mechanistic approaches developing new therapies, and better patient management.

2. Pathophysiology

RVH is the elevation of BP that follows the incomplete occlusion of one or both renal arteries. The progressive ischemia of kidney(s) is due to increasing reduction in lumen of stenotic renal artery which activates counterregulatory pathways, and leads to a sequence of events directed toward restoring kidney perfusion. Synthesis and secretion of renin and angiotensin II (Ang II), stimulation of sympathetic nervous system (SNS), endothelial dysfunction, increased aldosterone synthesis, oxidative stress and increased proinflammatory cytokine release, constitute pathways in the pathophysiology of RVH [17]. Figure 4-1 shows the major pathways of RVH and in figure 4-3 there is an integrative hypothesis accounting for the pathophysiology of RVH.

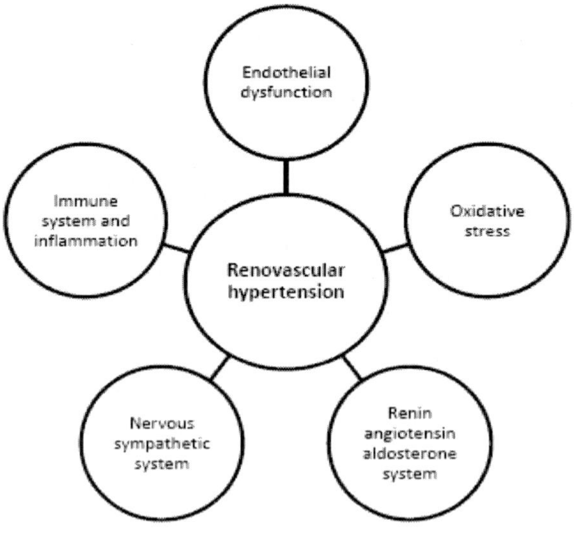

Figure 4-1. Major pathophysiological pathways of renovascular hypertension.

Harry Goldblatt in his study on dogs demonstrated the rise in BP associated with unilateral as well as bilateral clamping of renal artery [2]. These "one kidney-one clip"

(1K1C) and "two kidney one clip" (2K1C) are the fundamental models for understanding RVH. Classic Goldblatt's model of RVH indicates that mechanisms sustaining hypertension change over time [18], as it shown in figure 4-2.

The first phase of classic Goldblatt's hypertension model, is seen for approximately 4 weeks following clipping and is marked by immediate increase in BP, associated with an increase in plasma renin activity (PRA) and angiotensin levels. During this phase, removal of the clip or treatment with angiotensin convert enzyme inhibitor (ACEI) within 7- 10 days leads to immediate lowering of blood pressure. This phase is chiefly mediated by renin angiotensin aldosterone system (RAAS) activation as well as salt and water retention and volume expansion, the latter being more important in the 1K1C model [2,18].

The second phase of Goldblatt 2K1C hypertension occurs between weeks 5 to 8 following clipping and is marked by stable or increasing BP with salt-retention, volume expansion and downregulation of the RAAS. The removal of the clip or treatment with ACEI does reduce the BP to normal during this phase but a longer time is required to achieve this normal BP [19].

The third phase of Goldblatt hypertension model occurs 9 weeks or more after clipping. This phase is characterized by a decrease in PRA and in plasma Ang II levels with persistently elevated BP.

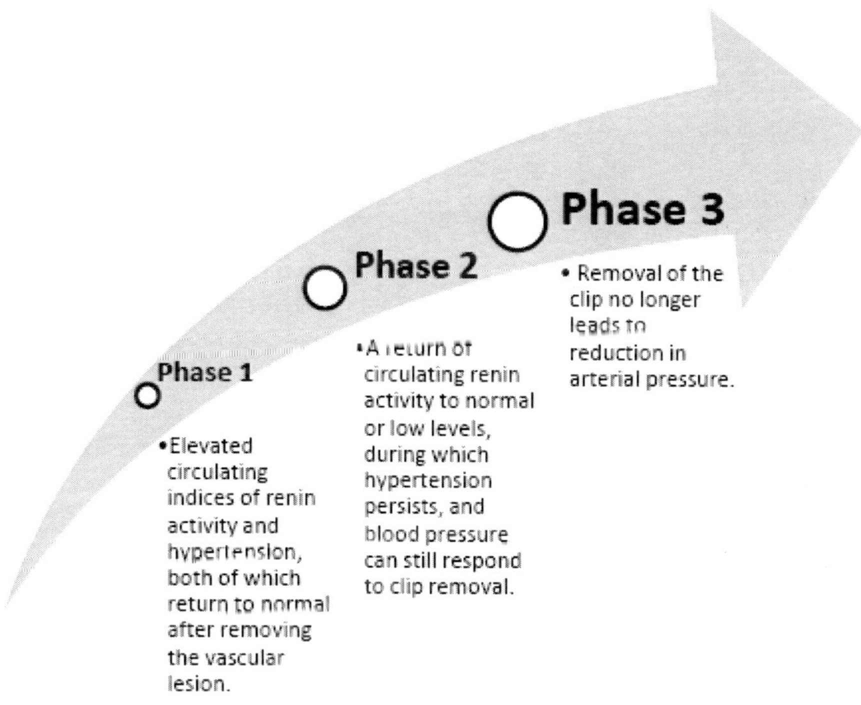

Figure 4-2. Classical phases of renovascular hypertension.

Although clip removal or ACEI in doses equal to those in Phase I and II do not reduce BP to normal, higher doses of ACEI as well as other anti-hypertensive medications are able to reduce the BP, sometimes to normal. In this phase, local vascular Ang II or intrarenal Ang II rather than the general renin angiotensin system may play an important role in the control of sympathetic neurotransmission [20].

This observation suggests that mechanisms producing RVH sometimes undergo a transition to an irreversible stage. Whether these phases apply directly to human renovascular disease is difficult to determine. Thus, it is suitable to present an updated mechanistic approach of pathophysiology of RVH for a better understanding.

2.1. Oxidative Stress

Oxidative stress constitutes a unifying mechanism of injury in many types of disease processes. It occurs when there is an imbalance between the generation of reactive oxygen species (ROS) and the antioxidant defense systems in the body. This process increases the presence and toxicity of ROS, which in turn can promote the formation of vasoactive mediators including endothelin-1 (ET-1), leukotriene, and prostaglandin F2α and isoprostane, which are products of lipid peroxidation. These mediators affect renal function and hemodynamics, both by inducing renal vasoconstriction and by changing glomerular capillary ultrafiltration characteristics [21].

Oxidative stress has been involved in the development of RVH [22]. Higher concentrations of ROS have been consistently implicated in vascular changes associated with clinical and experimental hypertension [23, 24]. As a matter of fact, the most important source of ROS in blood vessels is a superoxide-producing nicotinamide adenine dinucleotide phosphate-oxidase enzyme (NADPH oxidase), which is upregulated in many hypertensive conditions [25]. Activation of this enzyme, especially by Ang II, leads to functional and structural alterations in the vascular wall, which thus result in endothelial dysfunction, increased contractility and deposition of extracellular matrix proteins as well as vascular hypertrophy [26].

Recent evidence suggests that overactivity of NADPH oxidase-derived ROS, could contribute to hypertension [28]. Also reactive oxygen species activate several pathways that modulate renal microvascular function. Taken together, ROS increase renal vascular tone, sensitivity to vasoconstrictors, and tubuloglomerular feedback (TGF) that characterize pathophysiological conditions associated with increased oxidative stress [29]. The interaction of ROS with nitric oxide (NO) decreases bioavailability of the latter and, at the same time, it results in formation of the pro-oxidant peroxynitrite. These effects combine to impair intra-renal vascular, glomerular, and tubular function [30].

The most common cause of renal artery occlusive disease is atherosclerosis. Since renal artery stenosis (RAS) and atherosclerosis are both characterized by increased oxidative stress, their co-existence augments the production of ROS and impairs renal function. Actually, oxidative stress is increased in stenotic kidneys [31-33]. Furthermore, reduced endogenous nitric oxide may interfere with a spectrum of additional activities of the molecule, such as the loss of both its antithrombotic protection and inhibition of fibrosis related responses to injury [30]. The earliest and most pronounced pathologic features in renal ischemia consist of tubulointerstitial changes [34-37] that may mediate the progression of renal disease towards irreversible damage.

In addition, a recent study concludes that the development of RVH in RAS mice was associated with a rapid induction of NADPH oxidase subunits Ncf1 and Ncf2, which encode the NADPH oxidase subunits p47phox and p67phox, respectively [38]. Increased expressions of Ncf1 and Ncf2 have been described in several models of hypertension. In spontaneously hypertensive rats, Ncf1 and Ncf2 are highly expressed in vessels, the macula densa, distal tubules, cortical collecting ducts, and medullary collecting ducts [39]. A substantial rise of renal expression of Ncf1 has been reported in the Dahl salt-sensitive rat [40] as well as in spontaneously hypertensive rats [39]. In fact, a number of molecules targeted for oxidative stress pathways are being tested in animal models. HPP53 (a specific peroxisome proliferator-activated receptor δ agonist) showed prevention of necrosis and fibrosis in a 2 kidney 1 clip model in rats [41]. What is more, imperatorin, the active component of Radix Angelicae (Baizhi), showed antihypertensive and antioxidant effects in the renal injury of renovascular hypertensive rats, suggesting that IMP could be of therapeutic use in preventing renal injury related hypertension [42].

2.2. Immune System and Inflammation

There is enough evidence to suggest an important role of the immune system and inflammatory processes in the elevation of BP and the development of RVH [43]. Ang II and the SNS contribute to renovascular disease by promoting proinflammatory mechanisms within the vessel wall. Immune cells, particularly T-cells and macrophages can be activated by Ang II with subsequent cell recruitment into the vessel walls [44]. It has become increasingly clear that the central nervous system effects of Ang II are important for T-cell activation and vascular inflammation [45]. Recent evidence showed that RVH and renal damage may result from tissue inflammation [46]. In this sense, RAS, a major cause of RVH, exhibits increased expression of monocyte chemoattractant protein (MCP)-1, a chemokine that increases monocyte infiltration into inflamed tissues and an important inflammatory mediator [46]. Ang II can then increase macrophage infiltration [47].

Further, MCP-1 has been implicated in a variety of renal diseases [48, 49] and progressive renal damage, mediated through cognate receptors like CCR2 [49]. Activated macrophages and fibroblasts in the RAS kidney may directly induce NADPH oxidase activity, stimulating tumoral grow factor- β1 (TGF-β) production and triggering fibroblast proliferation and differentiation into collagen-secreting myofibroblasts [50]. Alternatively, a recent study showed that swine RAS kidneys exhibit increased levels of inflammation mediators [51, 33]. Hence, RAS may lead to microvascular remodeling and rarefaction in the stenotic kidney, probably consequent to ischemia, increased oxidative stress, and inflammation [51, 32].

2.3. Endothelial Dysfunction

Endothelial dysfunction may be defined as an impairment characterized by a shift of the actions of the endothelium toward reduced vasodilation, a proinflammatory state, and prothrombotic setting. The pathophysiology of endothelial dysfunction is complex and involves multiple mechanisms. It is characterized by unbalanced concentrations of vasodilating and vasoconstricting factors, the most important being represented by NO and Ang-II, respectively [52]. It is well known that diminished NO production and/or increased

ROS, in particular superoxide induced oxidative inactivation may lead to decrease NO availability, contributing to endothelial dysfunction and maintenance of hypertension. Endothelial NO is synthesized from L-arginine by a family of nitric oxide synthases and participates in the regulation of kidney function by counteracting the vasoconstrictor effects of Ang II [53]. In addition to its effects on the blood flow and tubular reabsorption of sodium, NO inhibits growth of vascular smooth muscle cells, mesangial cell hypertrophy and hyperplasia, and synthesis of extracellular matrix. Several studies have shown that endothelial nitric oxide synthase (eNOS) expression and/or NO concentration are significantly increased although endothelium-dependent vasorelaxation is decreased in spontaneously hypertensive (SHR), stroke-prone spontaneously hypertensive (SHRSP), and 2K1C renovascular hypertensive rats [54-57]. These results suggest that the sole inactivation of NO is responsible for endothelial dysfunction in these models. However, several evidence [58] reported that severe endothelial dysfunction occurred and caused not only an increase in NO inactivation, but also a decrease in its production from eNOS in SHRSP supplemented with a high-salt, high-fat diet. In fact, a link between high-fat or high-fat, high-sucrose diet mediated oxidative stress and a decrease in NO concentration has been recently demonstrated [59, 60].

In addition, a group of zinc-endopeptidases called matrix metalloproteinases (MMPs) plays an important role in vascular dysfunction and tissue remodeling in many cardiovascular conditions, including hypertension [61-62]. Increased MMP activation promotes excessive degradation of extracellular matrix components, vascular smooth muscle cell migration and proliferation; and monocyte invasion [63-64], thus contributing to hypertensive structural alterations. MMP-2, specifically, can also modulate vascular contractility via proteolysis of vasoactive peptides such as big ET-1 [65], calcitonin gene-related peptide. Actually, clinical and experimental studies have found increased expression and activity of MMP-2 (72-kDa gelatinase A) and MMP-9 (92-kDa gelatinase B) in plasma and vascular tissues of hypertensive patients [66] and animal models of hypertension [70-71]. Recent evidence showed that MMP-2 plays a major role in structural and functional vascular changes associated with 2K-1C hypertension. These vascular changes were attenuated by doxycycline, a nonspecific MMP inhibitor [72]. Along with this, other studies suggest that MMP-mediated vascular remodeling and dysfunction could result from increased oxidative stress [73-75]. ROS react with thiol groups, which preserve MMP latency [76], thus activating MMPs. In fact, it has been shown that ROS enhance the expression and activity of MMPs, especially MMP-2, via xanthine oxidase [76, 77, 34] and via mechanical stretch-induced vascular NADPH oxidase [35]. In addition to hypertension, ROS-induced MMP-2 activation has been reported to play a role in other pathophysiological cardiovascular conditions [36, 37, 73, 70]. Although increased oxidative stress and upregulation of MMPs (especially MMP-2) have been reported in animal models of hypertension, nevertheless, no previous study has examined whether antioxidants could prevent the increases in vascular MMP levels and the vascular dysfunction and remodeling associated with hypertension.

Moreover, endothelin peptides are potent and long-lasting vasoconstrictor peptides produced and released from endothelial cells. ET-1 production is augmented after simulation of renal endothelial cells with a variety of substances, such as thrombin and local cytokines, including TGF-β, interleukin- 1, tumor necrosis factor, and so on. It must be emphasized that renal ischemia is a potent stimulus for expression of the ET-1 gene in the kidney. This increase persists for days after resolution of the ischemic injury. Sustained vascular effects of

ET-1 may participate in the hypoperfusion, which lasts longer, beyond the vascular insult to postischemic kidneys [31].

2.4. Sympathetic Nervous System

There is mounting evidence that increased sympathetic nerve activity play important roles in RVH [22]. D'Elia JA & Weinraucuch [78], showed that studies by DiBona & Kopp [79, 80] demonstrated nerve endings in proximity to glomerular, tubular, and vascular structures. In addition, it has been shown that afferent impulses from the injured kidney may increase sympathetic nervous system activity in areas of the brain involved in noradrenergic regulation of blood pressure and contribute to the development and maintenance of hypertension associated with kidney disease [81]. Also, accumulated evidence indicates that human sympathetic nervous system deregulation contributes to the development of arterial hypertension [82]. Therefore, the crosstalk between the sympathetic nervous system and the kidneys plays a crucial role in hypertension. It thus influences several pathophysiological mechanisms such as the central sympathetic tone, the sodium balance and the systemic neurohumoral activation [83].

On the one hand, renal sympathetic nerve fibers critically influence renal function [84]. Adrenergic fibers innervate the most relevant renal structures such as the renal vasculature, the tubular epithelial cells throughout the nephron and the juxtaglomerular apparatus [85]. Increased renal sympathetic nerve activity results in a decrease in renal blood flow mediated by vasoconstriction, α1a adrenoceptors [85], increased renal tubular sodium and water reabsorption, α1b adrenoceptors [86], and an increased renin secretion rate, β1 adrenoceptors [87-88]. These effects are dependent on the degree of sympathetic activation and are considered to play a major part in the development and maintenance of hypertension [89].

Similarly, the kidneys can also influence the sympathetic system activity. Renal structures are richly innervated with baroreceptors and chemoreceptors. The afferent signaling from the kidneys is transmitted to the central nervous system and enhances sympathetic outflow, not only to the kidneys but also to other structures such as the heart and peripheral arterioles [90].

2.5. Renin Angiotensin Aldosterone System

RAAS have a major role in the development and maintenance of RVH [18]. The RAAS has an impressive pathophysiology and numerous systemic correlations, as it is a major regulatory system of vascular and renal function. RAAS is indeed an important player in the pathogenesis of RAS and ischemic nephropathy. Both the activation of the RAAS and sympathetic overactivity are highly responsible for the cardiovascular and renal morbidity in RAS patients [91]. The pathogenesis of RVH is complex, but it is mainly due to the over-activation of RAAS [92]. Activation of the renin-angiotensin system is an essential component for developing RVH, at least in the initial stages [93].

Studies in which animals are pre-treated with angiotensin-converting enzyme (ACE) inhibition indicate that development of hypertension is delayed so long as ACE inhibition continues. Genetic knockout animals without the angiotensin-1 receptor do not develop RVH.

Recent transplantation studies indicate that angiotensin receptors in both the systemic vasculature and kidney vasculature participate in this process [94, 95]. Measured components of the renin angiotensin system, e.g., plasma renin activity, are elevated only transiently in RVH [93].

Observations in both experimental animals and human subjects indicate that renin-release is eventually reduced partly related to the rise in systemic, and thereby renal, arterial pressures and/or sodium retention. Moreover, intrarenal Ang II against systemic RAAS has been described in the maintenance of RVH. Intrarenal Ang II is increased by means of receptor mediated internalization of circulating Ang II as well as by AT1 receptor mediated increase in intrarenal angiotensinogen [95, 96]. These observations describe the dual roles of Ang II, both for adaptation and maintenance of kidney function and for modulating many steps in the pathophysiology of renal injury in RVH.

2.6. Experimental Models

Hypertension is a multifactorial, polygenic disease that involves complex interactions between genetically determined homeostatic control mechanisms and environmental factors [98]. Its exploration thus requires availability of experimentally manipulable animal models. The ideal animal model for hypertension research should have human-like cardiovascular anatomy, hemodynamics, and physiology and develop human disease characteristics and complications in a timely or even accelerated fashion [99]. Inevitably, no species can consistently answer all of these needs, and experimental design and other constraints often dictate the choice of animal models for specific research applications. There are genetic and nongenetic models. Genetic models of hypertension were especially successful in rodents and have encouraged studies in human population with the candidate gene approach, as well as the development of new classes of drugs to decrease blood pressure and target organ injury. On the contrary, nongenetic approaches have resulted in development of extremely useful models that allow studying the effects of induced hypertension on end-organ damage in different species, including large animals possibly comparable with humans [7]. A most specific categorization of experimental models of RVH includes 2K1C, 1K1C, aortic coarctation, total occlusion and microembolization [7]. Genetic models that deserve attention are SHR, SHR-stroke prone, Dahl-salt-sensitive rat, among others. Table 4-2, contains a mechanistic approach of pathophysiological models of RVH. After that, there is a brief commentary about some important experimental models in this pathology.

Table 4-2. A mechanistic approach to the pathophysiology of renovascular hypertension

Pathway	Model	Comment	Reference
Oxidative Stress	Rat (nongenetic)	Overactivity of NAD(P)H oxidase-derived ROS.	[28]
	DOCA-salt hypertensive rats (genetic)	NADPH oxidase is upregulated in hypertensive conditions	[25]
	Pigs (nongenetic)	Pathogenic role of oxidative stress in renal injury	[33]
	Rat 2K1C(nongenetic)	Peroxisome proliferator-activated receptor δ agonist, HPP593, prevents renal necrosis under chronic ischemia.	[41]

Pathway	Model	Comment	Reference
	Rat 2K1C (nongenetic)	Effects of antioxidant on the blood pressure and oxidative stress in 2K1C hypertensive rats	[42]
Immune system and inflamamation	Human	T-cells and macrophages can be activated by Ang II with subsequent cell recruitment into the vessel walls	[100,101]
	Swine (Nongenetic)	Increased expression of monocyte chemoattractant protein (MCP)-1	[46]
	Rat (nongenetic)	Sustained renal interstitial macrophage infiltration following chronic angiotensin II infusions.	[47]
	Mice (genetic)	Blockade of CCR2 ameliorates progressive fibrosis in kidney.	[49]
Endothelial dysfunction	SHR (genetic)	Suppression of the development of hypertension by the inhibition of inducible nitric oxide synthase.	[54]
	SHRSP (genetic)	Impaired activities of antioxidant enzymes elicit endothelial dysfunction, despite enhanced vascular nitric oxide generation	[55]
	Human (genetic)	Glu298Asp variant of eNOS, genetic resistance to hypertension therapy.	[103]
	Human (genetic)	G11T polymorphism, variant of eNOS, is not associated with hypertension.	[104]
	SHR (genetic)	Vitamins reverse endothelial dysfunction through regulation of eNOS and NAD(P)H oxidase activities.	[136]
	Rat 2K1C (nongenetic)	Antihypertensive and antioxidant effects	[56]
	Human	MMP activation promotes excessive degradation of extracellular matrix components, vascular smooth muscle cell migration and proliferation, and monocyte invasion	[19]
Simpathetic nervous system	Human	Sympathetic neural activity in hypertension	[82]
	Rat (nongenetic)	Stimulatory action of phenol on the SNS could be mediated by downregulation of nNOS and IL-1beta in the brain.	[109]
	Rat 2K1C (nongenetic)	Increase in oxidative stress within the RVLM, PVN and in the ischaemic kidney plays a major role in the maintenance of sympathoexcitation and hypertension in 2K1C rats	[22]
Renin angiotensin aldosterone system	Human	Role of renin-angiotensin system blockade in atherosclerotic renal artery stenosis and renovascular hypertension	[110,111]
	Rat 2K1C (nongenetic)	The type 1a ATII receptors play a critical role in the development of 2K1C hypertension while the AT1b receptors play only a minor role	[94]
	Human	Role of the renin-angiotensin-aldosterone system in renal artery stenosis, renovascular hypertension	[91]
	Mice (genetic)	Regulation of blood pressure by the RAS is mediated by AT(1) receptors both within and outside the kidney	[95]

Oxidative Stress. Recent evidence have been demonstrated that NADPH oxidase is upregulated in hypertensive conditions [25], justifying the major role of this enzyme in the pathophysiology of oxidative stress in the pathophysiology of RVH. Accordingly, a pathogenic contribution in renal injury related with oxidative stress was informed [46]. In addition, several evidence support the idea that an increase in oxidative stress within the RVLM and systemically plays an relevant part in maintaining high arterial BP and sympathetic drive in 2K-1C hypertension [28].

Immune system and inflammation. Several studies have shown a relationship between immune system and RVH [100,101]. This study showed that T-cells and macrophages can be activated by Ang II with subsequent cell recruitment into the vessel walls. Furthermore, another study [46] demonstrated that increased expression of monocyte chemoattractant protein (MCP)-1 is related with RVH.

In terms of this, interstitial renal macrophage infiltration was informed following a chronic Ang II infusions [48]. Nevertheless, recent studies have been shown that blockade of CCR2 ameliorates progressive fibrosis in kidney, a classical hystopatological feature of RVH because of RAS [50].

Endothelial dysfunction. Glu298Asp variant of eNOS may be a genetic susceptibility factor for hypertension [102] or resistance to therapy [103], whereas G11T polymorphism is not associated with hypertension [104]. Mice deficient in the 3 NOS isoforms (neuronal, inducible, and endothelial) have been produced. In addition to the impaired vascular relaxation, eNOS knockout mice often have abnormal vascular remodeling [105] and microvascular density [106], alterations that likely contribute to hypertension in this model, as well as cardiac hypertrophy and endothelial dysfunction [107].

Sympathetic nervous system. Several animal models have been used to study the influence of renal sympathetic fibers on hypertension [108]. Ye et al., [109] demonstrated the importance of the renal sympathetic nervous system in hypertension. In this study, kidney damage was induced by intrarenal injection of phenol in rats, which caused a persistent elevation of the blood pressure and an increase in norepinephrine secretion in the hypothalamus, even in the absence of renal failure. In this model, performing renal denervation prevented the blood pressure increase.

The efficacy of renal denervation in several models and in multiple species established the key role of renal nerves in hypertension pathophysiology. As a matter of fact, recent studies showed an increase in oxidative stress within the RVLM, PVN and in the ischemic kidney plays a key role in the maintenance of sympathoexcitation and hypertension in 2K1C rats [22].

Renin Angiotensin aldosterone System. Blockade of the renin-angiotensin system is now established as an important element in the treatment of RVH [93].With the introduction of agents now capable of interrupting this system, such measures are rarely necessary. Based upon the potential adverse effects of angiotensin to magnify vascular injury, myocardial damage and remodeling and increase the risk of adverse cardiovascular outcomes, many argue that administration of ACEI should be part of managing nearly all patients with significant cardiovascular risk, based on data from the HOPE trial and others [110]. These observations have been extended to angiotensin-receptor blocking agents (ARB's) given the results from studies directly comparing ACE inhibition with angiotensin receptor blockade [111].

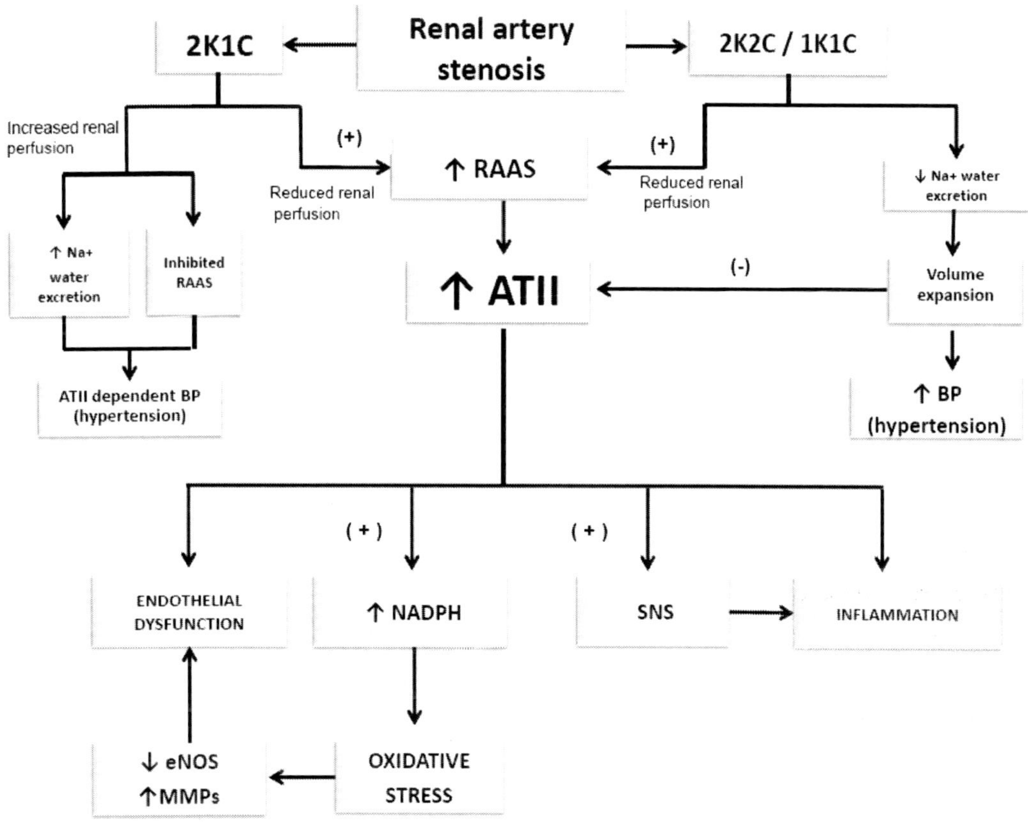

Figure 4-3. Hypothesis accounting for the pathophysiology of renovascular hypertension. 2K1C: two kidney – one clip, 1K1C: one kidney-one clip, eNOS: endothelial nitric oxide synthase, MMP's:matrix metalloproteinases, SNS: sympathetic nervous system, ATII: angiotensin II, BP: blood preasure, RAAS: renin angiotensin aldosterone system, NADPH: nicotinamide adenine dinucleotide phosphate-oxidase enzyme.

3. Diagnostic Approach and Therapy

3.1. Diagnostic Approach

For many years, clinical guidelines in hypertension treatment have stated that it is not recommended to use extensive testing for secondary hypertension in all patients. Most of them will have essential (idiopathic or primary) hypertension and these tests will bring more confusion than benefits. For this reason, considerable research was carried out in order to select the patients where the pretest likelihood of having secondary hypertension, and more specifically renovascular hypertension, would be higher. The most validated features are listed in table 4-3 [112-113].

Table 4-3. Suggestive clinical features of renovascular secondary hypertension

An rise in blood pressure over a previously well controlled patient
Severe or resistant hypertension
Age less than 30 or over 55 years old with no family history of hypertension and no obesity
An acute elevation in serum creatinine of at least 30 percent after administration of angiotensin-converting enzyme (ACE) inhibitor or angiotensin II receptor blocker (ARB)
Moderate to severe hypertension in a patient with diffuse atherosclerosis, a unilateral small kidney, or asymmetry in renal size of more than 1.5 cm that cannot be explained by another reason
Moderate to severe hypertension in patients with recurrent episodes of flash pulmonary edema
Abdominal bruit (not very sensitive)

Table 4-4. Methods for evaluating renovascular hypertension

Method	Rationale	Advantages	Drawbacks	References
Measurment of plasma renin	Measures how active renin is on plasma. In RVH it should be above normal	Non invasive	Low specificity. Influenced by sodium intake, volume status, etc.	[134]
Renal vein renin activity	Comparison of the renin release from two kidneys looking for asymmetry	Useful in diagnosis and prediction of outcomes with revascularization	Recent series show sensitivity <65% and PPV 18.5%	[137]
Split renal function test	Each kidney GFR measurement	Assesment of functional impact of lesions, providing information on the probability of benefit from revascularization	It requires urinary tract instrumentation and provides only indirect information	[114]
Captopril renography	Captopril amplifies differences in renal perfusion and 99m-Tc mercaptoacetyltriglycine is used as a marker	Highly specific, but it excludes RVH in normal studies	Limitations with advanced atherosclerosis or kidney disease. No anatomic information	[138]
Doppler Ultrasound	Stenosis leads to flow velocity augmentation on renal arteries. Waveform changes described	Inexpensive, highly available	Operator-dependent, difficult to assess fibromuscular dysplasia	[139]
CT angiography	Contrast milieu is used for imaging the anatomy of renal arteries and aorta by computed tomography	Excellent sensitivity and specificity. Stents do not cause artifacts	Expensive, potential nephrotoxicity	[140]
MRI angiography	Shows renal arteries and abdominal aorta using magnetic resonance technique	Not nephrotoxic; Excellent images	Expensive, gadolinium excluded in renal failure	[140]
Intraarterial angiography	Using contrast to reveal renal artery anatomy and lesions	Gold standard. Usually used during revascularization procedures	Invasive, not free from complications	[141]

The diagnosis tools used for detecting RVH have evolved through time. Noninvasive tests remain imperfect and the Gold Standard continues to be catheter based angiograms. The diagnostic tests fall into three categories: (1) physiologic and functional studies to evaluate the role of stenotic lesions particularly related to activation of the renin-angiotensin system, (2) perfusion and imaging studies to identify the presence and degree of vascular stenosis, and (3) studies to predict the likelihood of benefit from invasive maneuvers, including renal revascularization, the latter being probably the most important for clinical decision making [15,114].

A summary of the most commonly used tests, as well as their advantages and drawbacks are listed in table 4-4.

3.2. Therapy

The treatment of RVH is clearly under the premise of dealing with hypertensive patients. General recommendations found elsewhere on primary and secondary prevention apply as much as for essential hypertension patients [115]. The goal of treating patients with hypertension is to prevent morbidity and mortalilty associated with high BP [62]. This task may include the effort to simplify or potentially to eliminate long-term antihypertensive drug therapy. A further goal is to preserve kidney function and to prevent loss of kidney function related to impaired renal blood flow. In some instances, renal revascularization is undertaken to allow improved management of salt and water balance in the process of managing patients with congestive cardiac failure. This may allow safer use of diuretic agents and ACEI and ARB classes of medication in patients with critical renal artery lesions to the entire renal mass [15, 114].

The pathophysiology of RVH differs whether the disease is unilateral or bilateral as mentioned above. This is also a concern regarding therapy, since the potential hazards of any interventional procedure or the medical therapy differ as well. Patient survival is reduced in individuals with bilateral disease or a solitary functioning kidney and the development of faster GFR reduction is more likely in bilateral disease [116], although it is not predictable from patient to patient.

3.3. Medical Therapy

Since the introduction of agents blocking the renin-angiotensin system, most patients (86% to 92%) with unilateral renal artery disease can achieve blood pressure levels <140/90 mm Hg with medical regimens based on these agents. Recent treatment trials confirm that target blood pressure levels can regularly be achieved [117, 118] Even if a patient with RVH deteriorates his GFR due to the introduction of ACE inhibitors, long term outcomes and survival rates are better, probably due to the other mechanisms giving cardiovascular protection of these drugs. The experience with ACE inhibition in trials of congestive cardiac failure is reassuring in this regard. Thousands of patients with marginal arterial pressures and clinical heart failure have been treated over many years with a variety of ACE inhibitors, and more recently ARBs.

These patients are at high risk for undetected renal artery lesions as part of the atherosclerotic burden associated with coronary disease. Although a minor change in creatinine is observed in 8% to 10% of these individuals, an increase is sufficient to lead to withdrawal of these agents under trial when monitoring conditions that occur in only 1% to 2% of cases. Data from patients with high cardiovascular disease risk treated with ramipril included patients with creatinine levels up to 2.3 mg/dL. Those with creatinine between 1.4 and 2.3 mg/dL were at higher risk for cardiovascular mortality and had a major survival benefit from ACE inhibition [15, 114].

In terms of management and outcomes, reaching blood pressure goals in RVH could be more difficult, requiring a more intensive therapy. Progression to end stage renal disease is as common as taking a surgical approach. Results of prospective trials of medical versus surgical intervention started in the 1980s and extended to the 1990s. No differences in patient survival or renal function could be identified [119].

These studies indicate that progression of renovascular disease is not often fast nor predictable, having widely varying rates. More recent research has compared medical therapy alone versus endoluminal revascularization. Seven randomized controlled trials have been reported to date and none of them has found significant benefits over medical treatment for atherosclerotic renal artery stenosis [120-125]. A meta-analysis comprising of all them concluded that in patients with ARAS, percutaneous renal revascularization in addition to medical therapy may result in a lower requirement for antihypertensive medications, but not with improvements in serum creatinine or clinical outcomes, as compared with medical management alone [126].

3.4. Endovascular Interventions

The past two decades have been characterized by a major shift from surgical reconstruction toward preferential application of endovascular procedures [114]. The total volume of renal revascularization procedures registered for the U.S. Medicare population older than 65 years of age increased 62% from 13,380 to 21,600 between 1996 and 2000. This change reflects an increase in endovascular procedures by 2.4-fold, whereas surgical renovascular procedures decreased by 45% [127]. Carr et al., [128] in a review of stenting revascularization underline that the purpose of the procedure has shifted from treatment for RVH to a maneuver capable of recovering threatened renal function in patients with ischemic nephropathy and improving management of congestive heart failure, therefore widening its indications.

They also describe the criteria commonly used to offer stenting revascularization, when it is most likely to benefit patients with ARAS. These include: (a) new onset of hypertension that is not well controlled; (b) sudden worsening of previously stable hypertension; (c) patients with "flash pulmonary edema" with otherwise normal left ventricular function; and (d) patients with a recent (acute/subacute) deterioration in renal function who have the following anatomic findings: (1) a diameter stenosis of at least 60% in a kidney at least 8 cm in length; (2) bilateral ARAS, unilateral ARAS in a solitary kidney, or unilateral ARAS with contralateral renal artery occlusion (global ischemia); (3) minimal intrarenal nephrosclerotic changes at angiography or normal intrarenal resistive indexes at duplex sonography; (4) a renal biopsy revealing hyalinization of less than 50% of the glomeruli; or (5) asymmetrically delayed renal perfusion to the kidney ipsilateral to the ARAS shown by nuclear scintigraphy. However, even if these criteria are not fulfilled, revascularization may still be beneficial in a patient with renal insufficiency.

Consequently, there are no current clinical, anatomic, or diagnostic imaging factors that clearly define when revascularization will or will not be beneficial for patients with ARAS [128]. Technically, many advances have led to a safer procedure, with good results in terms of patency and restenosis. Technical success rates for renal artery stent placement approach 95%. In renal stent series with angiographic follow-up, recurrent diameter stenosis of greater than 50% occurred in 7-25% of patients at 6-24 months. Primary and secondary patency rates for renal stents approximate 70% and 90%, respectively, after 5 years of follow-up [129-135].

Conclusion and Perspectives

Up to date, none of the current available therapies have shown an impact in morbidity and mortality in randomized controlled trials, nor do they cover all the mechanisms involved.in the pathophysiology of renovascular hypertension. The pathophysiology of this disease is complex and involves at least, synthesis and secretion of renin and angiotensin II (Ang II), stimulation of sympathetic nervous system (SNS), endothelial dysfunction, increased aldosterone synthesis, oxidative stress and increased proinflammatory cytokine release. The evident anatomical preponderance of RVH defects should not discourage the attempt of discovering new drugs, going beyond from simply administering antihypertensive treatment that could prevent the effects of reduced blood flow in kidneys, without requiring invasive procedures. There is promising ongoing research that could provide newer tools to the available therapies, such as antioxidant agents, immune modulators, among others. Notably, a number of molecules targeted for oxidative stress pathways are being tested in animal models. HPP53 (a specific peroxisome proliferator-activated receptor δ agonist), showed prevention of necrosis and fibrosis in a 2 kidney 1 clip model in rats. Also, imperatorin, the active component of Radix Angelicae (Baizhi), showed antihypertensive and antioxidant effects in the renal injury of renovascular hypertensive rats, suggesting that IMP could be of therapeutic use in preventing renal injury related hypertension. The pendulum that led initially to excessive enthusiasm for renal revascularization appears to have swung to the opposite extreme.

Most criticism against the RCTs that presented to this date is directed to the fact that "average" values may obscure important individual differences. In this sense, developing more effective tools to identify viable kidneys and/or those at risk from irreversible vascular injury remains a top priority. This could lead to identify different profiles of RVH patients. As far as interventional procedures are concerned, more accurate endovascular techniques and imaging are getting better success rates. Nevertheless, they still fail in providing promising results in the long term.

Even in this pessimistic setting, the current recommendations of expert panels favoring adding renal revascularization to ARAS patients when there is (1) progressive decline in GFR during treatment of hypertension (2) failure to achieve adequate blood pressure control with optimal medical therapy (3) rapid or recurrent decline in the GFR in association with a reduction in systemic pressure (4) decline in GFR during therapy with ACE inhibitors or

ARBs and (5) recurrent congestive heart failure in a patient in whom the adequacy of left ventricular failure does not explain the cause, should prevail in spite of the poor results observed so far. This is based on our understanding of the disease and our belief in the possibility of rather saving or preserving a number of ischemic kidneys. This means that it is most likely that a set of patients successfully achieves a larger span of better quality life.

Interestingly, other types of interventional procedures are on sight. For instance, studies of nonsurgical renal sympathetic ablation by any modality will need to learn from past observation. Durability of effect cannot be assumed from short-term studies, and permanence of effect may have unanticipated consequences (postcardiovascular or neurological event hypotension or autonomic dysfunction). To this point, the discomfort of renal sympathetic ablation has only been reported as a brief procedural consequence. Surgical regional sympathetic nerve ablation has been associated with regional side effects. We will have to be alert for the possible existence of renal sympathetic dystrophic symptoms. Our current revision of the available literature regarding RVH has provided ground for much further research. Each of the mechanisms mentioned above, thought as contributors of hypertension and kidney injury have the potential of becoming targeted therapies.

References

[1] Goldblatt H, Lynch J, Hanzel RF, Summerville WW. Studies on experimental hypertension I: the production of persistent elevation of systolic blood pressure by means of renal ischemia. *J. Exp. Med.* 1934;59:347-379.

[2] Balk E, Raman G, Chung M, Ip S, Tatsioni A, Alonso A, Chew P, Gilbert SJ, Lau J. Effectiveness of management strategies for renal artery stenosis: a systemic review. *Ann. Intern. Med.* 2006;145:901–912.

[3] Basso N, Terragno NA. History about the discovery of the renin angiotensin system. *Hypertension* 2001; 38:1246-1249.

[4] Lewin A, Blaufox MD, Castle H, Entwisle G, Langford H. Apparent prevalence of curable hypertension in the Hypertension Detection and Follow-up Program. Arch. *Intern. Med.* 1985;145:424.

[5] Taler SJ, Textor SC, Augustine JE. Resistant hypertension: comparing hemodynamic management to specialist care. *Hypertension.* 2002;39: 982-988.

[6] Olin JW, Pierce M. Contemporary management of fibromuscular dysplasia. *Curr. Opin. Cardiol.* 2008; 23:527-536.

[7] Lerman LO, Textor SC, Grande JP. Mechanisms of Tissue Injury in Renal Artery Stenosis:Ischemia and Beyond. *Prog. Cardiovasc. Dis.* 2009;52: 196–203.

[8] Deal JE, Snell MF, Barratt TM, Dillon MJ. Renovascular disease in childhood. *J. Pediatr.* 1992;121:378-384.

[9] Piercy KT, Hundley JC, Stafford JM, Craven TE, Nagaraj SK, Dean RH, Hansen KJ. Renovascular disease in children and adolescents. *J. Vasc. Surg.* 2005;41:973-982.

[10] Pascual A, Bush HS, Copley JB Renal fibromuscular dysplasia in elderly persons. *Am. J. Kidney Dis.* 2005;45:63-66.

[11] Mousa AY, Campbell JE, Stone PA, Broce M, Bates MC, AbuRahma AF. Short- and long-term outcomes of percutaneous transluminal angioplasty/stenting of renal fibromuscular dysplasia over a ten-year period. *J. Vasc. Surg.* 2012;55:421-7.

[12] Estepa R, Gallego N, Orte L, Puras E, Aracil E, Ortuño J. Renovascular hypertension in children. *Scand. J. Urol. Nephrol.* 2001;35:388-392.

[13] Neymark E, LaBerge JM, Hirose R, Melzer JS, Kerlan RK Jr, Wilson MW, Gordon RL. Arteriographic detection of renovascular disease in potential renal donors: incidence and effect on donor surgery. Radiology. 2000;214:755-760.

[14] Lorenz EC, Vrtiska TJ, Lieske JC, Dillon JJ, Stegall MD, Li X, Bergstralh EJ, Rule AD Prevalence of renal artery and kidney abnormalities by computed tomography among healthy adults. *Clin. J. Am. Soc. Nephrol.* 2010;5:431-438.

[15] Textor SC. Renovascular hypertension update. *Curr. Hypertens. Rep.* 2006;8:521–527.

[16] Garovic V, Textor SC. Renovascular hypertension and ischemic nephropathy. *Circulation.* 2005;112:1362-1374.

[17] Krishna A, Kumar O, Kumar MS. Renovascular hypertension: A review article. Clinical queries: nephrology. 2013; 2: 38-48.

[18] Pradhan N, Rossi NF. Interactions between the sympathetic nervous system and Angiotensin system in renovascular hypertension. *Curr. Hypertens. Rev.* 2013;9:121-129.

[19] Martinez-Maldonado M. Pathophysiology of renovascular hypertension. *Hypertension* 1991; 17: 707-719.

[20] Naftilan AJ, Pratt RE, Eldridge CS, Lin HL, Dzau VJ. Angiotensin II induces c-fos expression in smooth muscle via transcriptional control. *Hypertension* 1989; 13: 706-711

[21] Rodrigo R, González J, Paoletto F. The role of oxidative stress in the pathophysiology of hypertension. *Hypertens. Res.* 2011;34:431-440.

[22] Campos RR, Oliveira-Sales EB, Nishi EE, Boim MA, Dolnikoff MS, Bergamaschi CT. The role of oxidative stress in renovascular hypertension. *Clin. Exp. Pharmacol. Physiol.* 2011;38:144-152.

[23] Brinckerhoff CE, Matrisian LM. Matrix metalloproteinases: a tail of a frog that became a prince. *Nat. Rev. Mol. Cell Biol.* 2002;3:207–214.

[24] Visse R, Nagase H. Matrix metalloproteinases and tissue inhibitors of metalloproteinases: structure, function, and biochemistry. *Circ. Res.* 2003;92:827–839

[25] Watts SW, Rondelli C, Thakali K, Li X, Uhal B, Pervaiz MH, Watson RE, Fink GD. Morphological and biochemical characterization of remodeling in aorta and vena cava of doca-salt hypertensive rats. *Am. J. Physiol. Heart, Circ. Physiol.* 2007;292:2438–2448.

[26] Derosa G, D'Angelo A, Ciccarelli L, Piccinni MN, Pricolo F, Salvadeo S, Montagna L, Gravina A, Ferrari I, Galli S, Paniga S, Tinelli C, Cicero AF.Matrix metalloproteinase-2, -9, and tissue inhibitor of metalloproteinase-1 in patients with hypertension. *Endothelium* 2006;13:227–231.

[27] Tallant C, Marrero A, Gomis-Rüth FX. Matrix metalloproteinases: fold and function of their catalytic domains. *Biochim. Biophys. Acta.* 2010;1803:20-28.

[28] Oliveira-Sales EB, Dugaich AP, Carillo BA, Abreu NP, Boim MA, Martins PJ, D'Almeida V, Dolnikoff MS, Bergamaschi CT, Campos RR. Oxidative stress contributes to renovascular hypertension. *Am. J. Hypertens.* 2008;21:98-104.

[29] Schnackenberg CG: Physiological and pathophysiological roles of oxygen radicals in the renal microvasculature. *Am. J. Physiol. Regul. Integr. Comp. Physiol.* 2002;282:335-342.

[30] Lerman LO, Nath KA, Rodriguez-Porcel M, Krier JD, Schwartz RS, Napoli C, Romero JC. Increased oxidative stress in experimental renovascular hypertension. *Hypertension* 2001;37:541-546.

[31] Chade AR, Best PJ, Rodriguez-Porcel M, Herrmann J, Zhu X, Sawamura T, Napoli C, Lerman A, Lerman LO. Endothelin-1 receptor blockade prevents renal injury in experimental hypercholesterolemia. *Kidney Int.* 2003;64:962-969.

[32] Zhu XY, Chade AR, Rodriguez-Porcel M, Bentley MD, Ritman EL, Lerman A, Lerman LO. Cortical microvascular remodeling in the stenotic kidney: role of increased oxidative stress. *Arterioscler. Thromb. Vasc. Biol.* 2004;24:1854-1859.

[33] Chade AR, Rodriguez-Porcel M, Herrmann J, Zhu X, Grande JP, Napoli C, Lerman A, Lerman LO. Antioxidant intervention blunts renal injury in experimental renovascular disease. *J. Am. Soc. Nephrol.* 2004;15:958–966.

[34] Viappiani S, Nicolescu AC, Holt A, Sawicki G, Crawford BD, León H, van Mulligen T, Schulz R. Activation and modulation of 72 kDa matrix metalloproteinase-2 by peroxynitrite and glutathione. *Biochem. Pharmacol.* 2009;77:826–834.

[35] Schulz R. Intracellular targets of matrix metalloproteinase-2 in cardiac disease: rationale and therapeutic approaches. *Annu. Rev. Pharmacol. Toxicol.* 2007;47:211–242.

[36] Arribas SM, Hinek A, Gonzalez MC. Elastic fibres and vascular structure in hypertension. *Pharmacol. Ther.* 2006;111:771–791.

[37] Rizzoni D, Muiesan ML, Porteri E, De Ciuceis C, Boari GE, Salvetti M, Paini A, Rosei EA.Vascular remodeling, macro- and microvessels: therapeutic implications. *Blood Press.* 2009;18:242–246.

[38] Hartono SP, Knudsen BE, Zubair AS, Nath KA, Textor SJ, Lerman LO, Grande JP. Redox signaling is an early event in the pathogenesis of renovascular hypertension. *Int. J. Mol. Sci.* 2013;14:18640-18656.

[39] Chabrashvili T, Tojo A, Onozato ML, Kitiyakara C, Quinn MT, Fujita T, Welch, W.J, Wilcox CS Expression and cellular localization of classic NADPH oxidase subunits in the spontaneously hypertensive rat kidney. *Hypertension* 2002; 39: 269–274.

[40] Tojo A, Onozato ML, Kobayashi N, Goto A, Matsuoka H Fujita T. Angiotensin II and oxidative stress in Dahl Salt-sensitive rat with heart failure. *Hypertension* 2002; 40: 834–839.

[41] Fedorova LV, Sodhi K, Gatto-Weis C, Puri N, Hinds TD Jr, Shapiro JI, Malhotra D. Peroxisome proliferator-activated receptor δ agonist, HPP593, prevents renal necrosis under chronic ischemia. *PLoS One.* 2013; 8:e64436.

[42] Cao YJ, He X, Wang N, He LC. Effects of imperatorin, the active component from Radix Angelicae (Baizhi), on the blood pressure and oxidative stress in 2K1C hypertensive rats. *Phytomedicine* 2013;20:1048-1054.

[43] Luft FC. Neural regulation of the immune system modulates hypertension-induced target-organ damage. *J. Am. Soc. Hypertens.* 2012; 6: 23-26.

[44] Guzik TJ, Hoch NE, Brown KA, McCann LA, Rahman A, Dikalov S, Goronzy J, Weyand C, Harrison DG. Role of the T cell in the genesis of angiotensin II induced hypertension and vascular dysfunction. *J. Exper. Med.* 2007; 204: 2449-2460.

[45] Marvar PJ, Thabet SR, Guzik TJ, Lob HE, McCann LA, Weyand C, Gordon FJ, Harrison DG. Central and peripheral mechanisms of T-lymphocyte activation and vascular inflammation produced by angiotensin II-induced hypertension. *Circ. Res.* 2010;107:263-270.

[46] Zhu XY, Chade AR, Krier JD, Daghini E, Lavi R, Guglielmotti A, Lerman A, Lerman LO. The chemokine monocyte chemoattractant protein-1 contributes to renal dysfunction in swine renovascular hypertension. *J. Hypertens.* 2009; 27:2063-73.

[47] Ozawa Y, Kobori H, Suzaki Y, Navar LG. Sustained renal interstitial macrophage infiltration following chronic angiotensin II infusions. *Am. J. Physiol. Renal Physiol.* 2007; 292:330–339.

[48] Eardley KS, Zehnder D, Quinkler M, Lepenies J, Bates RL, Savage CO, Howie AJ, Adu D, Cockwell P. The relationship between albuminuria, MCP-1/CCL2, and interstitial macrophages in chronic kidney disease. *Kidney Int.* 2006;69:1189–1197.

[49] Kitagawa K, Wada T, Furuichi K, Hashimoto H, Ishiwata Y, Asano M, Takeya M, Kuziel WA, Matsushima K, Mukaida N, Yokoyama H. Blockade of CCR2 ameliorates progressive fibrosis in kidney. *Am. J. Pathol.* 2004;165:237–246.

[50] Wynn T. Cellular and molecular mechanisms of fibrosis. *J. Pathol.* 2008;214:199–210.

[51] Chade AR, Zhu X, Mushin OP, Napoli C, Lerman A, Lerman LO. Simvastatin promotes angiogenesis and prevents microvascular remodeling in chronic renal ischemia. *Faseb. J.* 2006;20:1706–1708.

[52] Hink U, Li H, Mollnau H, Oelze M, Matheis E, Hartmann M, Skatchkov M, Thaiss F, Stahl RA, Warnholtz A, Meinertz T, Griendling K, Harrison DG, Forstermann U, Munzel T. Mechanisms underlying endothelial dysfunction in diabetes mellitus. *Circ. Res.* 2001 2;88:14-22.

[53] Meenakshi SR, Agarwal R. Nitric oxide levels in patients with chronic renal disease. *J. Clin. Diagn. Res.* 2013;7:1288-1290.

[54] Hong HJ, Loh SH, Yen MH. Suppression of the development of hypertension by the inhibitor of inducible nitric oxide synthase. *Br. J. Pharmacol.* 2000;131: 631–637.

[55] Ülker S, McMaster D, McKeown PP, Bayraktutan U. Impaired activities of antioxidant enzymes elicit endothelial dysfunction in spontaneous hypertensive rats despite enhanced vascular nitric oxide generation. *Cardiovasc. Res.* 2003; 59: 488–500.

[56] García-Saura, MF, Galisteo M, Villar IC, Bermejo A, Zarzuelo A, Vargas F, Duartel J, Effects of chronic quercetin treatment in experimental renovascular hypertension. *Mol. Cell. Biochem.* 2005; 270: 147–155.

[57] Ma XL, Gao F, Nelson AH, Lopez BL, Christopher TA, Yue TL, Barone FC. Oxidative inactivation of nitric oxide and endothelial dysfunction in stroke-prone spontaneous hypertensive rats. *J. Pharmacol. Exp. Ther.* 2001; 298: 879–885.

[58] Rodriguez-Rodriguez R, Herrera MD, de Sotomayor MA, Ruiz-Gutierrez V. Pomace Olive Oil improves endothelial function in spontaneously hypertensive rats by increasing endothelial nitric oxide synthase expression. *Am. J. Hypertens.* 2007; 20: 728–734.

[59] Yamamoto Y, Oue E. Antihypertensive effect of Quercetin in rats fed with a high-fat high-sucrose diet. *Biosci. Biotech. Bioch.* 2006;70:933–939.

[60] Chobanian AV, Bakris GL, Black HR, Cushman WC, Green LA, Izzo JL Jr, Jones DW, Materson BJ, Oparil S, Wright JT Jr, Roccella EJ; Joint National Committee on Prevention, Detection, Evaluation, and Treatment of High Blood Pressure. National

Heart, Lung, and Blood Institute; National High Blood Pressure Education Program Coordinating Committee. Seventh report of the Joint National Committee on Prevention, Detection, Evaluation, and Treatment of High Blood Pressure. *Hypertension*. 2003;42:1206-1252.

[61] Intengan HD, Schiffrin EL. Structure and mechanical properties of resistance arteries in hypertension: role of adhesion molecules and extracellular matrix determinants. *Hypertension* 2000;36:312–318.

[62] Intengan HD, Schiffrin EL. Vascular remodeling in hypertension: roles of apoptosis, inflammation, and fibrosis. *Hypertension* 2001;38:581–587.

[63] Dajnowiec D, Langille BL. Arterial adaptations to chronic changes in haemodynamic function: coupling vasomotor tone to structural remodelling. Clin Sci 2007;113:15–23.

[64] Humphrey JD. Mechanisms of arterial remodeling in hypertension: coupled roles of wall shear and intramural stress. *Hypertension* 2008;52: 195–200.

[65] Mulvany MJ. Small artery remodeling and significance in the development of hypertension. *News Physiol. Sci.* 2002;17:105–109.

[66] Nagase H, Visse R, Murphy G. Structure and function of matrix metalloproteinases and TIMPs. *Cardiovasc. Res.* 2006;69:562–573.

[67] Belo VA, Souza-Costa DC, Lana CM, Caputo FL, Marcaccini AM, Gerlach RF, Bastos MG, Tanus-Santos JE. Assessment of matrix metalloproteinase (mmp)-2, mmp-8, mmp-9, and their inhibitors, the tissue inhibitors of metalloproteinase (timp)-1 and timp-2 in obese children and adolescents. *Clin. Biochem.* 2009;42:984–990.

[68] Gonçalves FM, Jacob-Ferreira AL, Gomes VA, Casella-Filho A, Chagas AC, Marcaccini AM, Gerlach RF, Tanus-Santos JE. Increased circulating levels of matrix metalloproteinase (mmp)-8, mmp-9, and pro-inflammatory markers in patients with metabolic syndrome. *Clin. Chim. Acta* 2009;403:173–177.

[69] Palei AC, Sandrim VC, Cavalli RC, Tanus-Santos JE. Comparative assessment of matrix metalloproteinase (mmp)-2 and mmp-9, and their inhibitors, tissue inhibitors of metalloproteinase (timp)-1 and timp-2 in preeclampsia and gestational hypertension. *Clin. Biochem.* 2008;41:875–880.

[70] Brassard P, Amiri F, Schiffrin EL. Combined angiotensin ii type 1 and type 2 receptor blockade on vascular remodeling and matrix metalloproteinases in resistance arteries. *Hypertension* 2005;46:598–606.

[71] Ceron CS, Castro MM, Rizzi E, Montenegro MF, Fontana V, Salgado MC, Gerlach RF, Tanus-Santos JE. Spironolactone and hydrochlorothiazide exert antioxidant effects and reduce vascular matrix metalloproteinase-2 activity and expression in a model of renovascular hypertension. *Br. J. Pharmacol.* 2010;160:77–87.

[72] Flamant M, Placier S, Dubroca C, Esposito B, Lopes I, Chatziantoniou C, Tedgui A, Dussaule JC, Lehoux S. Role of matrix metalloproteinases in early hypertensive vascular remodeling. *Hypertension* 2007;50:212–218.

[73] Martinez ML, Castro MM, Rizzi E, Fernandes K, Demacq C, Bendhack LM, Gerlach RF, Tanus-Santos JE. Lercanidipine reduces matrix metalloproteinase-2 activity and reverses vascular dysfunction in renovascular hypertensive rats. *Eur. J. Pharmacol.* 2008;591:224–230.

[74] Ruddy JM, Jones JA, Stroud RE, Mukherjee R, Spinale FG, Ikonomidis JS. Differential effects of mechanical and biological stimuli on matrix metalloproteinase promoter activation in the thoracic aorta. *Circulation* 2009;120:262–268.

[75] Bode W, Maskos K. Structural basis of the matrix metalloproteinases and their physiological inhibitors, the tissue inhibitors of metalloproteinases. *Biol. Chem.* 2003;384:863–872.

[76] Okamoto T, Akaike T, Sawa T, Miyamoto Y, van der Vliet A, Maeda H. Activation of matrix metalloproteinases by peroxynitrite-induced protein s-glutathiolation via disulfide s-oxide formation. *J. Biol. Chem.* 2001;276:29596–29602.

[77] Yasmin, McEniery CM, Wallace S, Dakham Z, Pulsalkar P, Maki-Petaja K, Ashby MJ, Cockcroft JR, Wilkinson IB. Matrix metalloproteinase-9 (mmp-9), mmp-2, and serum elastase activity are associated with systolic hypertension and arterial stiffness. *Arterioscler. Thromb. Vasc. Biol.* 2005;25:372.

[78] D'Elia JA, Weinrauch LA. The autonomic nervous system and renal physiology. *Int. J. Nephrol. Renovasc. Dis.* 2013;6:149-160.

[79] DiBona GF. Neural control of the kidney: functionally specific renal nerve fibers. The Starling Lecture. *Am. J. Physiol. Regul. Integr. Comp. Physiol.* 2000;279:1517–1524.

[80] Kopp UC, Grisk O, Cicha MZ, Smith LA, Steinbach A, Schlüter T, Mähler N, Hökfelt T. Dietary sodium modulates the interaction between efferent renal sympathetic nerve activity and afferent renal nerve activity: role of endothelin. *Am. J. Physiol. Regul. Integr. Comp. Physiol.* 2009; 297: 337-351.

[81] Campese VM, Ku E, Park J. Sympathetic renal innervation and resistant hypertension. *Int. J. Hypertens.* 2011;2011:814354.

[82] Grassi G. Sympathetic neural activity in hypertension and related diseases. *Am. J. Hypertens.* 2010; 23: 1052-1060.

[83] Santos M, Carvalho H. Renal sympathetic denervation in resistant hypertension. *World J. Cardiol.* 2013;5:94-101.

[84] DiBona GF. Physiology in perspective: The Wisdom of the Body. Neural control of the kidney. *Am. J. Physiol. Regul. Integr. Comp. Physiol.* 2005; 289: 633- 641.

[85] DiBona GF, Sawin LL. Effect of renal denervation on dynamic autoregulation of renal blood flow. *Am. J. Physiol. Renal Physiol.* 2004; 286: 1209-1218.

[86] DiBona GF. Sympathetic nervous system and the kidney in hypertension. *Curr. Opin. Nephrol. Hypertens* 2002; 11: 197-200

[87] Clayton SC, Haack KK, Zucker IH. Renal denervation modulates angiotensin receptor expression in the renal cortex of rabbits with chronic heart failure. *Am. J. Physiol. Renal Physiol.* 2011; 300: 31-39.

[88] Hendel MD, Collister JP. Renal denervation attenuates longterm hypertensive effects of Angiotensin ii in the rat. *Clin. Exp. Pharmacol. Physiol.* 2006; 33: 1225-1230.

[89] Campese VM. Neurogenic factors and hypertension in renal disease. *Kidney Int. Suppl.* 2000; 75: 2-6.

[90] Hering D, Lambert EA, Marusic P, Walton AS, Krum H, Lambert GW, Esler MD, Schlaich MP. Substantial reduction in single sympathetic nerve firing after renal denervation in patients with resistant hypertension. *Hypertension* 2013; 61: 457-464.

[91] Covic A, Gusbeth-Tatomir P. The role of the renin-angiotensin-aldosterone system in renal artery stenosis, renovascular hypertension, and ischemic nephropathy: diagnostic implications. *Prog. Cardiovasc. Dis.* 2009;52:204-208.

[92] Yerram P, Karuparthi PR, Chaudhary K. Pathogenesis and management of renovascular hypertension and ischemic nephropathy.Minerva Urol Nefrol. 2012;64:63-72.

[93] Textor SC. Current approaches to renovascular hypertension. *Med. Clin. North Am.* 2009;93:717-732.

[94] Cervenka L, Horacek V, Vaneckova I, Hubacek JA, Oliverio MI, Coffman TM, et al. Essential role of AT1-A receptor in the development of 2K1C hypertension. *Hypertension* 2002;40:735–741.

[95] Crowley SD, Gurley SB, Oliverio MI, Pazmino AK, Griffiths R, Flannery PJ, et al. Distinct roles for the kidney and systemic tissues in blood pressure regulation by the renin-angiotensin system. *J. Clin. Invest.* 2005;115:1092–1099.

[96] Ingert C, Grima M, Coquard C, Barthelmebs M, Imbs JL. Contribution of angiotensin II internalization to intrarenal angiotensin II levels in rats. *Am. J. Physiol. Renal Physiol.* 2002; 283: 1003-1010.

[97] Navar LG, Nishiyama A. Why are angiotensin concentrations so high in the kidney? *Curr. Opin. Nephrol. Hypertension* 2004; 13: 107- 115.

[98] Takahashi N, Smithies O. Human genetics, animal models and computer simulations for studying hypertension. *Trends Genet.* 2004;20:136–145.

[99] White CJ, Ramee SR, Card HG, Abrahams LA, Svinarich JT, Wade CE, Rodkey WG, Virmani R Laser angioplasty: an atherosclerotic swine model. *Lasers Surg. Med.* 1988;8:318-321.

[100] Satokowa H, Hoshino S, Igari T, Iwaya F, Midorikawa H. The appearance of cytokines and adhesion molecules in saphenous vein valves in chronic venous insufficiency. *Phlebology* 2002;16:106–110.

[101] Takase S, Bergan JJ, Schmid-Scho¨nbein G. Expression of adhesion moleculesand cytokines on saphenous veins in chronic venous insufficiency. *Ann. Vasc. Surg.* 2000;14:427–435.

[102] Shoji M, Tsutaya S, Saito R, Takamatu H, Yasujima M. Positive association of endothelial nitric oxide synthase gene polymorphism with hypertension in northern Japan. *Life Sci.* 2000; 66:2557– 2562.

[103] Jáchymová M, Horký K, Bultas J, Kozich V, Jindra A, Peleska J, Martásek P. Association of the Glu298Asp polymorphism in the endothelial nitric oxide synthase gene with essential hypertension resistant to conventional therapy. *Biochem. Biophys. Res. Commun.* 2001;284:426 –430.

[104] Derebecka N, Holysz M, Dankowski R, Wierzchowiecki M, Trzeciak WH. Polymorphism in intron 23 of the endothelial nitric oxide synthase gene (NOS3) is not associated with hypertension. Acta Biochim Pol 2002;49:263– 268.

[105] Rudic RD, Shesely EG, Maeda N, Smithies O, Segal SS, Sessa WC. Direct evidence for the importance of endothelium-derived nitric oxide in vascular remodeling. *J. Clin. Invest.* 1998;101:731–736.

[106] Kubis N, Besnard S, Silvestre JS, Feletou M, Huang PL, Lévy BI, Tedgui A. Decreased arteriolar density in endothelial nitric oxide synthase knockout mice is due to hypertension, not to the constitutive defect in endothelial nitric oxide synthase enzyme. *J. Hypertens.* 2002;20:273– 280.

[107] Li W, Mital S, Ojaimi C, Csiszar A, Kaley G, Hintze TH. Premature death and age-related cardiac dysfunction in male eNOS-knockout mice. *J. Mol. Cell Cardiol.* 2004;37:671-680.

[108] DiBona GF, Esler M. Translational medicine: the antihypertensive effect of renal denervation. *Am. J. Physiol. Regu.l Integr. Comp. Physiol.* 2010; 298: 245-253.

[109] Ye S, Zhong H, Yanamadala V, Campese VM. Renal injury caused by intrarenal injection of phenol increases afferent and efferent renal sympathetic nerve activity. *Am. J. Hypertens.* 2002; 15: 717-724.

[110] Hackam DG, Spence JD, Garg AX, Textor SC. The role of renin-angiotensin system blockade in atherosclerotic renal artery stenosis and renovascular hypertension. *Hypertension* 2007;50:998– 1003.

[111] Yusuf S, Teo KK, Pogue J, Dyal L, Copland I, Schumacher H, et al. Telmisartan, ramipril, or both in patients at high risk for vascular events. *N. Engl. J. Med.* 2008;358:1547–1559.

[112] Missouris CG, Belli AM, MacGregor GA. "Apparent" heart failure: a syndrome caused by renal artery stenoses. *Heart.* 2000;83:152-155.

[113] Hirsch AT, Haskal ZJ, Hertzer NR, Bakal CW, Creager MA, Halperin JL, Hiratzka LF, Murphy WR, Olin JW, Puschett JB, Rosenfield KA, Sacks D, Stanley JC, Taylor LM Jr, White CJ, White J, White RA, Antman EM, Smith SC Jr, Adams CD, Anderson JL, Faxon DP, Fuster V, Gibbons RJ, Hunt SA, Jacobs AK, Nishimura R, Ornato JP, Page RL, Riegel B; American Association for Vascular Surgery; Society for Vascular Surgery; Society for Cardiovascular Angiography and Interventions; Society for Vascular Medicine and Biology; Society of Interventional Radiology. Practice Guidelines for the management of patients with peripheral arterial disease (lower extremity, renal, mesenteric, and abdominal aortic): a collaborative report from the American Association for Vascular Surgery/Society for Vascular Surgery, Society for Cardiovascular Angiography and Interventions, Society for Vascular Medicine and Biology, Society of Interventional Radiology, and the ACC/AHA Task Force on Practice Guidelines (Writing Committee to Develop Guidelines for the Management of Patients With Peripheral Arterial Disease): endorsed by the American Association of Cardiovascular and Pulmonary Rehabilitation; National Heart, Lung, and Blood Institute; Society for Vascular Nursing; TransAtlantic Inter-Society Consensus; and Vascular Disease Foundation. *Circulation* 2006; 113:463.

[114] Textor SC. Renovascular hypertension: is there still a role for stent revascularization? *Curr. Opin. Nephrol. Hypertens.* 2013;22:525-530.

[115] Fagard R, Narkiewicz K, Redon J, Zanchetti A, Böhm M, Christiaens T, Cifkova R, De Backer G, Dominiczak A, Galderisi M, Grobbee DE, Jaarsma T, Kirchhof P, Kjeldsen SE, Laurent S, Manolis AJ, Nilsson PM, Ruilope LM, Schmieder RE, Sirnes PA, Sleight P, Viigimaa M, Waeber B, Zannad F; ESH Scientific Council, Redon J, Dominiczak A, Narkiewicz K, Nilsson PM, Burnier M, Viigimaa M, Ambrosioni E, Caufield M, Coca A, Olsen MH, Schmieder RE, Tsioufis C, van de Borne P, ESC Committee for Practice Guidelines (CPG), Zamorano JL, Achenbach S, Baumgartner H, Bax JJ, Bueno H, Dean V, Deaton C, Erol C, Fagard R, Ferrari R, Hasdai D, Hoes AW, Kirchhof P, Knuuti J, Kolh P, Lancellotti P, Linhart A, Nihoyannopoulos P, Piepoli MF, Ponikowski P, Sirnes PA, Tamargo JL, Tendera M, Torbicki A, Wijns W, Windecker S; Document Reviewers, Clement DL, Coca A, Gillebert TC, Tendera M, Rosei EA, Ambrosioni E, Anker SD, Bauersachs J, Hitij JB, Caulfield M, De Buyzere M, De Geest S, Derumeaux GA, Erdine S, Farsang C, Funck-Brentano C, Gerc V, Germano G, Gielen S, Haller H, Hoes AW, Jordan J, Kahan T, Komajda M, Lovic D, Mahrholdt H, Olsen MH, Ostergren J, Parati G, Perk J, Polonia J, Popescu BA, Reiner Z, Rydén L, Sirenko Y, Stanton A, Struijker-Boudier H, Tsioufis C, van de Borne P,

Vlachopoulos C, Volpe M, Wood DA. 2013 ESH/ESC Guidelines for the management of arterial hypertension: The Task Force for the management of arterial hypertension of the European Society of Hypertension (ESH) and of the European Society of Cardiology (ESC). *Eur. Heart J.* 2013;34:2159-2219.

[116] Wright JR, Shurrab AE, Cheung C, Waldek S, O'Donoghue DJ, Foley RN, Mamtora H, Kalra PA.A prospective study of the determinants of renal functional outcome and mortality in atherosclerotic renovascular disease. *Am. J. Kidney Dis.* 2002;39:1153-1161.

[117] Kent D, Hayward R. When averages hide individual differences in clinical trials. *American Scientist* 2007;95:60–68.

[118] Textor SC, Lerman L, McKusick M. The uncertain value of renal artery interventions: where are we now? *JACC Cardiovasc. Interv.* 2009;2:175-82.

[119] Uzzo RG, Novick AC, Goormastic M, Mascha E, Pohl M. Medical versus surgical management of atherosclerotic renal artery stenosis. *Transplantation Proc.* 2002;34:723-725.

[120] ASTRAL Investigators, Wheatley K, Ives N, Gray R, Kalra PA, Moss JG, Baigent C, Carr S, Chalmers N, Eadington D, Hamilton G, Lipkin G, Nicholson A, Scoble J. Revascularization versus medical therapy for renal-artery stenosis. *N. Engl. J. Med.* 2009; 361:1953-1962.

[121] Bax L, Woittiez AJ, Kouwenberg HJ, Mali WP, Buskens E, Beek FJ, Braam B, Huysmans FT, Schultze Kool LJ, Rutten MJ, Doorenbos CJ, Aarts JC, Rabelink TJ, Plouin PF, Raynaud A, van Montfrans GA, Reekers JA, van den Meiracker AH, Pattynama PM, van de Ven PJ, Vroegindeweij D, Kroon AA, de Haan MW, Postma CT, Beutler JJ. Stent placement in patients with atherosclerotic renal artery stenosis and impaired renal function: a randomized trial. *Ann. Intern. Med.* 2009;150:840-848.

[122] Marcantoni C, Zanoli L, Rastelli S, Tripepi G, Matalone M, Mangiafico S, Capodanno D, Scandura S, Di Landro D, Tamburino C, Zoccali C, Castellino P. Effect of renal artery stenting on left ventricular mass: a randomized clinical trial. *Am. J. Kidney Dis.* 2012;60:39-46.

[123] van Jaarsveld BC, Krijnen P, Pieterman H, Derkx FH, Deinum J, Postma CT, Dees A, Woittiez AJ, Bartelink AK, Man in 't Veld AJ, Schalekamp MA The effect of balloon angioplasty on hypertension in atherosclerotic renal-artery stenosis. Dutch Renal Artery Stenosis Intervention Cooperative Study Group. *N. Engl. J. Med.* 2000;342:1007-1014.

[124] Plouin PF, Chatellier G, Darné B, Raynaud A. Blood pressure outcome of angioplasty in atherosclerotic renal artery stenosis: a randomized trial. Essai Multicentrique Medicaments vs Angioplastie (EMMA) Study Group. *Hypertension* 1998; 31:823-829.

[125] Webster J, Marshall F, Abdalla M, Dominiczak A, Edwards R, Isles CG, Loose H, Main J, Padfield P, Russell IT, Walker B, Watson M, Wilkinson R Randomised comparison of percutaneous angioplasty vs continued medical therapy for hypertensivepatients with atheromatous renal artery stenosis. Scottish and Newcastle Renal Artery StenosisCollaborative Group. *J. Hum. Hypertens.* 1998;15:329-335.

[126] Kumbhani DJ, Bavry AA, Harvey JE, de Souza R, Scarpioni R, Bhatt DL. Kapadia SR. Clinical outcomes after percutaneous revascularization versus medical management in patients with significant renal artery stenosis: a meta-analysis of randomized controlled trials. *Am. Heart J.* 2011; 161:622-630.

[127] Murphy TP, Soares G, Kim M. Increase in utilization of percutaneous renal artery interventions by Medicare beneficiaries 1996–2000. *AJR Am. J. Roentgenol.* 2004;183:561-568.

[128] Carr TM 3rd, Sabri SS, Turba UC, Park AW, Saad WE, Angle JF, Matsumoto AH. Stenting for atherosclerotic renal artery stenosis. *Tech. Vasc. Interv. Radiol.* 2010;13:134-145.

[129] Rundback JH, Gray RJ, Rozenblit G, Poplausky MR, Babu S, Shah P, Butt K, Tomasula J, Garrick R, Goodman A, Dolmatch B, Horton K. Renal artery stent placement for the management of ischemic nephropathy. *J. Vasc. Interv. Radiol.* 1998;9:413-420.

[130] Henry M, Henry I, Polydorou A, Polydorou AD, Hugel M. Recent advances in renal artery stenting. *J. Cardiovasc. Surg.* 2007;48:411-442.

[131] Blum U, Krumme B, Flügel P, Gabelmann A, Lehnert T, Buitrago-Tellez C, Schollmeyer P, Langer M. Treatment of ostial renal-artery stenoses with vascular endoprostheses after unsuccessful balloon angioplasty. *N. Engl. J. Med.*; 1997; 336:459-465.

[132] Bloch MJ, Trost DW, Sos TA. J Type B aortic dissection complicating renal artery angioplasty and stent placement. *Vasc. Interv. Radiol.* 2001;12:517-520.

[133] Harden PN, MacLeod MJ, Rodger RS, Baxter GM, Connell JM, Dominiczak AF, Junor BJ, Briggs JD, Moss JG. Effect of renal-artery stenting on progression of renovascular renal failure. *Lancet* 199719;349:1133-1136.

[134] Laragh JH, Sealey J, Brunner HR. The control of aldosterone secretion in normal and hypertensive man: abnormal renin-aldosterone patterns in low renin hypertension. *Am. J. Med.* 1972;53:649-663.

[135] Shesely EG, Maeda N, Kim HS, Desai KM, Krege JH, Laubach VE, Sherman PA, Sessa WC, Smithies O. Elevated blood pressures in mice lacking endothelial nitric oxide synthase. *Proc. Natl. Acad. Sci. USA* 1996;93:13176– 13181.

[136] Ülker S, McKeown PP, Bayraktutan U. Vitamins reverse endothelial dysfunction through regulation of eNOS and NAD(P)H oxidase activities. *Hypertension* 2003; 41: 534 539.

[137] Roubidoux MA, Dunnick NR, Klotman PE, Newman GE, Cohan RH, Kadir S, Svetkey LP. Renal vein renins: Inability to predict response to revascularisation in patients with hypertension. *Radiology* 1991;178:819-822.

[138] Reusz GS, Kis E, Cseprekál O, Szabó AJ, Kis E. Captopril-enhanced renal scintigraphy in the diagnosis of pediatric hypertension. *Pediatr. Nephrol.* 2010;25:185-189.

[139] Desberg AL, Paushter DM, Lammert GK, Hale JC, Troy RB, Novick AC, Nally JV Jr, Weltevreden AM. Renal artery stenosis: evaluation with color Doppler flow imaging. *Radiology* 1990 ;177:749-753.

[140] Rountas C, Vlychou M, Vassiou K, Liakopoulos V, Kapsalaki E, Koukoulis G, Fezoulidis IV, Stefanidis I. Imaging modalities for renal artery stenosis in suspected renovascular hypertension: prospective intraindividual comparison of color Doppler US, CT angiography, GD-enhanced MR angiography, and digital substraction angiography. *Ren. Fail.* 2007;29:295-302.

[141] Ziviello M. The risk in renal angiography. *Radiol. Med.* 1978;64:479-484.

In: Advances in Hypertension Research
Editor: Ramón Rodrigo
ISBN: 978-1-62948-857-8

Chapter 5

Hypertension in Metabolic Syndrome*

Cristóbal Orellana*†, *Felipe Parra and Roberto Brito
Molecular and Clinical Pharmacology Program, Institute of Biomedical Sciences,
Faculty of Medicine, University of Chile, Chile

Abstract

Metabolic syndrome (MS) is a highly prevalent pathological condition which can be defined as a cluster of metabolic disorders that are associated with increased risk of type 2 diabetes (T2D) and cardiovascular disease (CVD). One of the disorders occurring in MS is hypertension, which is by itself an important cardiovascular risk factor. There are mainly three mechanisms involved in the pathophysiology of MS`s hypertension: sympathetic hyperactivation, increased renin-angiotensin-aldosterone activity and endothelial dysfunction, being the later considered the most important. There has been an increasing interest in fully understanding the role of adipose tissue in MS-related hypertension, including the contribution of the perivascular adipose tissue, a new promising type of metabolic active adipocytes. The adipose tissue has the ability to release a large amount of mediators contributing to blood pressure modulation. Nowadays, there are several experimental model animals that allow researchers to study hypertension in MS. The animal models can be divided into two groups: genetic models and dietary-induced models of MS. Despite the fact that the animal models present mostly hypertension, they also have the other metabolic disorders of MS, allowing feasible the global study of this disease. Finally, nowadays the most widely accepted therapy of hypertension in MS is the same used in essential hypertension, including the use of beta-blockers and inhibitors of the renin-angiotensin-aldosterone system. New studies are trying to demonstrate the beneficial effects of antioxidant therapy in MS. Nevertheless, novel research lines are just emerging to generate pharmacological therapies with agents targeting specific mechanisms responsible for blood pressure elevation in MS. The development of new studies related with the complex processes

* Supported by FONDECYT, grant 1120594
† Corresponding Author: Lic. Cristóbal Orellana, Molecular and Clinical Pharmacology Program, Institute of Biomedical Sciences, Faculty of Medicine, University of Chile, Independencia 1027, C.P 8380453, Santiago 7, Chile, Telephone: 56-2-29786126 Fax: 56-2-29786126, E-mail: cristobalorellanagajardo@gmail.com.

involved in MS hypertension is currently improving the knowledge of this fascinating pathological condition, but new research efforts are still needed.

Keywords: Hypertension, metabolic syndrome, endothelial dysfunction

Abbreviations

ACE	Angiotensin I converting enzyme
ARB	Angiotensin Receptor Blocker
ATP	Adult Treatment Panel
BMI	Body Mass Index
CCK	Cholecystokinin
CHD	Coronary Heart Disease
CoQ10	Coenzyme Q10
CRP	C Reactive Protein
CVD	Cardiovascular Disease
EDHF	Endothelium Derived Hyperpolarizing Factor
eNOS	Endothelial Nitric Oxide Synthase
ET-1	Endothelin-1
FFA	Free Fatty Acids
FPG	Fasting Plasma Glucose
IDF	International Diabetes Federation
IL	Interleukin
IRS	Insulin receptor substrate
MS	Metabolic Syndrome
NCEP	National Cholesterol Education Program
NO	Nitric Oxide
NOS	Nitric Oxide Synthase
OLETF	Otsuka Long-Evans Tokushima Fatty Rats
PVAT	perivascular adipose tissue
RAAS	Renin-Angiotensin-Aldosterone System
ROS	Reactive Oxygen Species
SHROB	Spontaneously Hypertensive Obese Rat
T2D	Type 2 diabetes
TNF	Tumor Necrosis Factor
UT-II	Urotensin II
ZDF	Zucker Diabetic Fatty Rat

1. Introduction

Cardiovascular Disease (CVD) deaths are actually a huge problem worldwide. According to the World Health Organization's report, an estimated 17.3 million people died from CVD in 2008, representing 30% of all global deaths [1]. In relation to this, it has been estimated that the global mortality due to ischemic heart disease in developing countries, since 1990 will increase in 120% for women and in 137% for men by 2020, and 29% for women and 48% for men in developed countries [2]. It's for this reason that most of the efforts have been focused on determining the risk factors for CVD, to allow the prevention and management of this spectrum of diseases.

One of the most important CVD risk factor is the Metabolic Syndrome (MS), which is a multifactorial cluster of metabolic abnormalities. The analysis of a representative sample of United States of America adult population showed that MS affects approximately 24% of the individuals, being highly prevalent [3]. A more recent study found that approximately 34% of adults met the National Cholesterol Education Program (NCEP)-ATP III criteria for MS, showing an important increase of its prevalence [4]. On the other hand, Beltrán-Sánchez et al. found that, from 1999 to 2010, the prevalence of MS decreased from 25% to 23% in USA population, and so did hypertriglyceridemia prevalence and elevated blood pressure, possibly because of the increase of lipid-modifying and anti-hypertensive drugs, and also demonstrated that the prevalence of hyperglycemia and elevated waist circumference (WC) increased [5]. Other important aspect of MS is the following: It has been reported a high prevalence of MS in developing countries around the world [6]; for example: Venezuela (31.2%) [7], Mexico (26.6%) [8], Iran (33.7%) [9] and Turkey (33.4%) [10], among others. All the evidence mentioned above demonstrates the importance of the MS as a public health problem worldwide.

Several definitions of MS have been proposed. According to the ATP III of the NCEP, the diagnosis of MS requires the presence of at least three of the following risk factors: (i) Fasting plasma glucose (FPG) ≥ 100mg/dL (5.6mmol/L); (i) blood pressure ≥ 130/85 mmHg; (iii) triglyceride ≥ 150 mg/dL (1.7 mmol/L); (d) HDL cholesterol: men < 40mg/dL (1.03 mmol/L); women <50mg/dL (1.29 mmol/L); (e) men with WC > 102 cm. and women with WC >88 cm. [11]. Other MS criteria are those from the International Diabetes Federation (IDF). It says that a patient has MS if he/she has a WC ≥ 94 cm. in men and ≥ 80 cm. in women plus any two of these risk factors: (a) fasting plasma glucose (FPG) ≥ 100 mg/dL (5.6 mmol/L) or previously diagnosed impaired fasting glucose (b) blood pressure ≥ 130/85mmHg or treatment for hypertension; (c) Triglyceride ≥ 150 mg/dL (1.7 mmol/L); (d) HDL Cholesterol: men < 40 mg/dL (1.03 mmol/L); women < 50 mg/dL (1.29 mmol/L) or treatment for low HDL [12]. Despite the differences, all definitions of MS consider metabolic variables that depend largely on lifestyle. For example, the weight loss, mainly because of lifestyle changing instead of pharmacology treatment, has an important impact on reducing the prevalence of MS [13].

1.1. Metabolic Syndrome as a Risk Factor

A large amount of studies show that MS is an important risk factor for several diseases. For example, in an 11 years follow-up, men and women with the metabolic syndrome were 1.5 and 2 times more likely to develop coronary heart disease (CHD) than control subjects, respectively, while elevated blood pressure and low levels of HDL cholesterol exhibited the strongest associations with CVD [14]. Other study shows that MS is associated with a 2 fold increase in cardiovascular outcomes and a 1.5 fold increase in all-cause mortality [15]. Another interesting aspect is that rates for future cardiovascular events and coronary and carotid atherosclerosis were similar for subjects with the MS compared with CHD equivalent; and combined, the two conditions identified 70% of subjects who developed events [16], providing a new clinical tool for the management of CVD.

MS also increases the risk for Type 2 diabetes (T2D). Compared with persons without MS, those with the syndrome have an approximate 5-fold increase in diabetes risk [17]. In this regard, Lorenzo et al. demonstrated that the risk of T2D given by the presence of MS doesn't depend on concomitant impaired glucose tolerance, and when combined the two conditions, the risk is increased even more [18]. Recently, the analysis of two prospective studies showed that MS has a stronger association with new-onset T2D, rather than cardiovascular risk [19]. An important fact is that these studies considered only elderly population (individuals aged 60-82 years) [19].

Some studies have shown differences depending on the definition of MS used. For example, despite the fact that CVD prevalence was increased in patients with MS by using any of the existing definitions, Athyros et al. obtained a higher increase when the NCEP-ATP III criteria was implemented compared with the IDF definition [20]. Also, MS defined by the NCEP-ATP III criteria, when compared with the others definitions, is a strong predictor of uncontrolled hypertension and allows to identify patients at risk of poor blood pressure control [21], and the presence of MS, according to the NCEP-ATP III criteria but not the IDF definition, in T2D patients has a significant association with chronic kidney disease, allowing to recognize patients with higher risk [22]. Nevertheless, Mancia et al. demonstrated that the risk of cardiovascular events and T2D was similar for the different definitions of MS [23].

1.2. Metabolic Syndrome and Hypertension

Actually, 7.6 million premature deaths per year (13.5% of total) are attributable to high blood pressure [24]. Hypertension is considered to be the most important risk factor in the development of CVD worldwide [25], and the relationship between blood pressure and cardiovascular risk increases progressively [26]. High blood pressure induces structural changes in arterial system that affects mainly important organs, such as brain, heart, kidney, determining the principal complications of the disease [24].

Between all the components of MS, hypertension appears to be the strongest predictor of cardiovascular mortality [27]. Apparently, the concomitant presence of hypertension and MS would increase systemic organ damage caused by hypertension [28].

Considering the above, in this chapter we proposed to present new insight about the hypertension in the context of MS, including its pathophysiology, animal models and novel therapies, with the aim of encouraging the research in this not-yet fully elucidated field.

2. Pathophysiology

2.1. Metabolic Syndrome: General Overview

MS has multiple pathological mechanisms involved, which present a complex relationship between them. In this section, we will review the general mechanisms underlying

MS, giving the background to analyze new advances in pathophysiology of hypertension in MS.

2.1.1. Obesity, Free Fatty Acids and Cytokines in MS

Although not all obese develop insulin resistance and MS, obesity is the most prevalent component [5] of MS and is considered a key factor in the development of this syndrome and a major risk factor for CVD. In this sphere, intra-abdominal obesity has been found to associated with all the cluster of metabolic abnormalities in MS. Abnormalities in the structure and function of adipose tissue, mainly in visceral adipose tissue, have been identified as an early event in the development of MS [29].

In obese patients, it has been shown an increased free fatty acid (FFA) release from the adipocyte, mainly because hypertrophied adipocytes have a hyperlipolytic phenotype that is resistant to insulin [30, 31]. This high release of FFA produces a high flow of them to the liver, where they interfere with adequate hepatic metabolism, leading to an increase in hepatic glucose production. Another effect of FFA is the decrease in the availability of glucose in peripheral tissues [32, 33].

An early event, which follows adipose tissue increased metabolic activity, is the infiltration of macrophages in fat tissue [34], leading both an increase in the secretion of leptin and inflammatory mediators such as tumor necrosis factor (TNF)α and Interleukin (IL) 6, and also a decrease in the secretion of adiponectin [35, 36].

Selective hypothalamus leptin resistance has also been described in MS [37]. The principal consequence of the leptin-resistant state is enhanced insulin resistance. Additionally, the innate immune system can be stimulated by leptin, contributing to an increase inflammatory phenotype [38]. Adiponectin is a protein secreted by adipocytes, which has multiple functions, among which highlights its insulin sensitizing effect [39]. This effect is produced, among other mechanisms, by the increase in intracellular fatty acid oxidation in muscle and liver, by stimulation of AMP kinase. Due to its insulin sensitizing function, low levels of adiponectin enhance insulin resistance.

2.1.2. Insulin Resistance

Insulin resistance is established in the skeletal muscle and in the liver as a result of accumulation of diacylglycerol and acyl-CoAs in cytoplasm. This accumulation increases serine kinase activity, which leads to the suppression of insulin signaling by reducing Insulin receptor substrate (IRS)-1. This inhibits the glucose insulin-stimulated transport. Among the main mechanisms contributing to lipid accumulation in the liver and skeletal muscle, there is an increase in the release of FFA and cytokines from adipose tissue and a decrease in the oxidative capacity of the mitochondria [40].

Insulin resistance leads to disturbances in glucose tolerance and dyslipidemia. The dyslipidemic state associated with insulin resistance is characterized by elevated triglyceride and total cholesterol levels, normal or low plasma levels of LDL and low HDL plasma levels [33].

2.1.3. Metabolic Syndrome: A Systemic Oxidative Stress State

There is a large amount of studies that provide evidence about oxidative stress and its central role in the pathophysiology of MS. From a clinical point of view, reports from the

Third National Health and Nutrition Examination Survey indicate diminished concentrations of the antioxidants vitamins C and E and several carotenoids in participants with MS [41], indicating a possibly disrupted antioxidant defense system in MS. Animal models also reinforce the idea described above.

Studies in a diet-induced rat model of MS found increased oxidative stress and endothelial dysfunction, mainly by an increased NADPH oxidase activity and a downregulation of superoxide dismutase [42]. An interesting fact is that obese mice treated with apocynin, a NAD(P)H oxidase inhibitor, presented a reduction in reactive oxygen species (ROS) levels and an improvement in glucose and lipid metabolism, independent of body weight [43].

Considering the insulin resistance as a central mechanism underlying MS, it is important to mention that, despite it develops mainly secondary to obesity, increased ROS have also been shown to have a causal role insulin resistance [44]. In this regard, it can be mentioned that high doses of hydrogen peroxide [43] and reagents that accumulate ROS [45] can induce insulin resistance in adipocytes. It has been also demonstrated that the up-regulation of genes responsible for ROS production occurs in adipose tissue before the onset of insulin resistance and obesity in mice fed a high fat-diet [46], suggesting that oxidative stress could be the triggering factor that leads to an insulin resistance state in MS. A consequence of systemic oxidative stress present in MS is increased in oxidized LDL plasma levels in patients with the syndrome [47].

2.1.4. Metabolic Syndrome: A Systemic Proinflammatory State

Consistent with the above, MS has been described as a proinflammatory state, with increased levels of proinflammatory cytokines such as TNFα, (IL) 6, C Reactive Protein (CRP), (IL) 1, resistin, among others, and a decrease in levels of antiinflammatory molecules, mainly adiponectin [48, 49, 50, 51]. CRP is a general marker of inflammation, widely used in clinic and scientific research. Elevated levels of CRP are associated with increased Body Mass Index (BMI), WC, hyperglycemia and insulin resistance. Furthermore, CRP levels independently predicted the occurrence of future CVD events [52, 53].

TNFα mRNA levels are significantly higher in adipose tissue of obese patients than in lean subjects. Furthermore, they have been shown to be elevated in patients with MS [54]. The amount of TNFα mRNA correlates positively with plasma levels of insulin [54], and TNFα plasma levels are associated with increased WC, body weight and triglycerides [50].

2.2. Hypertension in Metabolic Syndrome

Hypertension in MS appears to have multifactorial causes, and its pathological mechanisms are not fully understood. Considering this, in this section we will comment new advances in pathophysiology of hypertension in the context of MS, emphasizing in alterations of regulatory systems and in vasoactive factors that contribute to endothelial dysfunction, the key mechanism underlying hypertension in MS.

2.2.1. Regulatory Systems

Sympathetic Nervous System

The sympathetic overactivity appears to a characteristic disturbance in MS. First of all, it has been shown that serum catecholamine concentrations and muscle sympathetic nervous activity are significantly increased in obese individuals as compared with lean individuals, and, also very important, muscle sympathetic nervous activity in subjects with central obesity is significantly greater than those in individuals with peripheral obesity [55]. This adrenergic overdrive could be a key pathological factor in hypertensive mechanisms of MS. Many causes have been proposed to explain this condition. One of the first of them proposed was the hyperinsulinemia itself. It has been demonstrated that the sympathetic system mediates the pathophysiologic link between hyperinsulinemia and hypertension [56]. Despite this, one of the most accepted theories is that the main cause of the sympathetic hyperactivity are the increased plasma levels of leptin, secondary to leptin resistance present in MS. Carlyle *et al.* proved that in a murine model, leptin-induced increases in blood pressure and tachycardia are mediated by increased adrenergic activity [57]. Leptin-induced increases in sympathetic activity and blood pressure, as occurs in obesity-related hypertension, are mediated by the ventromedial and dorsomedial hypothalamus [58]. Finally, other cause that can explain the sympathetic overactivity is the hyperlipidemia, particularly the high circulating levels of FFA in visceral obese individuals with MS. In relation to this, it has been proposed that the increased release of FFA into the portal vein from lipolysis in visceral fat depots could explain the association between visceral obesity and increased sympathetic nerve outflow, given that muscle sympathetic nerve activity is more closely associated with the level of abdominal visceral fat than total fat mass or abdominal subcutaneous fat [59]. Thus, all the mechanisms described above converge at the activation of the sympathetic system, contributing to the development of hypertension in the context of MS.

Renin-Angiotensin-Aldosterone System

The renin-angiotensin-aldosterone system (RAAS) plays a crucial role in blood pressure regulation, by affecting renal function and by modulating vascular tone. There is a large amount of evidence that suggests the idea that in subjects with MS there is an increased RAAS activity, and thereby contributes to the hypertension in the context of the syndrome. For example, aldosterone appears to be higher in obese subjects compared with lean patients and abdominal obesity correlates strongly with aldosterone levels in plasma [60]. Other study showed also increased plasmatic levels of aldosterone and also renin in patients with abdominal obesity and hyperinsulinemia [61]. And interesting fact is that aldosterone is associated with MS per se, independently of the association with its separate components [62]. Nowadays is also known that the adipose tissue also contributes to the activation of RAAS in MS. Murine models of MS have demonstrated increased activity of the adipose RAAS in obesity-related hypertension [63]. The activity of adipose tissue over RAAS would be mainly due to an increased local formation of angiotensin II [64]. Despite this, adipocyte also possesses aldosterone synthase, and adipocyte-derived aldosterone regulates adipocyte differentiation and vascular function in an autocrine and paracrine manner, respectively [65], and also secretes potent mineralocorticoid-releasing factors [66].

Although until recently it was believed that the main active secretory adipose tissue was the visceral fat. However, new research has shown the existence of another type of fat, which would have an important role in maintaining vascular homeostasis: the perivascular adipose tissue (PVAT) [67]. Lohn et al. described that PVAT presents an inhibitory effect on several pro-contractile agonists [68], while Gao et al. demonstrated that PVAT exerts its anti-contractile effects through two distinct mechanisms: by releasing a transferable relaxing factor which induces endothelium-dependent relaxation through nitric oxide (NO) release and by an endothelium-independent mechanism, possibly involving hydrogen peroxide [69]. Under pathological conditions, PVAT appears to release angiotensin-II, and thus contributing to hypertension in MS [70], but further studies are require to corroborate this. Considering the lack of evidence about the role of PVAT in hypertension in MS context, it brings new opportunities of promising research.

Besides the influence of adipose tissue in the increased activity of RAAS, other mechanism contributes to this, such as hyperinsulinemia [71], and the sympathetic overactivity present in MS.

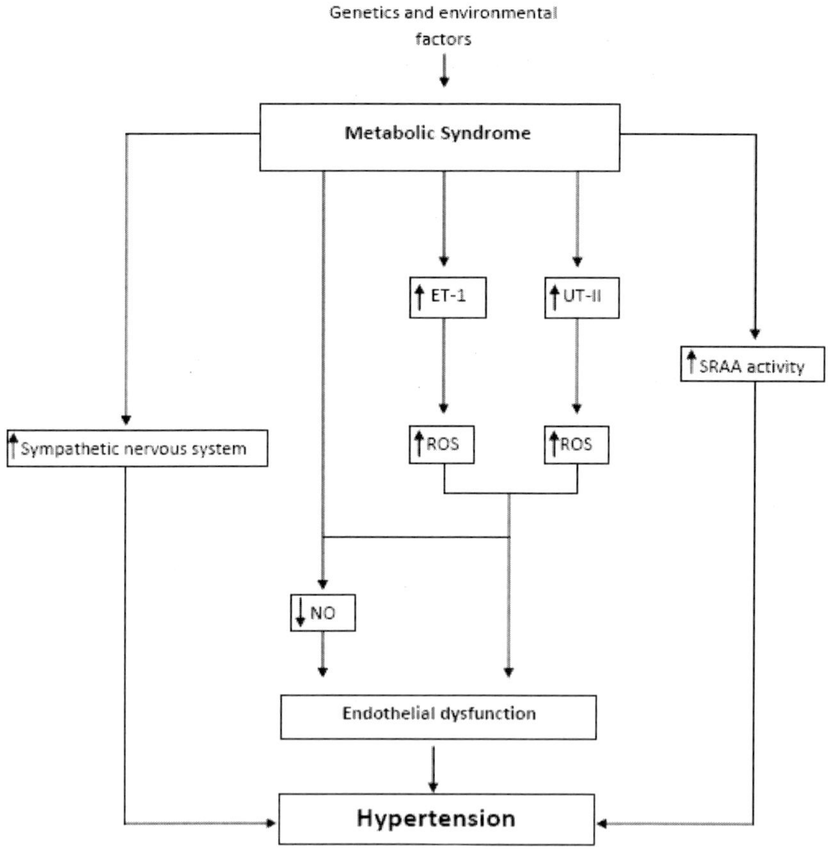

Figure 5-1. An schematic diagram illustrating the mechanism proposed of hypertension in the context of MS. Genetic and environmental factors involved in the development of the MS. Three main events are considered to be involved in the hypertension of MS: An enhanced sympathetic nervous system activity, an increased activity or renin angiotensin aldosterone system and endothelial dysfunction, which is caused by modifications in several key mediators for the vascular activity.

2.2.2. Vasoactive Factors

Nitric Oxide

It is well known that NO plays an important role as a key paracrine regulator of vascular tone and that the decrease in its bioavailability in the vasculature reduces vasodilatory capacity and contributes to hypertension. This explains the great interest generated by the study of this molecule in the context of the MS, and how can it be affected by all the alterations present in this syndrome. One aspect that is clearly not yet fully elucidated is the relation between insulin resistance, hyperinsulinemia and nitric oxide. It is well known that, under physiological conditions, insulin presents vasodilatory effects which are mediated by stimulation of NO release [72]. This mechanism allows insulin to recruits flow to the microvasculature in skeletal muscle and may be central in the regulation of glucose disposal [73].Considering this, it can be expected that in insulin resistance states, its vasodilatory effects will be diminished, and hyperinsulinemia could actually contribute to hypertension in MS. There are several studies that support this theory. For example, Kashyap *et al.* demonstrated that insulin-stimulated muscle nitric oxide synthase (NOS) activity is impaired in T2D subjects with insulin resistance, and the defect in insulin-stimulated NOS activity correlates with the severity of insulin resistance [74]. It has also has been shown that the insulin-induced increase of microvascular NO-dependent vasodilation is abolished in insulin resistance conditions [75]. Despite the facts mentioned above, new studies are required to fully understand the relation between insulin resistance and NO.

Besides insulin resistance, there are several other factors that contribute to the decrease in the bioavailability of NO in MS, and consequently to hypertension. One of the most important could be hypoadiponectinemia, which is characteristic of MS. Adiponectin has an important vascular action and directly stimulate production of NO in endothelial cells using phosphatidylinositol 3-kinase-dependent pathway [76], highlighting its importance in maintaining vascular tone under physiological conditions. Considering the above, several studies have shown that hypoadiponectinemia is implicated in genesis of hypertension. For example, Ohashi *et al.* demonstrated that adiponectin KO mice developed hypertension when maintained on a high-salt diet without insulin resistance, which was associated with reduced mRNA levels of endothelial nitric oxide synthase (eNOS) in aorta, and that adiponectin therapy lowered the elevated blood pressure [77]. A recent study shows also that adiponectin improves the redox state in human vessels by restoring eNOS coupling [78]. In this manner, all the evidence mentioned above establishes the hypoadiponectinemia as an important cause in the decrease in bioavailability of NO in MS.

Another factor that is gaining popularity is ghrelin, which is a hunger-stimulating peptide. A study made in MS patients shows that basal plasma ghrelin was significantly lower than in controls and ghrelin infusion resulted in a potentiation of the vasodilator response to acetylcholine, effect related to enhanced nitric oxide bioavailability [79]. Other study also demonstrate that in patients with MS, ghrelin has benefits to normalize the balance between vasoconstrictor mediators and NO, suggesting a protective role of ghrelin in vascular homeostasis [80]. Apparently, decreased levels of ghrelin in MS also affect NO bioavailability and contribute to the development of hypertension.

Finally, several others factors have been implied in the decrease in the bioavailability of NO in the vasculature, including hyperglycemia itself [81, 82], hyperleptinemia due to obesity-related leptin resistance [83], and mediators related to the proinflammatory and oxidative stress state characteristic of MS.

Endothelin-1

Endothelins are potent vasoconstrictor isopeptides produced in different vascular tissues, including vascular endothelium. Endothelin-1 (ET-1) is the main endothelin generated by the endothelium and the most important in the cardiovascular system. Despite the fact that ET-1 is mainly an endothelium-derived product, it is also produced by adipocytes and can be considered as an adipokine [84]. When Ferri et al. measured the circulating levels of this peptide in obese patients, their results showed significantly higher levels in patients compared with controls, and they were directly correlated with fasting insulin levels [85]. Other study showed that adipose tissue had a marked net release of ET-1 in vivo, which was 2.5-fold increase in obese patients when compared to lean subjects [86]. It has been also demonstrated that there is a significant correlation between BMI and the vasodilator response to endothelin blockade in obese-hypertensive subjects [87]. An interesting fact is that the effect of ET-1 could not be only due to its vasoconstrictor action. It has been shown that endogenous endothelin contributes directly to impair NO bioavailability in obesity [88]. All these evidence suggest that ET-1 plays an important in the pathophysiology of obesity-related hypertension. However, besides its role in hypertension, ET-1 could also contribute to insulin resistance in skeletal muscle of obese humans [89], generating a complex relation between this peptide and obesity-related disorders.

Urotensin-II

Urotensin-II (UT-II) is a potent vasoactive peptide [90], indeed the most potent vasoconstrictor identified, and acts trough activation of NADPH oxidase, increasing the levels of ROS. Recently, Gruson et al. demonstrated that UT-II plasma concentrations are significantly higher in T2D patients presenting with MS when compared with those who didn't have the syndrome [91]. Apparently, the role of UT-II in the pathogenesis of MS lies on its ability to modulate insulin resistance and inflammation [92]. Even though the epidemiological relation between MS and UT-II is yet clear, the role of UT-II in MS is not well elucidated and new studies are required.

Other Factors

Apart from the above factors, there are others that have been studied in essential hypertension, but its role in hypertension associated with MS has not been completely elucidated. Some of these are the eicosanoids and the endothelium dependent hyperpolarizing factor (EDHF). In relation to the first point, Wang et al. demonstrated that a high-fat diet causes the downregulation of CYP4A and CYP2C23 in renal tubules, which are responsible for renal 20-hydroxyeicosatetraenoic acid and epoxyeicosatrienoic acid formation [93]. The reduction in the synthesis of these eicosanoids may play an important role in the regulation of blood pressure in obesity-induced hypertension, being even a possible therapeutic target.

On the other hand is the EDHF. It has been suggested that endothelium-dependent relaxations, independent of the production of NO and PGI2, probably play an important role in cardiovascular physiology in the animal and in the human [94]. Therefore, a yet unidentified EDHF associated with the hyperpolarization of the vascular smooth-muscle cells was suggested [95]. There are several candidates proposed which may play this role, and over the last years its study has attracted much attention, mainly because of its likely contribution to hypertensive states. And MS it's not the exception. Beltowski et al. proposed that EDHF may be stimulated by leptin when NO becomes deficient, for example in short-term obesity, but leptin increases blood pressure in chronic obesity because its effect on EDHF is also attenuated [96]. This study is consistent with a more recent one, which demonstrated that the stimulation of EDHF by leptin is impaired in obesity due to excessive serine phosphorylation of IRS-1 [97]. Further studies are required to determine the role of this mediator in the pathophysiology of hypertension in the context of MS.

2.2.3. Endothelial Dysfunction in Metabolic Syndrome

Dysfunction of the endothelium has been implicated in the pathophysiology of different forms of cardiovascular disease, including hypertension. Endothelial dysfunction may be defined as impairment characterized by a shift of the actions of the endothelium toward reduced vasodilation, but its pathophysiology is complex and involves multiple mechanism. The main characteristic of this condition is the unbalanced concentrations of vasodilating and vasoconstricting factors, which may lead to hypertension. All the evidence mentioned above allows suggesting that MS is a condition in which all the metabolic alterations leads to endothelial dysfunction, and consequently to hypertension. One of the molecules that is most affected is NO, which is recognized is recognized as one of the major mediators of the maintenance of vascular homeostasis. Several mechanisms reduce the NO bioavailability in MS. Two of the most important are the proinlfammatory state and the oxidative stress present in MS. Metabolic alterations, such as hyperinsulinemia and hyperglycemia can also contribute to this NO-deficient state. Finally, the presence of hyperleptinemia, hypoadiponectinemia and reduced levels of ghrelin, conditions associated with visceral obesity, would also generate a reduction in NO-dependent blood vessel relaxation. This condition, added to the increased levels of potent vasoconstrictor factors such as ET-1, U-II and angiotensin II, generate endothelial dysfunction in MS, which could be the key mechanism underlying hypertension in this syndrome (Figure 5-1).

3. Animal Models

This following section presents the main models used in studies of MS, with assessment of hypertension.

3.1. Genetic Models

Genetic models of MS, that show hypertension as a sign, include Zucker Obese Rats, Zucker diabetic fatty rats, the Spontaneously Hypertensive Obese Rat and Otsuka Long-Evans Tokushima Fatty rats. These models are useful in evaluating specific molecular mechanisms that may be involved in development of MS-related hypertension in rodents. However, MS in humans is not a monogenetic disorder. Therefore, the relevant questions are whether these genetic changes mimic those observed in humans and whether these models show the range of signs that characterize MS, especially hypertension.

3.1.1. Zucker Obese Rats (fa/fa) and Zucker Diabetic Fatty Rats (ZDF)

The Zucker rat is probably the most commonly used rat model for MS. In 1961, L. M. Zucker and T. F. Zucker discovered that an autosomal recessive mutation in the fatty gene (fa) resulted in obesity [98]. The homozygotes for the mutation (fa/fa) develop obesity because of a defective leptin receptor [99, 100]. This mutation affects the extracellular part of the leptin receptor. In experiments using cells expressing wild-type or mutated leptin receptors, mutated receptors have shown weaker affinity for leptin, and an altered signal transduction [101, 102]. Zucker rats develop insulin resistance in addition to obesity, but glycemia remains normal, and they do not develop diabetes [103]. These rats have decreased plasma renin activity [104]. Moreover, sympathetic activity appears not to play a significant role in causing hypertension in this model. Endothelial function has been repetitively studied. The majority of studies report decreased endothelial function and decreased NO-dependent vasodilation.

ZDF rats are hyperglycemic [105] with hyperinsulinemia and hypertriglyceridemia, with diastolic and systolic dysfunction [106]. Serum cholesterol concentrations were slightly increased in ZDF young rats whereas the serum concentration of cholesterol was ~2.5 times higher in adult rats [107]. These rats also developed endothelial dysfunction [108]. ZDF rats showed only moderate increases in systolic blood pressure [109]. Also, ZDF rats show albuminuria [110] with thickening of basal membrane and glomerular fibrosis [110].

Increased hepatic triglyceride deposition was observed in ZDF rats [111]. ZDF rats also showed increased serum markers of inflammation such as TNFα and IL-1β [112].

3.1.2. The Spontaneously Hipertensive Obese Rat (SHROB)

Koletsky rat is a rat strain of spontaneous hypertension breeding origin that suffers a nonsense mutation of the leptin receptor gene [113, 114]. This mutation makes SHROB rats unable to respond to leptin [115]. The rat displays obesity, hypertension (although milder than that of their SHR ancestor), hyperinsulinemia, hyperlipidemia, and nephropathy, all superimposed on a hypertensive background. Thus, these rats exhibit all the symptoms of MS and are generally regarded as an adequate animal model of this disease [116]. Regarding cardiovascular function, SHROB rats develop diabetic retinopathy and other microvascular complication associated with MS. A study about diet and blood pressure reports that restrictive diets are not beneficial for blood pressure, likely because it is caused by sympathetic activation and cardiac hypertrophy [117].

Recently, studies have characterized the macrovascular and microvascular function in these rats. SHROB rats display a severely decreased endothelium relaxation with decreased NO production and an elevated release of vasoconstrictive prostanoids [118].

3.1.3. Otsuka Long-Evans Tokushima Fatty Rats

Otsuka Long-Evans Tokushima Fatty (OLETF) rats have been used as a rat model of human MS [119]. Pancreatic acini cells in OLETF rats were insensitive to the actions of cholecystokinin (CCK), which controls food intake [120], due to the absence of CCK-1 receptors [121]. Due to the lack of CCK-1 receptors, the average meal size and overall food intake were higher in OLETF rats [121]. OLETF rats presented with hyperglycemic with impaired glucose tolerance [122]. Plasma triglyceride concentrations in OLETF are increased and cholesterol concentrations are only slightly elevated [122]. OLETF rats show diffuse glomerulosclerosis [122]. Hearts from OLETF rats show cardiac hypertrophy with left ventricular systolic and diastolic dysfunction [123], and also showed higher blood pressure [124]. In OLETF rats, it has been showed decreased NO production, and L- arginine supplementation has improved hypertension [125]. This finding suggests that endothelial dysfunction play a key role in this model.

Table 5-1. Occurrence of metabolic syndrome components in the different study models

	Manifestation of Metabolic Syndrome						References
Animal Model	Obesity	Insuline Resistance	Glucose Intolerance	Hypertension	Dyslipidemia	Atherosclerosis	
fa/fa rats	+	+	-	controversial	+	+	98, 103, 116
ZDF rats	+	+	-	+	+	+	105-107, 109, 110
OLETF rats	+	adult	adult	+	+	+	119, 122, 123
SHROB rats	+	+	+	+	+	+	115,116
Fructose induced- MetS	+	+	+	+	+	+	127, 130-130, 134
Sucrose induced- MetS	+	+	+	+	+	+	140-142
High fat induced- MetS	+	+	+	+	+	+	144-151
Caffeteria diet induced- MetS	+	+	+	+	+	+	154, 155, 157, 158

3.2. Diet-Induced Metabolic Syndrome

Diet plays an important role in growth and development. The modern diet, especially in western countries, is rich in carbohydrates such as fructose and sucrose as well as saturated fat. This increased calorific intake has been associated with many diet-induced complications, including MS, renal and cardiovascular diseases [126]. Combinations of carbohydrate and fat-rich dietary components have been used in rodents to mimic these signs and symptoms of human MS, including hypertension.

3.2.1. Fructose-Induced Metabolic Syndrome

Fructose has become an important and pervasive ingredient in western diets [127, 128]. The world average per capita daily fructose intake increased by 16% between 1986 and 2007 [128], along with a proportionate increase in the incidence of obesity [129]. Unlike glucose, high-fructose feeding to rodents induced the development of symptoms of MS including high blood pressure, insulin resistance, impaired glucose tolerance and dyslipidemia [127, 130]. Fructose feeding induced ventricular dilatation, ventricular hypertrophy, decreased ventricular contractile function, infiltration of inflammatory cells in heart and hepatic steatosis [131,

132]. In the liver, fructose feeding induced both microvesicular and macrovesicular steatosis with periportal fibrosis and lobular inflammation [133]. Fructose has been reported to induce obesity [134], but this was not confirmed [131]. Fructose feeding in rats caused renal tubular injury, collagen deposition in interstitium and increased macrophage infiltration along with proliferation and hyperplasia of renal proximal tubules [135]. Increases in plasma uric acid and dyslipidemia take place not in all the studies [136].

3.2.2. High Carbohydrate-, High Fat-Induced Metabolic Syndrome

A diet high in carbohydrates together with fat, either of animal or plant origin, mimics the human diet more closely. Different combinations and amounts of carbohydrates and fats have been used in different studies [137-153]. The common carbohydrates used are fructose and sucrose whereas the source of fat varies in the different studies. Different combinations of sucrose and fat have been used to induce signs of MS. Rodents fed on high-sucrose, high-fat diet had increased body weight, abdominal fat deposition, hyperinsulinemia, hyperglycemia and hyperleptinemia [154, 155]. Combination of sucrose and fat also caused hepatic steatosis and increased hepatic lipogenic enzymes [156]. Fructose and fat have been used in combination to induce MS. Fructose and fat feeding increased body weight and the plasma concentrations of triglycerides, cholesterol, FFA and leptin [157, 158]. The combination of fructose and fat also caused hyperinsulinemia, insulin resistance, impaired glucose tolerance, increased abdominal fat deposition, hepatic steatosis and inflammation [157]. The rats fed with the high-fructose, high-fat diet showed cardiac hypertrophy, increased ventricular stiffness, ventricular dilatation, cardiac inflammation and fibrosis, hypertension, decreased cardiac function and endothelial dysfunction along with mild renal damage and increased pancreatic islet mass [157].

Regarding vascular function, in a cafeteria diet model, a negative association between plasma lipid levels and reduction in endothelial function, assessed by acetylcholine responses was found. PVAT exhibits a proinflammatory phenotype compared to other depots such as the subcutaneous one [159]. PVAT causes endothelial dysfunction via proinflammatory cytokines such as TNFα as well as through oxidative stress [160, 161]. A study has reported that increase in vascular oxidative stress is associated with increase in vascular NO production and NOS activity in rat model of obesity-induced hypertension [162].

In the table 5 - 1 we compared the different models of study of MS.

4. Therapy of Hypertension in Metabolic Syndrome

4.1. β-Blockers

β-Blockers reduce blood pressure by inhibiting sympathetic nervous system activity; however, individual agents within this class differ in terms of their mechanism of action and physiologic effects [163].

4.1.1. Traditional β-Blockers

Traditional β-blockers may reduce insulin sensitivity, lessen glycemic control, and increase the risk of new-onset diabetes [164].

Various mechanisms have been proposed to explain the negative effects of traditional β-blockers on glucose and lipid metabolism. Traditional β-blockers produce unopposed α1-adrenergic receptor activity, which may induce vasoconstriction, decrease skeletal blood flow, and reduce insulin-stimulated peripheral glucose uptake [165].

Also, β-blockers may not improve oxidative stress and NO production, impairing endothelial function [166]. Additionally, traditional β-blockers inhibit insulin secretion from pancreatic β-cells [167].

4.1.2. Vasodilating β-Blockers

Evidence suggests that nebivolol, a selective β1-blocker, mediates vasodilation via the stimulation of endothelium-derived NO release [168]. In patients with hypertension, nebivolol has been associated with improvements in glycemic control and dyslipidemia.

Labetalol, a nonselective β-blocker with α1-adrenergic receptor–blocking activity, is effective in the long-term management of mild, moderate, and severe hypertension and during hypertensive emergencies [169]. Although the effect of labetalol on glucose and lipid metabolism in hypertension has not been extensively studied, two small studies suggest that labetalol treatment is associated with neutral effects on glucose and lipid profiles [170].

Carvedilol is a nonselective β-blocker whose vasodilating activity has been attributed to α1- adrenergic receptor blockade [171]. A number of recent studies have reported that carvedilol exerts neutral effects on glucose and lipid metabolism.

Various mechanisms have been proposed to account for the favorable effects of vasodilating β-blockers on glucose and lipid metabolism, including α1-adrenergic receptor blockade and vasodilation, anti-inflammatory activity, reduced oxidative stress, and lack of weight gain.

Carvedilol and labetalol prevent norepinephrine binding to α1-adrenegric receptors, which decreases peripheral vascular resistance and increases peripheral blood flow and glucose uptake [163, 171]. Carvedilol and nebivolol also promote endothelial-dependent vasodilation by enhancing NO synthesis [168, 172].

Carvedilol possesses antioxidant properties, including the ability to scavenge ROS, suppress free radical generation, and prevent ferric ion-induced oxidation [173]. The antioxidant activity of carvedilol may also be related to stimulation of endothelial NO production or a reduction in NO inactivation [174]. Antioxidant activity is not limited to carvedilol, as nebivolol also decreases oxidative stress via a reduction in ROS generation and NO inactivation [175]. Vasodilating β-blockers have been shown to reduce proinflammatory mediators.

Nebivolol administration to patients with hypertension and dyslipidemia is associated with reduced levels of CRP [176], and carvedilol administration to patients with hypertension and diabetes is associated with reductions in CRP and monocyte chemotactic protein-1 [173].

4.2. Renin-Angiotensin-Aldosterone System Inhibitors

As mentioned above, angiotensin is overexpressed in obesity, directly contributing to obesity related hypertension and making the case to consider angiotensin-converting enzyme inhibitors (ACE) and angiotensin II-receptor blockers (ARB) as first-line agents. In comparison to ARB or ACE inhibitors, β-blockers and thiazide-based regimens increase insulin resistance and are associated with an increase in new cases of diabetes. In contrast, regimens based on RAAS inhibition are associated with significantly fewer cases of new diabetes [177-179].

This is of particular importance in the obese population, a group with an increased risk for the development of T2D [180]. In addition, ACE inhibitors and ARB have not been associated with weight gain or insulin resistance, and provide renal protection in diabetes, a highly prevalent disease among obese persons. The Second Australian National Blood Pressure (ANBP2) trial [181] reported slightly better outcomes in hypertensive white men (average BMI 27.4) treated with a regimen that began with an ACE inhibitor compared with a regimen that began with another type of diuretic. Calcium channel blockers are also effective in the treatment of obesity-related hypertension and have not been associated with weight gain or adverse changes in lipids [182, 183].

4.3. New Therapies

4.3.1. Vitamin C

The beneficial effects of antioxidant vitamins supplementation are attributed to their ability to scavenge ROS, control nitric oxide synthesis or release, inhibit ROS generation and upregulate antioxidant enzyme activities that metabolize these molecules [184]. In hypertensive rats, long term vitamin C administration significantly reduced systolic blood pressure and simultaneously reduced oxidative stress mediated by NADPH oxidase activation [185]. Vitamin C has beneficial effects not only on blood pressure but also on endothelial function in hypertensive and diabetic patients [186].

Vitamin C is a soluble compound and it prevents protein and lipid oxidation in the extracellular environment [187]. In vivo studies confirmed that vitamin C administration improves arterial vasodilatation by increasing NO production [188]. In addition, there is direct evidence that vitamin C has a beneficial effect on insulin sensitivity and some components of the antioxidant defense system in an animal model of insulin resistance [189].

Concerning the specific role of vitamin C in oxidative stress-associated arterial hypertension, mounting evidence suggest the importance of this vitamin in regulating endothelial function and vasodilation. In fact, vitamin C is known to improve elastic artery [190], by contrasting endothelial cell oxidation and by stimulating both endothelium-dependent and endothelium-independent arterial vasodilation [191]. In addition, vitamin C administration was able to restore endothelium-dependent vasodilation in hyperglycemic patients [192].

All the evidence mentioned above puts vitamin C as an important possibly pharmacology alternative for the treatment of hypertension in MS, but further studies are required.

4.3.2. Other Antioxidants

Systemic oxidative stress and nitrosative stress as well as inflammation increase with the development of MS-like components in SHR/cp rats, which display abdominal obesity, hypertension, hyperglycemia, insulin-resistance, and hyperlipidemia [193].

Coenzyme Q10 (CoQ10) is an endogenously synthesized compound that acts as an electron carrier in the mitochondrial respiratory chain [194]. In addition to its unique role in mitochondria, CoQ10 functions as an antioxidant, scavenging free radicals and inhibiting lipid peroxidation [195].

CoQ10 prevents vascular endothelial dysfunction seem to be linked to its hypotensive effect in SHR/cp rats. Furthermore, insulin resistance and the consequent hyperinsulinemia, important components of MS, are associated with endothelial dysfunction, probably due to increasing oxidative stress [196]. The physiological properties of insulin that cause enhancement of renal sodium reabsorption and stimulate SNS activity are believed to play a major role in the development of hypertension [197], although the underlying mechanisms in the setting of insulin resistance remain obscure [198]. Therefore, the hypotensive effect of CoQ10 observed in SHR/cp rats may be associated with its alleviation of hyperinsulinemia together with endothelial dysfunction. These findings suggest that the antioxidant properties of CoQ10 can be effective for ameliorating cardiovascular risk in MS.

Conclusion and Perspectives

The MS is a highly frequent condition and its prevalence is increasing around the world, mainly in developing countries. Knowing its prevalence, MS should be consider as a cluster of metabolic disorders whose importance lies in being one of the most important risk factor for the onset of T2D and CVD. At the same time, hypertension, one of the disorders that are included in the MS diagnostic criteria, is by itself considered to be the most important risk factor in the development of cardiovascular disease worldwide.

All the evidence presented in our review suggest that the visceral obesity appears to be the triggering condition of the serial of events involved in MS and hypertension, as well as the insulin resistance state would be the key pathological phenomenon underlying all the complex mechanisms that are involved in this highly prevalent syndrome, that includes the participation of a large amount of mediators and several pathological processes that are not fully yet elucidated.

Endothelial dysfunction appears to be the key mechanism underlying hypertension in MS, but there are several contributing factors that remain unknown. This is the reason why new studies are required to fully understand its pathophysiology and to generate new therapeutic strategies.

PVAT has demonstrated playing a crucial role in maintaining vascular homeostasis. In this manner, it appears to be a promising research field, because of its complex metabolic activity and its possibly role in the pathogenesis of elevated blood pressure in MS.

New pharmacological strategies should be directed against the metabolic disorders that explain the decreased NO bioavailability and endothelial dysfunction. In other words, hypertension in MS should be considered as a different pathological condition to essential hypertension

Finally, nowadays, despite the fact that there is an increased number of therapeutic alternatives for treat every single component of MS, efforts should focus on prevention and lifestyle changing, which has demonstrated to improve MS and to allow a better life quality.

References

[1] World Health Organization. Global atlas on cardiovascular disease prevention and control: policies, strategies and interventions. 2011.

[2] Yusuf S, Reddy S, Ounpuu S, Anand S. Global burden of cardiovascular diseases: part I: general considerations, the epidemiologic transition, risk factors, and impact of urbanization. *Circulation* 2001;104:2746–2753.

[3] Ford ES, Giles WH, Dietz WH. Prevalence of the Metabolic Syndrome among US Adults: Findings from the Third National Health and Nutrition Examination Survey. *JAMA* 2002; 287:356-359.

[4] Ervin RB. Prevalence of metabolic syndrome among adults 20 years of age and over, by sex, age, race and ethnicity, and body mass index: United States, 2003-2006. *Natl. Health Stat. Report* 2009;13:1-7.

[5] Beltrán-Sánchez H, Harhay MO, Harhay MM, McElligott S. Prevalence and Trens of Metabolic Syndrome in the Adult U.S. Population, 1999-2010. *J. Am. Coll. Cardiol.* 2013;62: 697-703.

[6] Misra A, Khurana L. Obesity and the Metabolic Syndrome in Developing Countries. *J. Clin. Endocrinol. Metab.* 2008; 93:9–30.

[7] Florez H, Silva E, Fernandez V, Ryder E, Sulbaran T, Campos G, Calmon G, Clavel E, Castillo-Florez S, Goldberg R. Prevalence and risk factors associated with the metabolic syndrome and dyslipidemia in White, Black, Amerindian and Mixed Hispanics in Zulia State, Venezuela. *Diabetes Res. Clin. Pract.* 2005;69:63–77.

[8] Aguilar-Salinas CA, Rojas R, Gomez-Perez FJ, Valles V, Rios-Torres JM, Franco A, Olaiz G, Rull JA, Sepulveda J. Analysis of the agreement between the World Health Organization criteria and the National Cholesterol Education Program-III definition of the metabolic syndrome: results from a population-based survey. *Diabetes Care* 2003;26:1635-1660.

[9] Azizi F, Salehi P, Etemadi A, Zahedi-Asl S. Prevalence of metabolic syndrome in an urban population: Tehran Lipid and Glucose Study. *Diabetes Res. Clin. Pract.* 2003;61:29–37.

[10] Ozsahin AK, Gokcel A, Sezgin N, Akbaba M, Guvener N, Ozisik L, Karademir BM. Prevalence of the metabolic syndrome in a Turkish adult population. *Diabetes Nutr. Metab.* 2004;17:230–234.

[11] National Cholesterol Education Program (NCEP) Expert Panel on Detection, Evaluation, and Treatment of High Blood Cholesterol in Adults (Adult Treatment Panel III). Third Report of the National Cholesterol Education Program (NCEP) Expert Panel on Detection, Evaluation, and Treatment of High Blood Cholesterol in Adults (Adult Treatment Panel III) final report. *Circulation* 2002;106:3143–3421.

[12] Alberti KG, Zimmet P, Shaw J. Metabolic syndrome — a new world-wide definition. A consensus statement from the International Diabetes Federation. *Diabet Med.* 2006;23:469–480.

[13] Phelan S, Wadden TA, Berkowitz RI, Sarwer DB, Womble LG, Cato RK, and Rothman R. Impact of weight loss on the metabolic syndrome. *Int. J. Obes.* (Lond) 2007;31:1442-1448.

[14] McNeill AM, Rosamond WD, Girman CJ, Golden SH, Schmidt MI, East HE, Ballantyne CM, Heiss G. The Metabolic Syndrome and 11-Year Risk of Incident Cardiovascular Disease in the Atherosclerosis Risk in Communities Study. *Diabetes Care* 2005;28:385-390.

[15] Mottillo S, Filion KB, Genest J, Joseph L, Pilote L, Poirier P, Rinfret S, Schiffrin EL, Eisenberg MJ. The Metabolic Syndrome and Cardiovascular Risk: A Systematic Review and Meta-Analysis. *J. Am. Coll. Cardiol.* 2010;56:1113-1132.

[16] Akosah KO, McHugh VL, Mathiason MA, Kulkarni A, Barnhart SI. Metabolic syndrome and coronary heart disease equivalent conditions in predicting cardiovascular events in young to middle-aged adults. *J. Cardiometab. Syndr.* 2006;1:173-177.

[17] Stern MP, Williams K, Gonzalez-Villalpando C, Hunt KJ, Haffner SM. Does the metabolic syndrome improve identification of individuals at risk of type 2 diabetes and/or cardiovascular disease? *Diabetes Care* 2004;27:2676–2681.

[18] Lorenzo C, Williams K, Hunt KJ, Haffner SM. The National Cholesterol Education Program–Adult Treatment Panel III, International Diabetes Federation, and World Health Organization Definitions of the Metabolic Syndrome as Predictors of Incident Cardiovascular Disease and Diabetes. *Diabetes Care* 2007;30:8-13.

[19] Sattar N, McConnachie A, Shaper AG, Blauw GJ, Buckley BM, de Craen AJ, Ford I, Forouhi NG, Freeman DJ, Jukema JW, Lennon L, Macfarlane PW, Murphy MB, Packard CJ, Stott DJ, Westendorp RG, Whincup PH, Shepherd J, Wannamethee SG. Can metabolic syndrome usefully predict cardiovascular disease and diabetes? Outcome data from two prospective studies. *Lancet* 2008;371:1927-1935.

[20] Athyros VG, Ganotakis ES, Elisaf MS, Liberopoulos EN, Goudevenos IA, Karagiannis A. Prevalence of vascular disease in metabolic syndrome using three proposed definitions. Int J Cardiol 2007;117:204-210.

[21] Cortez-Dias N, Martins SR, Belo A, Fiuza M. Association of metabolic risk factors with uncontrolled hypertension: comparison of the several definitions of metabolic syndrome. *J. Hypertens.* 2013;31:1991-1997.

[22] Luk AO, Ma RC, So W-Y, Yang X-L, Kong AP, Ozaki R, Ko GT, Chow C-C, Cockram CS, Chan JC, Tong PC. The NCEP-ATPIII but not the IDF criteria for the metabolic syndrome identify Type 2 diabetic patients at increased risk of chronic kidney disease. *Diabet Med.* 2008;25:1419-1425.

[23] Mancia G, Bombelli M, Facchetti R, Casati A, Ronchi I, Quarti-Trevano F, Arenare F, Grassi G, Sega R. Impact of different definitions of the metabolic syndrome on the prevalence of organ damage, cardiometabolic risk and cardiovascular events. *J Hypertens.* 2010;28:999-1006.

[24] Lawes CM, Vander Hoorn S, Rodgers A, International Society of Hypertension. Global burden of blood-pressure-related disease, 2001. *Lancet* 2008;371:1513-1518.

[25] Yusuf S, Hawken S, Ounpuu S, Dans T, Avezum A, Lanas F, McQueen M, Budaj A,Pais P, Varigos J, Lisheng L. Effect of potentially modifiable risk factors associated

with myocardial infarction in 52 countries (the INTERHEART Study): case control study. *Lancet* 2004;364:937–952.

[26] Antikainen R, Jousilahti P, Tuomilehto J. Systolic blood pressure, isolated systolic hypertension and risk of coronary heart disease, strokes, cardiovascular disease and all-cause mortality in the middle-aged population. *J. Hypertens.* 1998;16:577-583.

[27] Shin CY, Yun KE, Park HS. Blood pressure has a greater impact on cardiovascular mortality than other components of metabolic syndrome in Koreans. *Atherosclerosis* 2009;205:614-619.

[28] Leoncini G, Ratto E, Viazzi F, Vaccaro V, Parodi D, Parodi A, Falqui V, Tomolillo C, Deferrari G, Pontremoli R. Metabolic syndrome is associated with early signs of organ damage in nondiabetic, hypertensive patients. *J. Intern. Med.* 2005;257:454–460.

[29] Engstrom G, Hedblad B, Stavenow L, Lind P, Janzon L, Lindgarde F. Inflammation-sensitive plasma proteins are associated with future weight gain. *Diabetes* 2003;52:2097–101.

[30] Mittelman SD, Van Citters GW, Kirkman EL, Bergman RN. Extreme insulin resistance of the central adipose depot in vivo. *Diabetes* 2002;51:755–761.

[31] Mauriège P, Marette A, Atgié C, Bouchard C, Thériault G, Bukowiecki LK, Marceau P, Biron S, Nadeau A, Després JP. Regional variation in adipose tissue metabolism of severely obese premenopausal women. *J. Lipid.* 1995;36:672–684.

[32] Wine KL. Free fatty acids and type 2 diabetes mellitus. Am J Med 2003;115:29–36.

[33] Redon J, Cifkova R, Laurent S, Nilsson P, Narkiewicz K, Erdine S, Mancia G. Mechanisms of hypertension in the cardiometabolic syndrome. *J. Hypertens.* 2009;27:441-451.

[34] Weisberg SP, McCann D, Desai M, Rosenbaum M, Leibel RL, Ferrante AW Jr. Obesity is associated with macrophage accumulation in adipose tissue. *J. Clin. Invest.* 2003;112:1796-1808.

[35] Bremer AA, Jialal I. Adipose tissue dysfunction in nascent metabolic syndrome. *J. Obes. 2013*;2013:393192.

[36] Rajala MW, Scherer PE. Minireview: The adipocyte--at the crossroads of energy homeostasis, inflammation, and atherosclerosis. *Endocrinology*. 2003;144:3765-3773.

[37] Flier JS. Obesity wars: molecular progress confronts an expanding epidemic. *Cell* 2004;116:337–350.

[38] Lord G. Role of leptin in immunology. *Nutr. Rev.* 2002;60:33–58.

[39] Pajvani UB, Scherer PE. Adiponect systemic contributor to insulin sensitivity. *Curr. Diab. Rep.* 2003;3:207–213.

[40] Lowell BB, Shulman GI. Mitochondrial dysfunction and type 2 diabetes. *Science* 2005;307:384-387.

[41] Ford ES, Mokdad AH, Giles WH, Brown DW. The metabolic syndrome and antioxidant concentrations: findings from the Third National Health and Nutrition Examination Survey. *Diabetes* 2003;52:2346–2352.

[42] Roberts CK, Barnard RJ, Sindhu RK, Jurczak M, Ehdaie A, Vaziri ND. Oxidative stress and dysregulation of NAD(P)H oxidase and antioxidant enzymes in diet-induced metabolic syndrome. *Metabolism* 2006;55:928-934.

[43] Furukawa S, Fujita T, Shimabukuro M, Iwaki M, Yamada Y, Nakajima Y, Nakayama O, Makishima M, Matsuda M, Shimomura I. Increased oxidative stress in obesity and its impact on metabolic syndrome. *J. Clin. Invest.* 2004;114:752–61.

[44] Houstis N, Rosen ED, Lander ES. Reactive oxygen species have a causal role in multiple forms of insulin resistance. *Nature* 2006;440:944–948.

[45] Lin Y, Berg AH, Iyengar P, Lam TK, Giacca A, Combs TP, Rajala MW, Du X, Rollman B, Li W, Hawkins M, Barzilai N, Rhodes CJ, Fantus IG, Brownlee M, Scherer PE. The hyperglycemia-induced inflammatory response in adipocytes: the role of reactive oxygen species. *J. Biol. Chem.* 2005;280:4617-26.

[46] Coenen KR, Hasty AH. Obesity potentiates development of fatty liver and insulin resistance, but not atherosclerosis, in high-fat diet-fed agouti LDLR-deficient mice. *Am. J. Physiol. Endocrinol. Metab.* 2007;293:492-499.

[47] Holvoet P, Kritchevsky S, Tracy R, Mertens A, Rubin S, Butler J, Goodpaster B, Harris T. The metabolic syndrome, circulating oxidized LDL, and risk of myocardial infarction in well-functioning elderly people in the health, aging, and body composition cohort. *Diabetes* 2004;53:1068-1073.

[48] Norata GD, Ongari M, Garlaschelli K, Raselli S, Grigore L, Catapano AL. Plasma resistin levels correlate with determinants of the metabolic syndrome. Eur J Endocrinol 2007;156:279–284.

[49] Bahia L, Aguiar LG, Villela N, Bottino D, Godoy-Matos AF, Geloneze B, Tambascia M, Bouskela E. Relationship between adipokines, inflammation, and vascular reactivity in lean controls and obese subjects with metabolic syndrome. *Clinics* 2006;61:433–440.

[50] Xydakis AM, Case CC, Jones PH, Hoogeveen RC, Liu MY, Smith EO, Nelson KW, Ballantyne CM. Adiponectin, inflammation, and the expression of the metabolic syndrome in obese individuals: the impact of rapid weight loss through caloric restriction. *J. Clin. Endocrinol. Metab.* 2004;89:2697–2703.

[51] Van Guilder GP, Hoetzer GL, Greiner JJ, Stauffer BL, Desouza CA 2006 Influence of metabolic syndrome on biomarkers of oxidative stress and inflammation in obese adults. *Obesity* (Silver Spring) 2006;14:2127–2131.

[52] Ridker PM, Buring JE, Cook NR, Rifai N. C-reactive protein, the metabolic syndrome, and risk of incident cardiovascular events: an 8-year follow-up of 14,719 initially healthy American women. *Circulation* 2003;107:391–397.

[53] Cornier MA, Dabelea D, Hernandez TL, Lindstrom RC, Steig AJ, Stob NR, Van Pelt RE, Wang H, Eckel RH. The metabolic syndrome. *Endocr. Rev.* 2008;29:777-822.

[54] Hotamisligil GS, Arner P, Caro JF, Atkinson RL, Spiegelman BM. Increased adipose tissue expression of tumor necrosis factor-α in human obesity and insulin resistance. *J. Clin. Invest.* 1995;95:2409–2415.

[55] Grassi G, Dell'Oro R, Facchini A, Quarti Trevano F, Bolla GB, Mancia G. Effect of central and peripheral body fat distribution on sympathetic and baroreflex function in obese normotensives. *J. Hypertens.* 2004;22:2363-2369.

[56] Lembo G, Napoli R, Capaldo B, Rendina V, Iaccarino G, Volpe M, Trimarco B, Saccà L. Abnormal sympathetic overactivity evoked by insulin in the skeletal muscle of patients with essential hypertension. *J. Clin. Invest.* 1992;90:24-29.

[57] Carlyle M, Jones OB, Kuo JJ, Hall JE. Chronic cardiovascular and renal actions of leptin: role of adrenergic activity. *Hypertension* 2002;39:496-501.

[58] Marsh AJ, Fontes MA, Killinger S, Pawlak DB, Polson JW, Dampney RA. Cardiovascular responses evoked by leptin acting on neurons in the ventromedial and dorsomedial hypothalamus. *Hypertension* 2003;42:488-493.

[59] Alvarez GE, Beske SD, Ballard TP, Davy KP. Sympathetic neural activation in visceral obesity. *Circulation* 2002;106:2533-2536.

[60] Goodfriend TL, Egan BM, Kelley DE. Aldosterone in obesity. *Endocr. Res.* 1998; 24: 789-96.

[61] Egan BM, Stepniakowski K, Goodfriend TL. Renin and aldosterone are higher and the hyperinsulinemic effect of salt restriction greater in subjects with risk factors clustering. *Am. J. Hypertens.* 1994;7:886-893.

[62] Bochud M, Nussberger J, Bovet P, Maillard MR, Elston RC, Paccaud F, Shamlaye C, Burnier M. Plasma aldosterone is independently associated with the metabolic syndrome. *Hypertension* 2006;48:239-245.

[63] Boustany CM, Bharadwaj K, Daugherty A, Brown DR, Randall DC, Cassis LA. Activation of the systemic and adipose renin-angiotensin system in rats with diet-induced obesity and hypertension. *Am. J. Physiol. Regul. Integr. Comp. Physiol.* 2004;287:943-949.

[64] Engeli S, Schling P, Gorzelniak K, Boschmann M, Janke J, Ailhaud G. The adipose-tissue renin-angiotensin-aldosterone system: role in the metabolic syndrome? *Int. J. Biochem. Cell Biol.* 2003;35:807-825.

[65] Briones AM, Nguyen Dinh Cat A, Callera GE, Yogi A, Burger D, He Y, Corrêa JW, Gagnon AM, Gomez-Sanchez CE, Gomez-Sanchez EP, Sorisky A, Ooi TC, Ruzicka M, Burns KD, Touyz RM. Adipocytes produce aldosterone through calcineurin-dependent signaling pathways: implications in diabetes mellitus-associated obesity and vascular dysfunction. *Hypertension* 2012;59:1069-1078.

[66] Ehrhart-Bornstein M, Lamounier-Zepter V, Schraven A, Langenbach J, Willenberg HS, Barthel A, Hauner H, McCann SM, Scherbaum WA, Bornstein SR. Human adipocytes secrete mineralocorticoid-releasing factors. *Proc. Natl. Acad. Sci. USA* 2003;100:14211-14216.

[67] Gao YJ. Dual modulation of vascular function by perivascular adipose tissue and its potential correlation with adiposity / lipoatrophy-related vascular function. *Curr. Pharm. Des.* 2007; 13: 2185–2192.

[68] Lohn M, Dubrovska G, Lauterbach B, Luft FC, Gollasch M, Sharma AM. Periadventitial fat releases a vascular relaxing factor. *FASEB J.* 2002;16:1057–1063.

[69] Gao YJ, Lu C, Su LY, Sharma AM, Lee RMKW. Modulation of vascular function by perivascular adipose tissue: The role of endothelium and hydrogen peroxide. *Br. J. Pharmacol.* 2007;151: 323–331.

[70] Soltis EE, Cassis LA. Influence of perivascular adipose tissue on rat aortic smooth muscle responsiveness. *Clin. Exp. Hypertens.* A 1991;13:277-296.

[71] Petrasek D, Jensen G, Tuck M, Stern N. In vitro effects of insulin on aldosterone production in rat zona glomerulosa cells. *Life Sci.* 1992;50:1781-1787.

[72] Scherrer U, Randin D, Vollenweider P, Vollenweider L, Nicod P. Nitric oxide release accounts for insulin's vascular effects in humans. *J. Clin. Invest.* 1994;94:2511-2515.

[73] Vincent MA, Barrett EJ, Lindner JR, Clark MG, Rattigan S. Inhibiting NOS blocks microvascular recruitment and blunts muscle glucose uptake in response to insulin. Am *J. Physiol. Endocrinol. Metab.* 2003;285:123-129.

[74] Kashyap SR, Roman LJ, Lamont J, Masters BS, Bajaj M, Suraamornkul S, Belfort R, Berria R, Kellogg DL, Liu Y, DeFronzo RA. Insulin resistance is associated with

impaired nitric oxide synthase activity in skeletal muscle of type 2 diabetic subjects. *J. Clin. Endocrinol. Metab.* 2005;90:1100-1105.

[75] deJongh RT, Serné EH, IJzerman RG, de Vries G, Stehouwer CD. Impaired microvascular function in obesity: implications for obesity-associated microangiopathy, hypertension, and insulin resistance. *Circulation* 2004;109:2529-2535.

[76] Chen H, Montagnani M, Funahashi T, Shimomura I, Quon MJ. Adiponectin stimulates production of nitric oxide in vascular endothelial cells. *J. Biol. Chem.* 2003;278:45021–45026.

[77] Ohashi K, Kihara S, Ouchi N, Kumada M, Fujita K, Hiuge A, HibuseT, Ryo M, Nishizawa H, Maeda N, Maeda K, Shibata R, Walsh K, Funahashi T, Shimomura I. Adiponectin replenishment ameliorates obesity-related hypertension. *Hypertension* 2006;47:1108-1116.

[78] Margaritis M, Antonopoulos AS, Digby J, Lee R, Reilly S, Coutinho P, Shirodaria C, Sayeed R, Petrou M, De Silva R, Jalilzadeh S, Demosthenous M, Bakogiannis C, Tousoulis D, Stefanadis C, Choudhury RP, Casadei B, Channon KM, Antoniades C. Interactions between vascular wall and perivascular adipose tissue reveal novel roles for adiponectin in the regulation of endothelial nitric oxide synthase function in human vessels. *Circulation* 2013; 127: 2209-2221.

[79] Tesauro M, Schinzari F, Iantorno M, Rizza S, Melina D, Lauro D, Cardillo C.Ghrelin improves endothelial function in patients with metabolic syndrome. *Circulation* 2005;112:2986-2992.

[80] Tesauro M, Schinzari F, Rovella V, Di Daniele N, Lauro D, Mores N, Veneziani A, Cardillo C. Ghrelin restores the endothelin 1/nitric oxide balance in patients with obesity-related metabolic syndrome. *Hypertension* 2009; 54:995-1000.

[81] Taylor PD, McCarthy AL, Thomas CR, Poston L. Endothelium-dependent relaxation and noradrenaline sensitivity in mesenteric resistance arteries of streptozotocin induced diabetic rats. *Br. J. Pharmacol.* 1992;107:393–399.

[82] Akbari CM, Saouaf R, Barnhill DF, Newman PA, LoGerfo FW, Veves A. (1998 Oct). Endothelium-dependent vasodilatation is impaired in both microcirculation and macrocirculation during acute hyperglycemia. *J. Vasc. Surg.* 1998; 28: 687-94.

[83] Bełtowski J, Wójcicka G, Jamroz A. Stimulatory effect of leptin on nitric oxide production is impaired in dietary-induced obesity. *Obes. Res.* 2003;11:1571-1580.

[84] Fain JN, Tagele BM, Cheema P, Madan AK, Tichansky DS.Release of 12 adipokines by adipose tissue, nonfat cells, and fat cells from obese women. *Obesity* (Silver Spring) 2010;18:890-896.

[85] Ferri C, Bellini C, Desideri G, Baldoncini R, Properzi G, Santucci A, De Mattia G. Circulating endothelin 1 levels in obese patients with the metabolic syndrome. *Exp. Clin. Endocrinol. Diabetes* 1997;105:38-40.

[86] vanHarmelen V, Eriksson A, Aström G, Wåhlén K, Näslund E, Karpe F, Frayn K, Olsson T, Andersson J, Rydén M, Arner P. Vascular peptide endothelin-1 links fat accumulation with alterations of visceral adipocyte lipolysis. *Diabetes* 2008;57:378-386.

[87] Cardillo C, Campia U, Iantorno M, Panza JA. Enhanced vascular activity of endogenous endothelin-1 in obese hypertensive patients. *Hypertension* 2004;43:36–40.

[88] Mather KJ, Lteif A, Steinberg HO, Baron AD. Interactions between endothelin and nitric oxide in the regulation of vascular tone in obesity and diabetes. *Diabetes* 2004;53:2060-2066.

[89] Lteif A, Vaishnava P, Baron AD, Mather KJ. Endothelin limits insulin action in obese/insulin-resistant humans. *Diabetes* 2007;56:728-734.

[90] Djordjevic T, BelAiba RS, Bonello S, Pfeilschifter J, Hess J, Görlach A. Human urotensin II is a novel activator of NADPH oxidase in human pulmonary artery smooth muscle cells. *Arterioscler. Thromb. Vasc. Biol.* 2005;25:519-525.

[91] Gruson D, Rousseau MF, Ketelslegers JM, Hermans MP. Raised plasma Urotensin II in type 2 diabetes patients is associated with the metabolic syndrome phenotype. *J. Clin. Hypertens.* (Greenwich) 2010;12:653–660.

[92] Barrette PO, Schwertani AG. A closer look at the role of urotensin II in the metabolic syndrome. *Front Endocrinol.* (Lausanne) 2012;3:165.

[93] Wang MH, Smith A, Zhou Y, Chang HH, Lin S, Zhao X, Imig JD, Dorrance AM. Downregulation of renal CYP-derived eicosanoid synthesis in rats with diet-induced hypertension. *Hypertension* 2003;42:594–599.

[94] Félétou M, Vanhoutte PM. EDHF: the complete story. First edition. Boca Raton: Taylor & Francis CRC press; 2006.

[95] Quinn MT, Parthasarathy S, Steinberg D. Endothelial cell-derived chemotactic activity for mouse peritoneal macrophages and the effects of modified forms of low density lipoprotein. *Proc. Natl. Acad. Sci. USA* 1985;82:5949-5953.

[96] Bełtowski J, Wójcicka G, Jamroz-Wiśniewska A. Role of nitric oxide and endothelium-derived hyperpolarizing factor (EDHF) in the regulation of blood pressure by leptin in lean and obese rats. *Life Sci.* 2006;79:63-71.

[97] Bełtowski J, Wójcicka G, Jamroz-Wiśniewska A, Marciniak A. Resistance to acute NO-mimetic and EDHF-mimetic effects of leptin in the metabolic syndrome. *Life Sci.* 2009;85:557-567.

[98] Zucker LM, Zuker TF. Fatty, a new mutation in the rat. *J. Hered.* 1961;52:275-278.

[99] Chua SC Jr, Chung WK, Wu-Peng XS, Zhang Y, Liu SM, Tartaglia L, Leibel RL Phenotypes of mouse diabetes and rat fatty due to mutations in the OB (leptin) receptor. *Science* 1996;271:994-996.

[100] Phillips MS, Liu Q, Hammond HA, Dugan V, Hey P, Caskey CJ, Jess JF. Leptin receptor missense mutation in the fatty Zucker rat. *Nat. Genet.* 1996;13:18-19.

[101] White DW, Wang DW, Chua SC Jr, Morgenstern JP, Leibel RL, Baumann H, Tartaglia LA. Constitutive and impaired signaling of leptin receptors containing the Gln→Pro extracellular domain fatty mutation. *Proc. Natl. Acad. Sci. USA* 1997;94:10657-10662.

[102] Yamashita T, Murakami T, Lida M, Kuwajima M, Shima K. Leptin receptor of Zucker fatty rat performs reduced signal transduction. Diabetes 1997;46:1077-1080.

[103] Bray GA. The Zucker fatty rat: a review. *Fed. Proc.* 1997;36:148-153.

[104] Alonso-Galicia M, Brands MW, Zappe DH, Hall JE. Hypertension in obese Zucker rats: role of angiotensin II and adrenergic activity. *Hypertension* 1996;28:1047-1054.

[105] Mizuno M, Sada T, Kato M, Koike H. Renoprotective effects of blockade of angiotensin II AT1 receptors in an animal model of type 2 diabetes. *Hypertens. Res.* 2002;25:271-278.

[106] van de Brom CE, Huisman MC, Vlasbom R, Boontje NM, Duijst S, Lubberink M, Molthoff CF, Lammertsma AA, van der Velden J, Boer C, Ouwens DM, Diamant M.

Altered myocardial substrate metabolism is associated with myocardial dysfunction in early diabetic cardiomyopathy in rats: studies using positron emission tomography. *Cardiovasc. Diabetol.* 2009;8:39.

[107] Sparks JD, Phung TL, Bolognino M, Cianci J, Khurana R, Peterson R G, Sowden MP, Corsetti JP, Sparks CE. Lipoprotein alterations in 10- and 20-week-old Zucker diabetic fatty rats: Hyperinsulinemic versus insulinopenic hyperglycemia. *Metabolism* 1998;47:1315-1324.

[108] Serpillon S, Floyd BC, Gupte RS, George S, Kozicky M, Neito V, Recchia F, Stanley W, Wolin MS, Gupte SA. Superoxide production by NAD(P)H oxidase and mitochondria is increased in genetically obese and hyperglycemic rat heart and aorta before the development of cardiac dysfunction. The role of glucose-6-phosphate dehydrogenase-derived NADPH. *Am. J. Physiol. Heart Circ. Physiol.* 2009;297:153-162.

[109] Suzaki Y, Ozawa Y, Kobori, H. Intrarenal oxidative stress and augmented angiotensinogen are precedent to renal injury in zucker diabetic fatty rats. *Int. J. Biol. Sci.* 2006;1:40-46.

[110] Schafer S, Schimidts HL, Bleich M, Busch AE, Linz W. Nephroprotection in Zucker diabetic fatty rats by vasopeptidase inhibition is partly bradykinin B2 receptor dependent. *Br. J. Pharmacol.* 2004;143:27-32.

[111] Xu KZ, Zhu C, Kim MS, Yamahara J, Li Y. Pomegranate flower ameliorates fatty liver in an animal model of type 2 diabetes and obesity. *J. Ethnopharmacol.* 2009;22:280-287.

[112] Ferreira L, Teixeira-de-Lemos E, Pinto F, Parada B, Mega B, Vala H, Pinto R, Garrido P, Sereno J, Fernandes R, Santos P, Velada I, Melo A, Nunes S, Teixeira F, Reis F. Effects of sitagliptin treatment on dysmetabolism, inflammation, and oxidative stress in an animal model of type 2 diabetes (ZDF rat). *Mediators Inflamm.* 2010;2010:592760.

[113] Ernsberger P, Koletsky RJ, Friedman JE. Molecular pathology in the obese spontaneous hypertensive Koletsky rat: a model of Syndrome X. *Ann. NY Acad. Sci.* 1999;892:272-288.

[114] Hiraoka J, Hosoda K, Ogawa Y, Ikeda K, Nara Y, Masuzaki H, Takaya K, Nakagawa K, Mashimo T, Sawamura M, Koletsky RJ, Yamori Y, Nakao K. Augmentation of obese (ob) gene expression and leptin secretion in obese spontaneously hypertensive rats (Obese SHR or Koletsky rats). *Biochem. Biophys. Res. Commum.* 1997;231:582-585.

[115] Takaya K, Ogawa Y, Hiroaka J, Hosoda K, Yamori Y, Nakao K, Koletsky RJ. Nonsense mutation of leptin receptor in the obese spontaneously hypertensive Koletsky rat. *Nat. Genet.* 1996;14:130-131.

[116] Alexaindre de Artiñano A, Miguel Castro, M. Experimental rat models to study the metabolic syndrome. *Br. J. Nutr.* 2009;102:1246-1253.

[117] Ernsberger P, Koletsky RJ, Baskin, JS, and Foley, M. Refeeding hypertension in obese spontaneously hypertensive rats. *Hypertension* 1994;24:699-705.

[118] Mendizabal Y, Llorens, S, and Nava, E. Reactivity of the aorta and mesenteric resistance arteries from the obese spontaneously hypertensive rat: effects of glitazones. *Am. J. Physiol. Heart Circ. Physiol.* 2011;301;1319-1330.

[119] Shima K, Zhu M, Mizuno A. Pathoetiology and prevention of NIDDM lessons from the OLETF rat. *J. Med. Invest.* 1999;46:121-129.

[120] Antin J, Gibbs J, Holt J, Young RC, Smith, G. P. Cholecystokinin elicits the complete behavioral sequence of satiety in rats. *J. Comp. Physiol. Psychol.* 1975; 89:784-790.

[121] Moran TH, Bi S. Hyperphagia and obesity in OLETF rats lacking CCK-1 receptors. *Dev. Psychobiol.* 2006;48:360-367.

[122] Kawano K, Hirashima T, Mori S, Natori T. OLETF (Otsuka Long-Evans Tokushima fatty) rat: a new NIDDM rat strain. *Diabetes Res. Clin. Pract.* 1994;24:317-320.

[123] Karakikes, I Kim, M, Hadri L, Sakata, Sun Y, Zhang W, Chemaly ER, Hajjar RJ, Lebeche D. Gene remodeling in type 2 diabetic cardiomyopathy and its phenotypic rescue with SERCA2a. *PLoS One* 2009;4:6474.

[124] Yagi K, Kim S, Wanibuchi H, Yamashita T, Yamamura Y, Iwao H.Characteristics of diabetes, blood pressure, and cardiac and renal complications in Otsuka Long-Evans Tokushima Fatty rats. *Hypertension* 1997;29:728-735.

[125] Kawano T, Nomura M, Nisikado A, Nakaya Y, Ito S. Supplementation of L-arginine improves hypertension and lipid metabolism but not insulin resistance in diabetic rats. *Life Sci.* 2003;73:3017-3026.

[126] Massiera F, Barbry P, Guesnet P, Joly A, Luguet S, Moreilhon-Brest C, Mohsen-Kanson T, Amri EZ, Ailhaud GA. Western-like fat diet is sufficient to induce a gradual enhancement in fat mass over generations. *J. Lipid Res.* 2010;51:2352-2361.

[127] Le K A, Tappy L. Metabolic effects of fructose. *Curr. Opin. Clin. Nutr. Metab. Care* 2006;9:469-475.

[128] Tappy L, Le KA. Metabolic effects of fructose and the worldwide increase in obesity. *Physiol. Rev.* 2010;90:23-46.

[129] Bray GA, Nielsen S J, Popkin, BM. Consumption of high-fructose corn syrup in beverages may play a role in the epidemic of obesity. *Am. J. Clin. Nutr.* 2004;79:537-543.

[130] Tran LT, Yuen VG, McNeill JH. The fructose fed rat: a review on the mechanisms of fructose-induced insulin resistance and hypertension. *Mol. Cell Biochem.* 2009;332:145-159.

[131] Patel J, Iyer A, Brown L. Evaluation of the chronic complications of diabetes in a high fructose diet in rats. *Indian J. Biochem. Biophys.* 2009;46:66-72.

[132] Chang KC, Liang Jt, Tseng CD, Wu, ET, Hsu KL, Wu MS, Lin YT, Tseng YZ. Aminoguanidine prevents fructose-induced deterioration in left ventriculararterial coupling in Wistar rats. *Br. J. Pharmacol.* 2007;151:34-36.

[133] Kawasaki T, Igarash, K koeda, T, Sugimoto K, Nakagawa K, Hayashi S, Ymaji R, Iyi, H, Fukusato, T, and Yamanouchi, T. Rats fed fructose- enriched diets have characteristics of nonalcoholic hepatic steatosis. *J. Nutr.* 2009;139:2067-2071.

[134] Bocarsly ME, Powell ES, Avena, NM, Hoebel, BG. High-fructose corn syrup causes characteristics of obesity in rats: increased body weight, body fat and triglyceride levels. *Pharmacol. Biochem. Behav.* 2010;97:101-106.

[135] Nakayama T, Kosugi T, Gersch M, Connor T, Sanchez-Lozada LG, Lanaspa MA, Roncal C, Perez-Pozo SE, Johnson R J, Nakagawa T. Dietary fructose causes tubulointerstitial injury in the normal rat kidney. *Am. J. Physiol. Renal. Physiol.* 2010;29:712-720.

[136] Miatello R, Vazquez M, Renna, Cruzado M, Zumino, A P, and Risler, N. Chronic administration of resveratrol prevents biochemical cardiovascular changes in fructose fed rats. *Am. J. Hypertens.* 2005;18:864-870.

[137] Panchal SK, Poudyal H, Lyer A, Nazer R, Alam MA, Diwan V, Kauter K, Sernia C, Campbell F, Ward L, Gobe G, Fenning A, Brown L. High carbohydrate high fat diet-induced metabolic syndrome and cardiovascular remodeling in rats. *J. Cardiovasc. Pharmacol.* 2011;57:611-624.

[138] Kanarek R B, Aprille JR, Hirsh E, Gualtiere L, Brown CA. Sucrose-induced obesity: effect of diet on obesity and brown adipose tissue. *Am. J. Physiol.* 1987;253:158-166.

[139] Santure M, Pitre M, Marette A, Deshaies Y, Lemieux C, Lariviere R, Nadeau A, Bachelard H. Induction of insulin resistance by high-sucrose feeding does not raise mean arterial blood pressure but impairs haemodynamic responses to insulin in rats. Br *J. Pharmacol.* 2002;137:185-196.

[140] Coehlo MS, Lope KL, Freitas RA, de Oliveira-Sales EB, Bergasmaschi CT, Campos RR, Casarini DE, Carmona AK, Araujo MS, Heimann JC, Dolnikoff MS. High sucrose intake in rats is associated with increased ACE2 and angiotensin-(1–7) levels in the adipose tissue. *Regul. Pept* 2010;162:61-67.

[141] Lombardo YB, Drago S, Chicco A, Fainstein-Day P, Gutman R, Gagliardino JJ, Gomez Dumm CL. Long-term administration of a sucrose-rich diet to normal rats: Relationship between metabolic and hormonal profiles and morphological changes in the endocrine pancreas. *Metabolism* 1996;45:1527-1532.

[142] Sharma N, Okere IC, Barrows BR, Lei B, Duda MK, Yuan CL, Previs SF, Sharov VG, Azimzadeh AM, Ernsberger P, Hoit BD, Sabbah H, Stanley WC. High-sugar diets increase cardiac dysfunction and mortality in hypertension compared to low-carbohydrate or high-starch diets. *J. Hypertens.* 2008;26:1402-1410.

[143] Huang W, Metlakunta A, Dedousis N, Zhang P, Sipula I, Dube JJ, Scott, DK, O'Doherty RM. Depletion of liver kupffer cells prevents the development of diet-induced hepatic steatosis and insulin resistance. *Diabetes* 2010;59:347-357.

[144] Woods SC, Seeley RJ, Rushing PA, D'Alessio D, Tso PA. Controlled high-fat diet induces an obese syndrome in rats. *J. Nutr.* 2003;133:1081-1087.

[145] Kobayasi R, Akamine EH, Davel AP, Rodrigues MA, Carvalho CR, Rossoni LV. Oxidative stress and inflammatory mediators contribute to endothelial dysfunction in high-fat diet-induced obesity in mice. *J. Hypertens.* 2010;28:2111-2119.

[146] Deji N, Kume S, Araki S, Soumura M, Sugimoto T, Isshiki K, Chin-Kanasaki M, Sakaguchi M, Koya D, Haneda M, Kashiwagi A, Uzu T. Structural and functional changes in the kidneys of high-fat diet-induced obese mice. *Am. J. Physiol. Renal. Physiol.* 2009;296:118-126.

[147] Buettner R, Parhofer KG, Woenckhaus M, Wrede CE, Kunz-Schughart LA, Scholmerich J, Bolheimer LC. Defining high-fat-diet rat models: metabolic and molecular effects of different fat types. *J. Mol. Endocrinol.* 2006;36:485-501.

[148] Sutherland LN, Capozzi LC, Turchinsky NJ, Bell RC, Wright DC. Time course of high-fat diet-induced reductions in adipose tissue mitochondrial proteins: potential mechanisms and the relationship to glucose intolerance. *Am. J. Physiol. Endocrinol. Metab.* 2008;295:1076-1083.

[149] Lei F, Zhang XN, Wang W, Xing DM, Xie WD, Su H, Du LJ. Evidence of antiobesity effects of the pomegranate leaf extract in high-fat diet induced obese mice. *Int. J. Obes.* 2007;31:1023-1029.

[150] Sweazea KL, Lekic M, Walker BR. Comparison of mechanisms involved in impaired vascular reactivity between high sucrose and high fat diets in rats. *Nutr. Metab.* 2010;4:7-48.

[151] Kim SM, Rico CW, Lee SC, Kang MY. Modulatory effect of rice bran and phytic acid on glucose metabolism in high fat-fed C57BL/6N mice. *J. Clin. Biochem. Nutr.* 2010;47:12-17.

[152] Hsu CL, Wu CH, Huang SL, Yen GC. Phenolic compounds rutin and o-coumaric acid ameliorate obesity induced by high-fat diet in rats. *J. Agric. Food Chem.* 2009;57:425-431.

[153] Kohli R, Kirby M, Xanthakos SA, Softic S, Feldstein AE, Saxena V, Tang PH, Miles L, Miles MV, Balistreri WF, Woods SC, Seeley RJ. High-fructose, medium chain trans fat diet induces liver fibrosis and elevates plasma coenzyme Q9 in a novel murine model of obesity and nonalcoholic steatohepatitis. *Hepatology* 2010;52:934-944.

[154] Murase T, Mizuno T, Omachi T, Onizawa K, Komine Y, Kondo H, Hase T, Tokimitsu I. Dietary diacylglycerol suppresses high fat and high sucrose diet-induced body fat accumulation in C57BL/6J mice. *J. Lipid Res.* 2001;42:372-378.

[155] Parekh PI, Petro AE, Tiller JM, Feinglos MN, Surwit RS. Reversal of diet-induced obesity and diabetes in C57BL/6J mice. *Metabolism* 1998;47:1089-1096.

[156] Sato A, Kawano H, Notsu T, Ohta M, Nakakuki M, Mizuguchi K, Itoh M, Suganami T, Ogawa Y. Antiobesity effect of eicosapentaenoic acid in high-fat/high-sucrose diet-induced obesity: importance of hepatic lipogenesis. *Diabetes* 2010;59:2495-2504.

[157] Hsu CL, Wu CH, Huang SL, Yen GC. Phenolic compounds rutin and o-coumaric acid ameliorate obesity induced by high-fat diet in rats. *J. Agric. Food Chem.* 2009;57:425-431.

[158] Wada T, Kenmochi H, Miyashita Y, Sasaki M, Ojima M, Sasahara M, Koya D, Tsuneki H, Sasaoka T. Spironolactone improves glucose and lipid metabolism by ameliorating hepatic steatosis and inflammation and suppressing enhanced gluconeogenesis induced by high-fat and high-fructose diet. *Endocrinology* 2010;151:2040-9.

[159] Chatterjee TK, Stoll LL, Denning GM, Harrelson A, Blomkalns AL, Idelman G, Rothenberg FG, Neltner B, Romig-Martin SA, Dickson EW, Rudich S, Weintraub NL. Proinflammatory phenotype of perivascular adipocytes: influence of high-fat feeding. *Circ. Res.* 2009;104:541-549.

[160] Dobrian AD, Davies MJ, Schriver SD, Lauterio TJ, Prewitt RL. Oxidative stress in a rat model of obesity-induced hypertension. *Hypertension* 2001;37:554-560.

[161] Ketonen J, Shi J, Martonen E, Mervaala E. Periadventitial adipose tissue promotes endothelial dysfunction via oxidative stress in diet-induced obese C57BL/6 mice. *Circ. J. 2010*;74:1479-1487.

[162] Elizalde M, Ryden M, van Harmelen V, Eneroth P, Gyllenhammar H, Holm C, Ramel S, Olund A, Arner P, Anderson K. Expression of nitric oxide synthases in subcutaneous adipose tissue of non obese and obese humans. *J. Lipid Res.* 2000;41:1244-1251

[163] Packer M. Beta-adrenergic blockade in chronic heart failure: principles, progress, and practice. *Prog. Cardiovasc. Dis.* 1998;41:39-52.

[164] Jacob S, Rett K, Wicklmayr M, Agrawal B, Augustin HJ, Dietze GJ. Differential effect of chronic treatment with two beta-blocking agents on insulin sensitivity: the Carvedilol–Metoprolol study. *J. Hypertens.* 1996;14:489-494.

[165] Lund-Johansen P, Omvik P, Nordrehauq JE. Long-term hemodynamic effects of antihypertensive treatment. *Clin. Investig.* 1992;70-58-64.

[166] Agabiti-Rosei E, Porteri E, Rizzoni D. Arterial stiffnes, hypertension, and rational use of nebivolol. *Vasc. Health Risk Manag.* 2009;5:353-360.

[167] DeFronzo RA, Mandarino L, Ferranini E. Metabolic and molecular pathogenesis of type 2 diabetes mellitus. In: DeFronzo RA, Ferrannini E, Keen H, Zimmet P, eds. International Textbook of Diabetes Mellitus, Vol 1, 3rd ed. Chichester: John Wiley & Sons Ltd; 2004:389–438.

[168] Agabiti Rosei E, Rizzoni D. Metabolic profile of nebivolol, a beta-adrenoceptor antagonist with unique characteristics. *Drugs* 2007;67:1097-1107.

[169] Louis WJ, McNeill JJ, Drummer OH. Pharmacology of combined alpha-beta-blockade. *Drugs* 1984;28:16-34.

[170] Siwach SB, Dahiya SS, Seth S, Seth RK, Sharma D. Effect of atenolol and labetalol on serum lipids. *J. Assoc. Physicians India* 1993;41:293-294.

[171] Pedersen ME, Cockcroft JR. The vasodilatory beta-blockers. *Curr. Hypertens. Rep.* 2007;9:269-277.

[172] Kozlovski VI, Lomnicka M, Chlopicki S. Nebivovol and carvedilol induce NO-dependent coronary vasodilatation that is unlikely to be mediated by extracellular ATP in the isolated guinea pig heart. *Pharmacol. Rep.* 2006;58:103-110.

[173] Dandona P, Ghanim H, Brooks DP. Antioxidant activity of carvedilol in cardiovascular disease. *J. Hypertens.* 2007;25:731-741.

[174] Toda N. Vasodilating beta-adrenoceptor blockers as cardiovascular therapeutics. *Pharmacol. Ther.* 2003;100:215-234.

[175] Fratta Pasini A, Garbin U, Nava MC, Stranieri C, Davoli A, Sawamura T, Lo Cascio V, Cominacini L. Nebivolol decreases oxidative stress in essential hypertensive patients and increases nitric oxide by reducing its oxidative inactivation. *J. Hypertens.* 2005;23:589-596.

[176] Rizos E, Bairaktari E, Kostoula A, Hasiotis G, Achimastos A, Ganotakis E, Elisaf M, Mikhailidis DP. The combination of nebivolol plus pravastatin is associated with a more beneficial metabolic profile compared to that of atenolol plus pravastatin in hypertensive patients with dyslipidemia: a pilot study. *J. Cardiovasc. Pharmacol. Ther.* 2003;8:127-134.

[177] Jandeleit-Dahm KA, Tikellis C, Reid CM, Johnston CI, Cooper ME. Why blockade of the renin-angiotensin system reduces the incidence of new-onset diabetes. *J. Hypertens.* 2005;2:463–473.

[178] Lindholm LH, Ibsen H, Borch-Johnsen K, Olsen MH, Wachtell K, Dahlöf B, Devereux RB, Beevers G, de Faire U, Fyhrquist F, Julius S, Kjeldsen SE, Kristianson K, Lederballe-Pedersen O, Nieminen MS, Omvik P, Oparil S, Wedel H, Aurup P, Edelman JM, Snapinn S; LIFE study group. Risk of new-onset diabetes in the Losartan Intervention For Endpoint reduction in hypertension study. *J. Hypertens.* 2002;20:1879–1886.

[179] Gupta AK, Dahlof B, Dobson J, Sever PS, Wedel H, Poulter NR; Anglo-Scandinavian Cardiac Outcomes Trial Investigators. Determinants of new-onset diabetes among 19.257 hypertensive patients randomized in the Anglo-Scandinavian Cardiac Outcomes Trial – Blood Pressure Lowering Arm and the relative influence of antihypertensive medication. *Diabetes Care* 2008;31:982–988.

[180] Lardizabal JA, Deedwania PC. The role of renin-angiotensin agents in altering the natural history of type 2 diabetes mellitus. *Curr. Cardiol. Rep.* 2010;12:464–471.

[181] Wing LM, Reid CM, Ryan P, Beilin LJ, Brown MA, Jennings GL, Johnston CI, McNeil JJ, Macdonald GJ, Marley JE, Morgan TO, West MJ; Second Australian National Blood Pressure Study Group. A comparison of outcomes with angiotensin-converting – enzyme inhibitors and diuretics for hypertension in the elderly. *N. Engl. J. Med.* 2003;348:583–592.

[182] Redon J, Cifkova R, Laurent S, Nilsson P, Narkiewicz K, Erdine S, Mancia G; Scientific Council of the European Society of Hypertension. The metabolic syndrome in hypertension: European Society of Hypertension position statement. *J. Hypertens.* 2008;26:1891–1900.

[183] Grimm C, Köberlein J, Wiosna W, Kresimon J, Kiencke P, Rychlik R. New-onset diabetes and antihypertensive treatment. *GMS Health Technol. Assess.* 2010;6:3.

[184] Flora S. Role of free radicals and antioxidants in health and disease. *Cell. Mol. Biol.* 2007:53:1–2.

[185] Zhan CD, Sindhu RK, Vaziri ND. Up-regulation of kidney NAD(P)H oxidase and calcineurin in SHR: reversal by lifelong antioxidant supplementation. *Kidney Int.* 2004;65:219–227.

[186] Antoniades C, Tousoulis D, Tentolouris C, Toutouzas P, Stefanadis C. Oxidative stress, antioxidant vitamins, and atherosclerosis. From basic research to clinical practice. *Herz* 2003;28:628–638.

[187] Duarte TL, Lunec J. Review: when is an antioxidant not an antioxidant? A review of novel actions and reactions of vitamin C. *Free Radic. Res.* 2005;39:671–686.

[188] Ulker S, McKeown PP, Bayraktutan U. Vitamins reverse endothelial dysfunction through regulation of eNOS and NAD(P)H oxidase activities. *Hypertension* 2003;41:534-549.

[189] Faure P, Barclay D, Joyeux-Faure M, Halimi S. Comparison of the effects of zinc alone and zinc associated with selenium and vitamin E on insulin sensitivity and oxidative stress in high-fructose-fed rats. *J. Trace Elem. Med. Biol.* 2007;21:113-119.

[190] Moreau KL, Gavin KM, Plum AE, Seals DR. Ascorbic acid selectively improves large elastic artery compliance in postmenopausal women. *Hypertension* 2005;45:1107–1112.

[191] Schneider MP, Delles C, Schmidt BM, Oehmer S, Schwarz TK, Schmieder RE, John S. Superoxide scavenging effects of N-acetylcysteine and vitamin C in subjects with essential hypertension. *Am. J. Hypertens.* 2005;18:1111–1117.

[192] Beckman JA, Goldfine AB, Gordon MB, Creager MA. Ascorbate restores endothelium dependent vasodilation impaired by acute hyperglycemia in humans. *Circulation* 2001;103:1618–1623.

[193] Shimamoto K, Ura N. Mechanisms of insulin resistance in hypertensive rats. *Clin. Exp. Hypertens. 2006*;28:543-552.

[194] Quinzii CM, López LC, Naini A, DiMauro S, Hirano M. Human CoQ10 deficiencies. *Biofactors* 2008;32:113-118.

[195] Lankin VZ, Tikhaze AK, Kapel'ko VI, Shepel'kova GS, Shumaev KB, Panasenko OM, Konovalova GG, Belenkov YN. Mechanisms of oxidative modification of low density lipoproteins under conditions of oxidative and carbonyl stress. *Biochemistry* (Mosc) 2007;72:1081-1090.

[196] Picchi A, Gao X, Belmadani S, Potter BJ, Focardi M, Chilian WM, Zhang C. Tumor necrosis factor-alpha induces endothelial dysfunction in the prediabetic metabolic syndrome. *Circ. Res.* 2006;99:69–77.

[197] Ginsberg HN. Insulin resistance and cardiovascular disease. *J. Clin. Invest.* 2000;106:629–631.

[198] Ceriello A, Motz E. Is oxidative stress the pathogenic mechanism underlying insulin resistance, diabetes and cardiovascular disease? The common soil hypothesis revisited. *Arterioscler. Thromb. Vasc. Biol.* 2004;24:816–823.

In: Advances in Hypertension Research
Editor: Ramón Rodrigo
ISBN: 978-1-62948-857-8

Chapter 6

Hypertension and Chronic Kidney Disease*

María Fernanda Galleguillos†, Catherine Céspedes and Diego Saa
Molecular and Clinical Pharmacology Program, Institute of Biomedical Sciences, Faculty of Medicine, University of Chile, Chile

Abstract

Chronic kidney disease (CKD) has been defined as a permanent kidney damage, resulting in diminished glomerular filtration rate (GFR) and presence of albuminuria. It is becoming an increasingly important public health issue owing in part to its steadily increasing prevalence due to an aging population and increases in hypertension, diabetes mellitus and obesity. On the other hand, despite advances in chronic renal replacement therapies (CRRT) including dialysis and kidney transplantation, these patients are at an increased risk of cardiovascular morbidity and mortality. Furthermore, CRRT have important associated economic costs, such that the burden on health care systems has forced the attention of clinical physicians on researching prevention strategies. Thus, treatment of hypertension has become of increasing interest to researchers around the world, because the cause-effect relationship of CKD and hypertension is cyclic. Hypertension is a risk factor and one of the leading causes of CKD worldwide, while most of patients with CKD present hypertension due to progressive renal failure and subsequently volume expansion and increased systemic vascular resistance. Therefore, many different clinical guidelines emphasize the importance of decreasing blood pressure to slow progression of renal disease and reduce cardiovascular morbidity and mortality. In order to accomplish such an objective; however, a better understanding of the pathophysiology and the mechanisms of hypertension in context of CKD is needed, to

* Supported by FONDECYT, grant 1120594
† Corresponding author: María Fernanda Galleguillos Elgueta, Molecular and Clinical Pharmacology Program, Institute of Biomedical Sciences, Faculty of Medicine, University of Chile, Independencia 1027, C.P. 8380453, Santiago, Chile, Telephone: 56-2-29786126 Fax: 56-2-29786126, E-mail: fernanda.galleguillos.e@gmail.com.

develop better drugs that allow aiming multiple important targets and thus optimizing current treatment interventions and lowering the costs.

Keywords: Chronic kidney disease, hypertension, chronic renal replacement therapies, renin-angiotensin-aldosterone system, oxidative stress, sympathetic nervous system.

Abbreviations

AASK	African American Study of Kidney Disease
ABP	Ambulatory blood pressure
ACE	Angiotensin-converting enzyme
ACEIs	ACE inhibitors
ADA	American Diabetes Association
ADMA	Asymmetric dimethylarginine
Ang II	Angiotensin II
ANP	Atrial natriuretic peptide
ARBs	Angiotensin II receptor blockers
AT_1-R	Angiotensin II type 1 receptor
CAT	Catalase
CKD	Chronic kidney disease
CRRT	Chronic renal replacement therapies
CuZnSOD	Copper–zinc superoxide dismutase
CVD	Cardiovascular disease
DA	Dopamine
ED	Endothelial dysfunction
ESRD	End stage renal disease
ET-1	Endothelin-1
GFR	Glomerular filtration rate
GPx	Glutathione peroxidase
GSH	Glutathione
H_2O_2	Hydrogen peroxide
ICV:	Intracerebroventricular
JNC-7	Joint National Committee's seventh report
K/DOQI	Kidney Disease Outcomes Quality Initiative
KDIGO	Kidney Disease Improving Global Outcomes
KEEP	Kidney Early Evaluation Program
L-NAME	L-arginine analog N-nitro-L-arginine methylester
MSNA	Muscle sympathetic nerve activity
NADP or NADPH	Nicotinamide adenine dinucleotide phosphate
NADP/NADPH oxidase	Nicotinamide adenine dinucleotide phosphate-oxidase
NE	Norepinephrine
NHANES	National Health and Nutrition Examination Survey
NKF	National Kidney Foundation
NO	Nitric oxide
NOS	Nitric oxide synthase

$\bullet O_2^-$	Superoxide anion
OE :	Oxidative stress
$^\cdot OH$	Hidroxyl radical
$ONOO^-$	Peroxynitrite
PAI-1	Plasminogen activator inhibitor-1
PH	Posterior hypothalamus
PSNS	Parasympathetic nervous system
PTH	Parathyroid hormone
PVN	Paraventricular nucleus of hypothalamus
RAAS	Renin-angiotensin-aldosterone system
ROS	Reactive oxygen species
RSNA	Renal sympathetic nervous system activity
RVLM	Rostral ventrolateral medulla
SNA	Sympathetic nerve activity
SNS	Sympathetic nervous system
TGF-β	Transforming growth factor-β
TLH	Thick ascending loop of Henle
TNF-α	Tumor necrosis factor α
UII	Urotensin II

1. Introduction

Chronic kidney disease (CKD) is becoming an important public health issue [1–3], because it is associated with all-cause and cardiovascular disease mortality [4]. Furthermore, CKD may progress to end-stage renal disease (ESRD) which in the United States alone affects up to 570,000 people, including nearly 400,000 dialysis patients and over 17,000 transplant recipients [5]. However, ESRD is only the tip of the iceberg, since the prevalence of earlier stages of CKD has been estimated to be as high as 80 times greater than ESRD prevalence [2]. The prevalence of CKD in the United States has been steadily increasing, as manifested by a study by Coresh et al. where they compared the prevalence of CKD over 2 decades; 10.0% between 1988–1994 versus 13.1% between 1999–2004 [6]. Similar prevalence rates has been obtained in different epidemiologic studies in England, Korea and India, with prevalence rates of CKD ranging from 13% to 17% [4, 7, 8].

Theoretically, the reasons to explain this steady increase in CKD prevalence are multiple, not only due to its increasingly high incidence, but also because it has been associated with poor outcomes [2], despite the advances in chronic renal replacement therapies (CRRT). In addition, from an economic perspective, the substantial costs during earlier stages of CKD depend on stage and include among other costs up to 1.9-2.5 times more prescriptions, 1.3-1.9 times more outpatient visits, and 1.6-2.2 times more probability of inpatient stay [9]. Finally, as disease severity progresses into CRRT, costs increase markedly and remain elevated thereafter. Therefore, more proactive management in earlier stages may lead to improved clinical and economic outcomes through the slowing of disease progression and prevention of comorbidities [10]. Thus, as mentioned previously, CKD-associated all-cause and cardiovascular disease (CVD) morbid-mortality risk are mainly attributed to myocardial infarction, heart failure, stroke, or sudden cardiac death, as well as many chronic diseases, such as diabetes [1, 2, 4, 5]. Therefore, management of high risk patients who develop either hypertension and/or diabetes is particularly important, since elevated blood pressure (BP) is closely associated with CKD progression, and lowering of BP may slow down GFR decline [4], as shown by a number of studies reporting that hypertension is involved in CKD, emphasizing the importance of BP control in improving kidney function. Both Kidney Early Evaluation Program (KEEP) and National Health and Nutrition Examination Survey (NHANES) data showed a strong association between hypertension and kidney disease [12].

In 2002, the National Kidney Foundation (NKF) Kidney Disease Outcomes Quality Initiative (K/DOQI) guidelines proposed a definition and classification system for CKD [13]. These definitions and classification systems were later adopted with some minor clarifications in 2004 by the international guideline group Kidney Disease Improving Global Outcomes (KDIGO) [14].

Finally, current definition of CKD corresponds to: (a) kidney damage for more than 3 months, as defined by structural or functional abnormalities of the kidney manifested by either pathological abnormalities and/or markers of kidney damage including abnormalities in the composition of the blood or urine (such as albuminuria), or abnormalities in imaging test, or (b) by a GFR below 60 mL/min/1.73m^2 for at least three months, irrespective of the cause [13, 14].

On the other hand, hypertension is a common comorbidity in 65–95% of patients with CKD and a major risk factor for progressive deterioration of renal function [11, 15]. Hypertension is a chronic non transmittable disease that affects more than 67.5 million adults in the United States.

According to the National Health and Nutrition Examination Survey (NHANES) data, antihypertensive medication use among US adults with hypertension has increased from 63.5% to 77.3% during the past decade (2001–2010) [12]. However, there continues to be a gap between hypertension treatment and control, as BP was controlled in only 47% of all hypertensive patients and 60% of treated hypertensive patients [16]. Thus, the vast majority of patients remain uncontrolled, with office BP >130/80 mmHg [11, 15, 17]. As mentioned earlier, BP control is an important therapeutic target in this population. However, BP control in patients with CKD and hypertension mare a specific subset of patients who may impose a difficult challenge: on one hand they might benefit from tight BP control, but they might also suffer detrimental effects from it, due to worsening renal function, orthostasis, and low DBP due to a large pulse pressure [16]. Poorly controlled hypertension is a major risk factor in non-dialysis CKD patients.

Current guidelines for CKD patients along with the Seventh Report of the Joint National Committee on High BP (JNC-7) recommend an office BP target <130/80 mm Hg [4, 18, 19]. These recommendations, largely extrapolated from post hoc analysis of renal trials, are being debated, because recent trials and cohort studies have in fact disclosed a lack of association between more aggressive treatment or achieved BP and prognosis. The absence of a predictive role of office BP in treated CKD might relate, at least in part, to the high prevalence of white coat hypertension (i.e., high office BP and normal ambulatory blood pressure [ABP]), which might also explain why ABP better predicts mortality and ESRD than office BP [18].

Considering all of the arguments presented previously, novel strategies that are aimed at identifying, preventing, and treating CKD and its related risk factors are urgently needed and under extensive research [2]. Thus, pharmaceutical industries have focused their efforts mainly on the key pathophysiologic role of both hypervolemia and activation of the renin-angiotensin-aldosterone system (RAAS) in hypertension and CKD. As a result, lifestyle modifications and pharmacologic therapeutic strategies for patients with hypertension and CKD have mostly focused on interventions in these two pathways. It has been extensively demonstrated that RAAS inhibition decreases the progression of both worsening renal function and proteinuria [11]. In addition, it has been demonstrated that they are also effective interventions to prevent or delay CKD progression, which results in less ESRD and cardiovascular comorbidity [3]. Furthermore, accumulating evidence shows that activation of the sympathetic nervous system (SNS) contributes to the pathophysiology of numerous chronic cardiovascular diseases, including essential hypertension, heart failure, obstructive sleep apnea, metabolic syndrome, and diabetes, as well as CKD [20]. This last fact has been demonstrated in patients undergoing haemodialysis, who show increased sympathetic activity.

Thus, sympathetic activation induces renal vasoconstriction and increased renin secretion with enhanced sodium and water reabsorption. Hyperactivation of the sympathetic nervous system aggravates hypertension and it is related to left ventricular hypertrophy, heart failure, arrhythmias and atherogenesis. Other studies were conducted where correction of uraemia by renal transplantation did not result in the normalization of sympathetic activity, suggesting that sympathetic activation is driven by the native kidney [21]. In this chapter, we will review the major mechanisms that play an important role in hypertension in context of CKD, focusing on recent research studies pointing towards novel therapeutic targets.

2. Pathophysiology

Kidney and high blood pressure are intimately related, both pathophysiologically and pathogenically. Uncontrolled long-standing elevated BP is well recognized as both a manifestation and a contributor to CKD. Uncontrolled hypertension is an independent predictor of CKD progression and increased risk of ESRD as noted in multiple retrospective studies of individuals with and without baseline CKD [22]. Traditionally this hypertension has been viewed as largely volume-dependent. More than three decades ago, Kim et al. [23] showed that hypertensive and normotensive hemodialysis patients differ in peripheral vascular resistance and not in cardiac output. Importantly, after bilateral nephrectomy blood pressure was reduced by a decrease in resistance and not in cardiac output. This provided direct evidence that the diseased kidneys were somehow involved in the genesis of increased vascular resistance and therefore hypertension in CKD. Nowadays there is evidence demonstrating that the pathogenesis in the development and maintenance of hypertension related to CKD is complex and multifactorial, especially in the late stages of renal disease. In addition to the classical factors, such as increased intravascular volume and excessive activity of the RAAS, new recognized mechanisms have been gaining growing attention, such as the sympathetic nervous system hyperactivity, endothelial dysfunction and alterations of several humoral and neural factors that promote increased blood pressure [24-27] (Table 6-1).

2.1. Blood Volume and Sodium Homeostasis

During the last decades, a bulk of evidence shows that volume expansion is the first and major pathogenic mechanism for hypertension in CKD. The fundamental role of the kidney in the control of sodium and water homeostasis is well acknowledged [24].

Table 6-1. Factors that may cause hypertension in chronic kidney disease

Factor	Dominant mechanism
Impaired sodium excretion	Expansion of ECF volume
Activation of RAAS	Direct vasoconstriction Sympathetic activation
Sympathetic activation	Direct vasoconstriction Stimulation of renin release
Imbalance in prostaglandins or kinins	Vasoconstriction
Endothelin	Direct vasoconstriction Renal injury
Reduced nitric oxide	Loss of vasodilator effect
Urotensin II	Vasoconstriction/Vasodilatation Inotropic effects
Uric acid	Inflammation Endothelial dysfunction

ECF: extracellular fluid;
RAAS: renin-angiotensin-aldosterone system.

The kidneys play such a vital role in long-term blood pressure regulation that Guyton argued that sustained hypertension could not occur in the absence of impairment of renal handling of sodium [28]. The total body sodium content is the main determinant of extracellular volume, so that alterations in sodium balance will result in clinical situations of volume depletion or excess. In physiological conditions, the volume expansion is followed by an increase in natriuresis, thus maintaining a constant ratio between the volume of the intravascular space and vascular capacitance. These changes can be achieved by suppression of RAAS, inactivation of the sympathetic nervous system (SNS) and eliciting intrarenal hemodynamic changes.

As kidney function progressively decreases in CKD, in order to maintain sodium balance the fraction of sodium excretion of functioning nephrons increases proportional to the loss of glomerular filtration. Thus, there is a proportional increase in the excretion of sodium, to the decrease in functioning nephrons. This increase has been partly attributed to increased circulating natriuretic factor secretion inhibiting sodium´s distal reabsorption [29]. Atrial natriuretic peptide (ANP) is released in response to the expansion of extracellular space and increases sodium excretion through a variety of mechanisms, including increased glomerular capillary hydraulic pressure and increased glomerular ultrafiltration coefficient [30]. Add to this the increased insulin resistance, elevated parathyroid hormone (PTH), inappropriate activation of the RAAS and SNS, and the vascular endothelium, the result is an increase in the peripheral vascular resistance.

According to the Guyton's whole-body auto-regulation concept, many organs, including the kidney, have the ability to maintain a relatively constant blood flow in the presence of variations of the perfusion pressure [27]. Guyton proposed that this auto-regulation could be responsible for the secondary increase of the peripheral resistance in the presence of blood volume expansion, as occurring in CKD [24]. (Table 6-2)

When kidney failure progresses to later stages, total sodium excretion decreases despite the renal and extrarenal mechanisms of adaptation [31], leading to a positive sodium and fluid balance.

Table 6-2. Mechanisms of adaptation to sodium balance in chronic kidney disease

Increased fractional excretion of sodium Expansion of volume Increased natriuretic peptides Decline in mineralocorticoid activity Release of renal vasoactive substances (prostaglandins, kinins, catecholamines) Hyperfiltration in functioning nephrons
Extrarenal mechanisms
Accumulation of intracellular sodium due to alterations in the activity of Na-K-ATPase and metabolic acidosis Increase in plasma volume Increase in interstitial fluid

Taken to the extreme, this positive sodium balance causes extracellular volume expansion, which can lead to acute pulmonary edema and/or anasarca. However, the most common manifestation of the extracellular space expansion in patients with end stage renal disease (ESRD) is hypertension (figure 6-1).

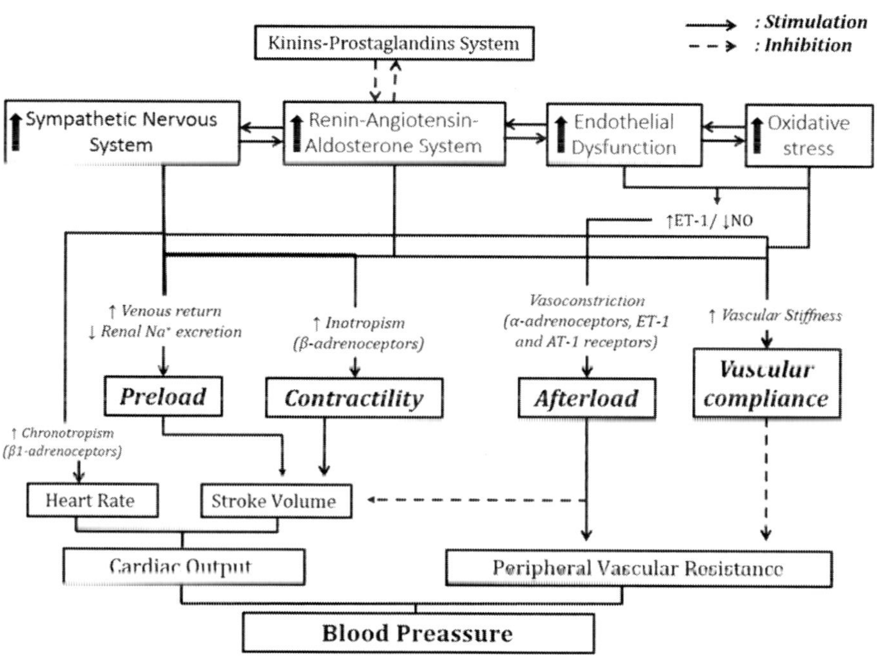

Figure 6-1. Pathophysiology of CKD: Blood volume and sodium homeostasis. ET-1: endothelin 1, NO: nitric oxide, ET-1 receptor: endothelin 1 receptor and AT-1 receptor: angiotensine 1 receptor.

2.2. Symphathetic Nervous System

The autonomic nervous system plays a key position in the normal regulation of the cardiovascular system. This is primarily achieved through the effects of the SNS on the function of the heart, arteries, arterioles, veins and kidneys. The parasympathetic nervous system (PSNS), through vagus nerve regulation of the heart rate, plays a subsidiary role [32]. Accumulating evidence has shown that the SNS plays an important role in the pathophysiology and progression of several chronic disorders, e.g., arterial hypertension, cardiac arrhythmias, heart failure, and in particular CKD [11]. In 1972, Kim et al. [24] provided indirect evidence for the existence of sympathetic activation in patients with ESRD and hypertension. They showed that hypertension in ESRD is caused by an increased peripheral resistance. In 1983, Ishii et al. [33] documented elevated concentrations of plasma catecholamines and enhanced sensitivity to norepinephrine (NE) in patients with CKD, indicating increased sympathetic activity in this group. Subsequently, increased muscle sympathetic nerve activity (MSNA) has been reported in patients with ESRD undergoing haemodialysis [34].

Sympathetic hyperactivity plays an important and distinct role in hypertension associated with CKD. This was recognized as an early pathophysiological element of CKD initiated by various forms of renal damage via afferent signals through sensory renal nerves [35]. In 2011, Grassi et al. [36] demonstrated that increased adrenergic activation is detectable in the early stages of CKD (mean estimated glomerular filtration rate: 40.7 ml/min per 1.73 m^2, MDRD formula) despite adequate BP control. They showed that the magnitude of the adrenergic overdrive parallels the severity of CKD and is inversely related ($p<0.0001$) to the GFR [36]. Penne et al. [37] found that the severity of CKD correlates positively with MSNA. These clinical data provide solid support for the view that sympathetic activity is increased in CKD, but the exact pathophysiological responsible mechanisms are not yet fully defined. Renal ischemia, elevated angiotensin II (Ang II), and suppressed brain nitric oxide (NO) all stimulate sympathetic activity [38, 39]. Furthermore, other factors like chemoreflex activation and asymmetric dimethylarginine (ADMA) also activate the SNS in CKD. The most important are explained below:

2.2.1. Angiotensin II

The activation of the SNS in CKD may be related to the effects of circulating Ang II released from the kidneys. Ang II can stimulate the SNS by a direct effect on the vasomotor center in the brain stem. In addition, Ang II increases the NE release at the adrenergic nerve terminal and inhibits the presynaptic reuptake of NE. In 2002, Campese et al. [40] showed that intracerebroventricular (ICV) infusion of Ang II raises BP, renal sympathetic nervous system activity (RSNA), and NE secretion from the posterior hypothalamus (PH) compared to control rats. Pretreatment with losartan, an AT1 receptor blocker, given as an ICV infusion 20 min prior to the infusion of Ang II completely abolished the effects of Ang II on BP, RSNA, and NE secretion from the PH. Antagonists of the RAAS, such as angiotensin-converting enzyme (ACE) inhibitors and angiotensin II AT1 receptor antagonists, inhibit the production of Ang II or its ability to bind to its receptor, resulting in partial inhibition of the SNS activity in humans with CKD [41]. Same results were shown in 5/6 nephrectomized rats [42], and in the phenol-renal injury model [43].

2.2.2. Oxidative Stress

Reactive oxygen species (ROS) are involved in the regulation of SNS activity [44]. Different studies have found increased oxidative stress (OE) in different areas of the brain related with hypertension and sympathetic over-activity [45]. More details on this particular topic will be discussed later in another section.

2.2.3. Hypoxia and Renal Injury

The main factor is probably renal ischemia [46]. Substantial evidence suggests that kidney ischemia may be responsible for SNS activation in renal hypertension. This is supported by studies in conscious rats with acute renal artery stenosis where it was found hemodynamic changes, renin-dependent hypertension and increased vasoconstrictor tone when plasma renin activity increased. Besides, induced hypertension in these rats is not only renin-dependent but it is also associated with inappropriately high neurogenic vasoconstrictor tone. In the experiment, the renin-angiotensin system was removed with ACE inhibitor undergoing a sharp reduction in renal blood flow, but not the systemic vasoconstrictor tone, which makes us thinking that hypertension is also mediated by renal afferent stimulation that activates SNS [46]. Restoration of renal perfusion in humans with renovascular hypertension reduces MSNA to control levels and leads to normalization of BP [38]. In rats, induction of renal artery stenosis [47], partial renal ablation by arterial ligation [48] or intrarenal phenol injection [49] cause excitation of the renal afferent nerves, this results in neurogenic hypertension. In other experimental model of phenol-induced acute renal injury, even minimal renal damage that did not alter the GFR induced permanent neurogenic hypertension, which could be prevented by renal sympathectomy [50]. Additionally, in the phenol hypertension model, nephrectomy of the injured kidney several weeks after the induction of renal damage results in normalization of BP [51]. Recovery of renal function after kidney transplantation does not result in significant reductions in MSNA in transplant recipients with intact native kidneys, whereas bilateral nephrectomy in transplant recipients restores MSNA to the levels seen in normal control individuals [35]. These findings indicate that in injured kidneys afferent signals to central integrative structures in the brain lead to increased sympathetic activation [52]. Thus, diseased kidneys themselves, independent of renal function, contribute to sympathetic overdrive in ESRD. Furthermore, more recent studies show that afferent renal nerves provide tonic sympathetic inhibition, which seems to be mediated by neurokinin release acting via neurokinin 1 receptor pathways [53].

Renal ischemia and renal injury activate the SNS via mechano- and chemoreceptors-mediated release of adenosine, a potent activator of afferent neurons. Katholi RE et al. [54] found that adenosine evokes an increase in afferent renal nerve traffic, as can be shown during adenosine infusion in the renal artery of uninephrectomized dogs. Independently of the sympathetic effects, renal ischemia also leads to an increase in Ang II through RAAS activation, thus further contributing to sustained sympathetic stimulation [55, 56].

2.2.4. Nitric Oxide

Recent studies have provided compelling evidence that nitric oxide synthase (NOS) is present in specific areas of the brain involved in the neurogenic control of BP [46]. In normal rats, the basal activity of the central SNS is regulated by local NO production. Evidence also indicates that local production of NO may modulate sympathetic activity in brain nuclei involved in the neurogenic regulation of BP [57], and thus chronically reduced NO bioavailability in these nuclei results in sympathetic overactivity and hypertension.

In animals, the sympathoexcitatory effect of NO inhibition has been clearly demonstrated during systemic administration of NO synthesis inhibitors and is greatly attenuated by sympathectomy or by renal denervation (RD) [58]. Basal activity of central sympathetic activity is inhibited by central NO production [58]. NO synthesis inhibition by L-arginine analog N-nitro-L-arginine methylester (L-NAME) results in an increase of central sympathetic activity, thereby increasing MSNA activity [59]. Patients with CKD and ESRD have impaired NO bioavailability caused by a variety of mechanisms, e.g., inflammation, OE, and uremic toxins, which interfere with renal NOS activity and accumulation of endogenous inhibitors of NOS, including ADMA, which is a common finding in patients with CKD [60 – 62]. In addition, ADMA levels correlate positively with MSNA and plasma NE levels, left ventricular hypertrophy, and left ventricular dysfunction, that may contribute to cardiovascular morbidity and mortality [63, 64]. These findings suggest that ADMA plays a major role in reducing NO levels, leading to enhanced sympathetic nervous activation. However, ADMA cannot be the only element involved because its levels are very low [65]. Moreover, direct effects of uremia cannot be the whole story, because SNS activity is already increased at earlier stages when renal function is not or only slightly impaired [41] and sympathetic hyperactivity remains after correction of uremia by renal transplantation [35].

The central SNS provides the kidneys with efferent fibers and receives information from the kidneys via afferent fibers [32]. The efferent fibers innervate predominantly the renal vasculature, the proximal tubular segment of the nephron, and juxtaglomerular renin-containing granular cells [66]. Efferent nerve terminals co-release a variety of neurotransmitters, specifically NE, neuropeptide Y and adenosine triphosphate [67]. The principal mechanisms by which the renal efferent nerves stimulation influence the regulation of BP are:

- *Increasing efferent arteriolar vasoconstriction (mediated through α-receptors),* causing a greater fraction of plasma to traverse the glomerulus and be filtered [68]. This relative increase in filtration of plasma leaves a greater concentration of proteins present when plasma finishes its course through the glomerulus and then enters the network of capillaries surrounding the proximal tubule. Because of this protein enrichment, this plasma has a greater oncotic pressure, so that it can reabsorb more sodium filtered at the glomerulus while it passes through the peritubular capillaries and tubules. This leads to overall sodium retention, primarily obtained from glomerular filtrate [69].
- *Increasing tubular sodium reabsorption via β1-adrenoceptor-mediated stimulation of adluminalbasolateral Na/K adenosine triphosphatase* [66].
- *Reducing renal blood flow via α1-adrenoreceptor stimulation* [66], increasing arterial stiffness. But there are more factors that lead to an excess of vasoconstriction, including RAAS, endothelin and endothelial dysfunction (ED) [70].
- *Increasing renin release from the juxtaglomerular apparatus via β1-adrenoceptor stimulation* [66]. Release of renin initiates the cascade of RAAS, which results in an increase in circulating angiotensin II [68], which will exert their corresponding responses, like inflammation, fibrosis, increase of arterial stiffness [70] and

enhancement of sympathetic nerve activity (SNA), mediated by ROS [26] (figure 6-2). An increased activity of SNS could be related to upregulated renal sodium reabsorption [71].

Dopamine (DA), a precursor of norepinephrine, has a natriuretic effect by inhibiting Na-K-ATPase in proximal tubular segments. Patients with CKD have reduced urinary excretion of DA and decreased activity of the renal dopaminergic system, which correlates well with the degree of renal dysfunction [72]. These data show that the reduced activity of renal dopaminergic system in CKD, by decreasing the sodium excretion, may be another factor connected with the hypertension of CKD [24].

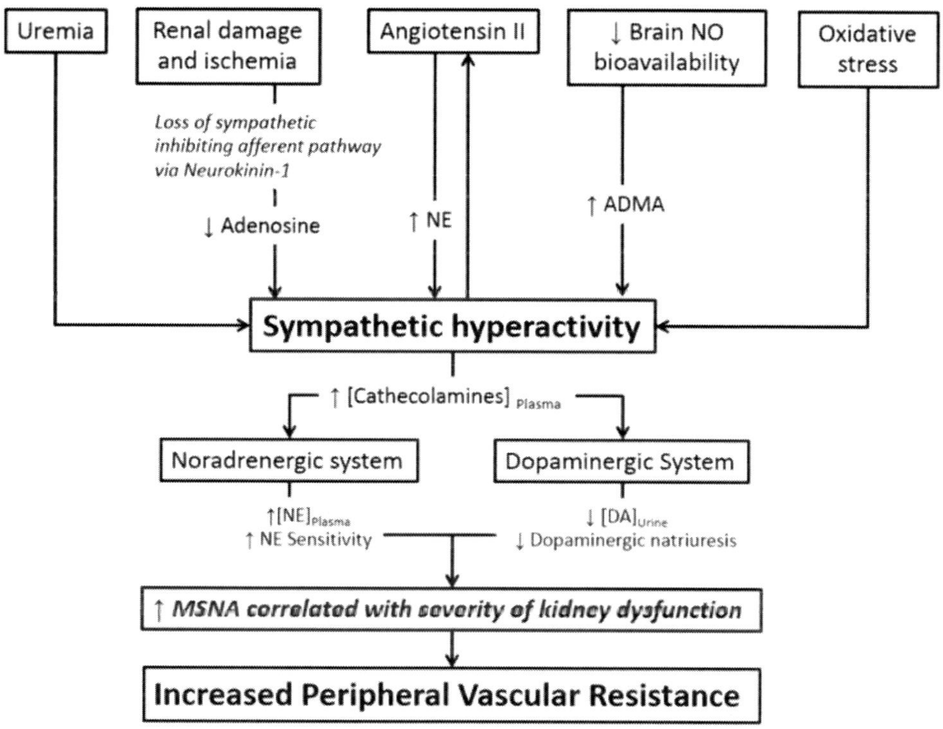

Figure 6-2. Pathophysiology of CKD: Symphathetic hyperactivity. NE: Norepinephrine, ADMA: Asymmetric dimethylarginine, DA: Dopamine.

2.3. The Renin-Angiotensin-Aldosterone System

Evidence suggests the importance of tissue RAAS in the brain, heart, adrenal glands, and vasculature, as well as in the kidney. Recent studies highlight an important role of the RAAS in the progression of kidney disease [73, 74]. The relevance of the RAAS, in physiological terms, is based on its capacity to regulate arterial pressure and sodium balance [24]. This system is often activated in hypertensive patients with CKD [46]. In presence of hypotension, hypoperfusion and/or sympathetic hyperactivity, the juxtaglomerular cells react by secreting renin, which cleaves angiotensinogen, leading to an increase in angiotensin I, which is further cleaved into Ang II in the lungs by ACE. Ang II directly causes vasoconstriction, has trophic effects, stimulates the SNS vasomotor center in the brainstem and plays an important role in the water and chloride reabsorption in proximal tubule [55]. Ang II acts mainly on the type 1 Ang II receptors (AT1 receptors) in the vasculature, leading to vasoconstriction and on the zona glomerulosa, where it stimulates the secretion of aldosterone [24]. The ability of Ang II to generate ROS through activation of the reduced nicotinamide adenine dinucleotide phosphate (NADPH) oxidase after binding to angiotensin receptor, suggesting a role in creating OE in vascular tissue. Regarding the role of aldosterone, it has been established that the hormone participate in the process of tissue fibrogenesis [75, 76].

Several non-hemodynamic effects of Ang II also contribute to kidney disease. Ang II stimulates mesangial cell proliferation, induces expression of transforming growth factor-β (TGF-β), and stimulates production of plasminogen activator inhibitor-1 (PAI-1), all of which enhances inflammation in the kidney, leading to glomerular and tubulointerstitial fibrosis. Increased arterial stiffness also plays a role in hypertension in kidney disease [70].

Factors that lead to excess vasoconstriction include overactivity of the SNS, activation of the RAAS, and smooth muscle hypertrophy mediated by Ang II and potent vasoconstrictors including endothelin. Impaired ability to vasodilate is often mediated by ED and prostaglandin deficiency [70]. Besides its peripheral actions, experimental research suggests that Ang II contributes to the regulation of arterial pressure and intravascular volume through actions on several brain sites [77]. Indeed acute increases in circulating Ang II concentration affect the SNS through actions on the brain, sympathetic ganglia, and sympathetic nerve endings [55] (figure 6-3).

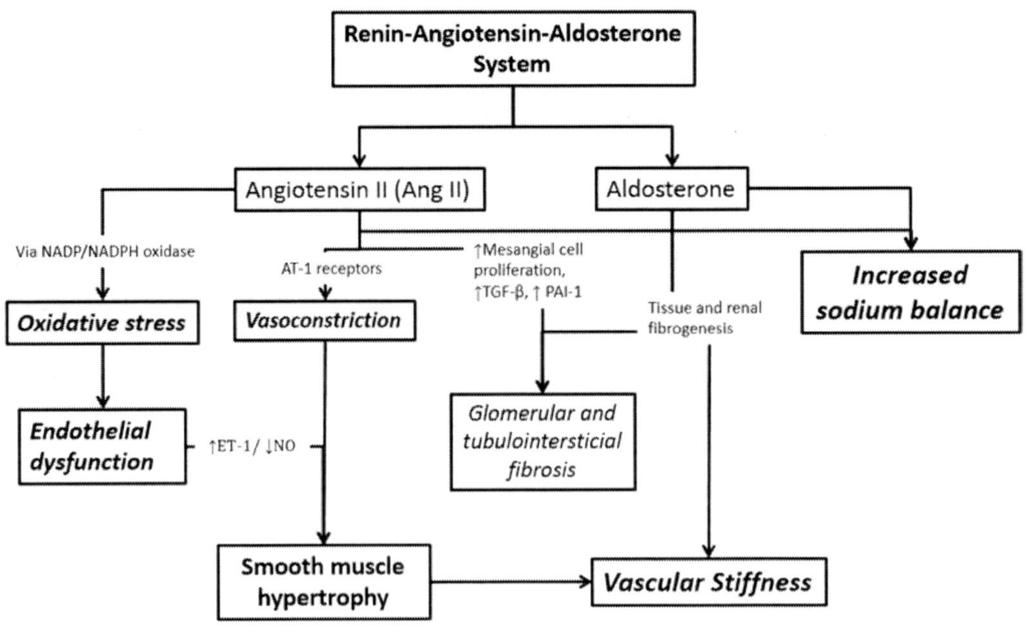

Figure 6-3. Pathophysiology of CKD: Renin-Angiotensin-Aldosterone System (RAAS). NADP/NADPH oxidase: Nicotinamide adenine dinucleotide phosphate-oxidase, AT-1 receptors: angiotensin 1 receptors, TGF-β: Transforming growth factor-β, PAI-1: Plasminogen activator inhibitor-1, ET-1: endothelin 1, NO: Nitric oxide.

2.4. Oxidative Stress

There is a close relationship between renal OE and hypertension. The OE and the damage caused by ROS and reactive nitrogen species in kidney disease are now recognized as major participants not only in the multiple complications related with CKD [78 – 80], but also in the development and maintenance of the hypertension by Ang II central and peripheral actions, mediated by ROS, ED, and renal damage [45, 81, 82]. OE can occur as a result of increased ROS generation, depressed antioxidant system, or both. The enzymes copper–zinc superoxide dismutase (CuZnSOD), catalase (CAT), and glutathione peroxidase (GPx) constitute the main antioxidant system. CuZnSOD converts O_2^-, a highly reactive and cytotoxic agent, to hydrogen peroxide (H_2O_2), and H_2O_2 is converted to water and molecular oxygen by either CAT or GPx. In CKD animal models (two-kidney one clip (2K-1C) rat model), the activity of these enzymes is reduced in the kidney´s cortex [83]. Moreover, the excretion of OE biomarkers like malondialdehyde [84] and 8-isoprostane are increased [85]. Also, in CKD patients it has been found elevated levels of OE biomarkers [86]. The OE related to CKD is induced by diverse vasoconstrictor mechanisms, including blockade of NOS [87, 88], and activation of Ang II type 1 and thromboxane receptors [89, 90]. The involvement whereby OE takes part of the development and maintenance of the hypertension is by 3 ways:

2.4.1. Endothelial Dysfunction

In healthy vessels, endothelial cells produce NO and ROS, where they play a role in cellular signaling related to the control of endothelial function and maintenance of vascular integrity. In CKD, increased ROS production, reduces NO bioavailability [44, 87, 88], and both of these, are associated with inflammation, ED and vascular remodeling.

Exposure of endothelium to high concentrations of ROS induces hypertrophy and expression of adhesion molecules with infiltration of inflammatory cells. ROS also activates profibrotic, proliferative and apoptotic pathways leading to increased extracellular matrix accumulation (fibrosis) [91]. These effects are mediated through redox-sensitive signaling pathways including MAPK, PTP, tyrosine kinases, proinflammatory genes, ion channels, and Ca^{2+} [92 – 94].

These changes in vascular function and structure (related to the oxidative-induced ED), reduces vasodilation, increases contraction, vascular inflammation and structural remodeling, causing increased peripheral resistance and elevated BP [94].

The consequences of endothelial injury is amplified by the exaggerated systemic response of complement factor D, CD40 and its ligand system, prothrombotic state and others, which contribute to further vascular damage [95].

2.4.2. Renal Damage

The kidney, and particularly the renal medullary circulation, plays a fundamental role in modulating long-term blood pressure control and fluid balance [96, 97]. ROS are important regulators of medullary blood flow [97].

Elevation of $\bullet O_2^-$ or reduction of NO in the renal medulla decreases medullary blood flow and Na excretion, resulting in sustained hypertension. OE within the renal medulla makes the kidney functionally more vulnerable to effects of Ang II and salt, and promotes renal dysfunction [98]. Superoxide ($\bullet O_2^-$) and H_2O_2 increase afferent arterial tone and reactivity and enhance renal vascular resistance. Renal ROS influence GFR, tubuloglomerular feedback response and Na+ transport. NO inhibits reabsorption of NaCl in the thick ascending limb, whereas $\bullet O_2^-$enhances NaCl reabsorption. Moreover, pro-oxidant agents attack lipid membranes of renal cell, causing peroxidation of these. This lipid peroxidation compromises the integrity of the basement membrane and the epithelium of the organs, which may also affect transport functions performed in the renal tubule [80, 99]. Ang II and OE also promote mesangial cell proliferation, mesangial matrix accumulation, and podocyte injury, thus favoring hypertension [100].

2.4.3. Ang II Central and Peripheral Actions

ROS are involved in the regulation of SNS activity [44]. The 2K-1C animal model reflects the renovascular Ang II-dependent form of arterial hypertension (CKD). This model is characterized by increased sympathetic vasomotor hyperactivity and baroreflex dysfunction. The mechanism by which Ang II enhances SNA are mediated, in part, by ROS [26, 57]. In experimental models of renovascular hypertension, the activation of Ang II type I receptor increases NAD(P)H oxidase enzyme activity which have subunits in the renal cortex, medulla and renal vessels [101, 102], thereby enhancing $\bullet O_2^-$ production [103], and it engaging the central autonomic nervous system [45, 81, 82]. 2K-1C animal models, have demonstrated sympathetic hyperactivity [81], which is reduced after vitamin C treatment. These effects might be mediated by the interaction of vitamin C with $\bullet O_2^-$, enhancing central NO bioavailability, which exerts a tonic and chronic inhibition on the central SNS [57]. The central Ang II effects seem to be mediated by increased OE in brain regions involved in the noradrenergic control of BP. It was found increased OE in central regions implicated in the tonic sympathetic vasomotor outflow, the rostral ventrolateral medulla (RVLM), and the paraventricular nucleus of hypothalamus (PVN) [45, 81]. Kishi T et al. [104] found that increased levels of OE in key brain nuclei mediate the activation of the SNS in phenol-renal injury model of hypertension. Same results were found in stroke-prone spontaneously hypertensive rats [105].

Increased OE within the RVLM and PVN was associated with hypertension and sympathetic overactivity in the 2K 1C Goldblatt model of renovascular hypertension [45], and superoxide signaling in the RVLM was found to play a major role in sustained hypertension and SNS activation in this model. ROS are also involved in the intracellular signaling mechanisms of Ang II in the brain, in central SNS activation and BP elevation in experimental models of obesity-induced hypertension [82, 106, 107], renovascular hypertension, and salt-sensitive hypertension (figure 6-4). The treatment with acute intravenous infusion of vitamin C reduced arterial pressure and SNA in renovascular-animal models. Moreover, chronic antioxidant therapy also shows to improve OE and BP in these models [45]. Despite these experimental data, antioxidants currently have no a definitive role in the management of hypertension in CKD patients [104].

2.5. Urotensin II

Urotensin II (UII) is a potent 11-amino acid vasoactive peptide that produces vasodilatation and inotropic effects in addition to its powerful vasoconstrictive effect [108]. Is part of a family of vasoactive peptides first isolated from various fish species nearly 30 years ago [109] and later from frogs, rodents, pigs, primates and humans [110].

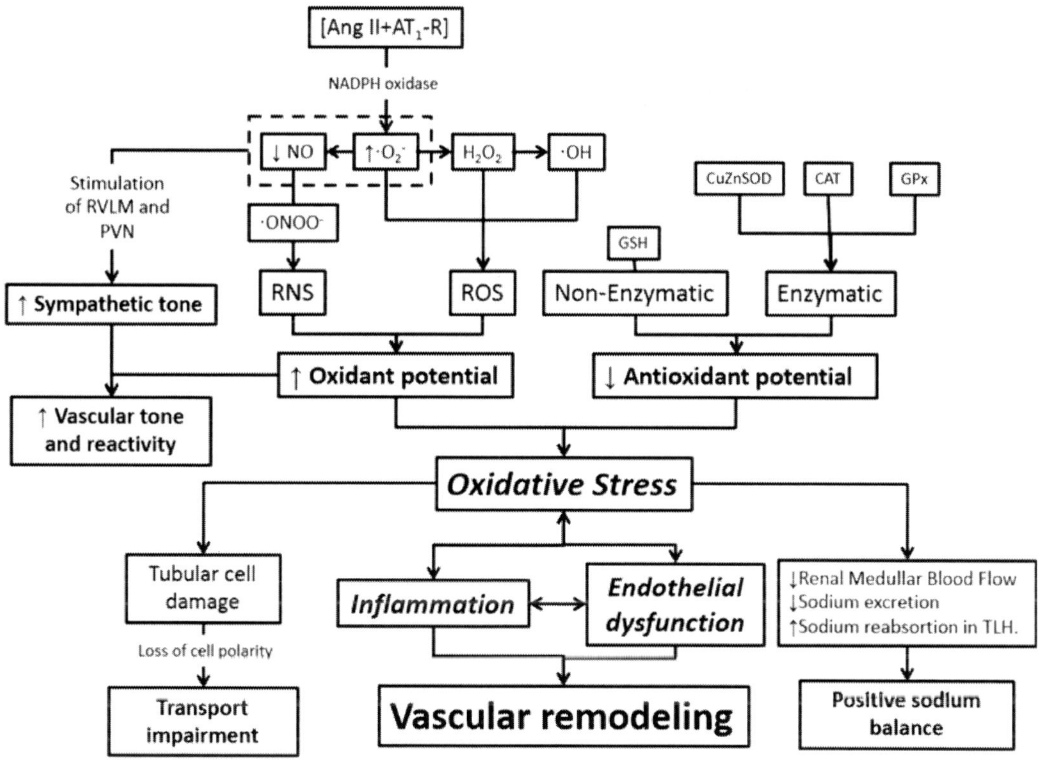

Figure 6-4. Pathophysiology of CKD: Oxidative stress. Ang II: Angiotensin II, AT1-R: Angiotensin 1 receptor, NADPH oxidase: Nicotinamide adenine dinucleotide phosphate-oxidase, NO: Nitric oxide. O2-: Oxide ion, H2O2: Hydrogen peroxide. OH: Hidroxyl radical, RVLM: Rostral ventrolateral medulla, PVN: Paraventricular nucleus of hypothalamus. ONOO-: Peroxynitrite, CuZnSOD: Copper–zinc superoxide dismutase, CAT: Catalase, GPx: Glutathione peroxidase, GSH: Glutathione, RNS: Reactive nitrogen species, ROS: Reactive oxygen species, TLH: Thick ascending loop of Henle.

The vasomotor effects of UII vary greatly, depending on the species studied, interactions with other vasoactive molecules and the vascular bed used [111]. Recent studies have shown increased expression of UII and its receptors in animals and patients with hypertension, heart failure, atherosclerosis, diabetic nephropathy and CKD [112 – 117]. Thus, UII has been implicated in the pathophysiology of the above-mentioned disorders and as a possible therapeutic target. However, a lot of conflicting results have been reported. The kidney plays a major role in UII production, which may contribute to its hemodynamic effects [118]. The administration of UII has an anti-natriuretic effect that is independent of blood pressure, suggesting a direct tubular action and a possible role in the pathogenesis of hypertension [119, 120]. Song W. et al. demonstrated that an injection of UII induced a reduction in the glomerular filtration rate, urine out flow, and sodium excretion in normal rats, whereas injection of Urantide, a UII antagonist, resulted in increases in these variables [121]. Immunohistochemistry of the kidney showed positive UII staining in the renal tubular cells, blood vessels and epithelial cells [116]. Furthermore, UII receptors are expressed in glomerular arterioles, thin ascending limbs, and inner medullary collecting ducts [121]. Totsune K. et al. demonstrated that plasma concentrations of UII are elevated in patients with CKD [117], same results were found in patients with congestive heart failure [122, 123], hypertension [124], and diabetes mellitus [125, 126]. Also studies shown an increased excretion of UII in urine of hypertensive patients [127], and patients with reduced renal function due to diabetic nephropathy [126], suggesting that UII may therefore contribute to cardiovascular regulation and be involved in the pathophysiology of cardiovascular and renal diseases. However, Mosenkis et al. observed a positive correlation between UII concentration and renal function, UII concentrations were lower in subjects with proteinuria, a history of hypertension or a diagnosis of diabetes [128]. Also, more researchers have reported conflicting results about UII blood and urine concentrations in patients with kidney disease. Totsune et al. reported higher plasma UII concentrations in patients with CKD and ESRD compared with control subjects, although the concentrations did not correlate with serum creatinine levels [117]. The same investigators later found no differences in plasma UII concentrations of diabetic patients with and without proteinuria or the presence of hypertension [125]. Matsushita et al. reported higher urine UII concentrations in hypertensive subjects, although, again, the UII concentrations did not correlate with serum creatinine [127]. Cheung et al. demonstrated high plasma UII concentrations in 62 hypertensive subjects compared with 62 normotensive controls [124], whereas others found no differences between the plasma concentrations of UII in hypertensive versus normotensive subjects [129]. Targeting UII receptors as a new antihypertensive therapy was first considered when Abdel-Razik AE et al. demonstrated that spontaneously hypertensive rats were sensitive to UII, causing an increase in their blood pressure [119]. Supporting this, are in vitro studies of UII in human vessels showing potent vasoconstriction [130] and synergy with Ang II [131]. However, in vivo administration of UII has produced conflicting haemodynamic results. These range from cutaneous vasodilation [132] to potent vasoconstriction [133, 134, 135], and some studies show no haemodynamic changes [136]. A pathophysiological role for UII has been implicated in CKD and hypertension although it is not yet clear whether it has a causative or protective influence. More studies are needed to define their dominant mechanism.

2.6. Uric Acid

Uric acid is an end product of purine metabolism. It is produced mainly by the liver and intestines, but also by other tissues, such as muscles, kidneys and the endothelium [137]. Under normal conditions, two-thirds of the uric acid produced is eliminated in the urine and one-third is removed by the biliary tree [138]. When it develops a uric acid overproduction, undersecretion or both, occurs a hyperuricemia that is defined as the accumulation of serum uric acid beyond its solubility point in water (6.8 mg/dl) [139]. Hyperuricemia is common in CKD. Experimental evidence suggests that uric acid itself may harm patients with CKD by contributing to increase inflammation, CKD progression and therefore hypertension. Although controversial, these observations are supported by many large prospective observational studies that show increased serum uric acid levels that predict the development and progression of CKD in various populations [137]. Traditionally, hyperuricemia associated with hyperuricosuria has been postulated to cause kidney disease by depositing intraluminal crystal in the collecting duct of the nephron in a manner reminiscent of gouty arthropathy [140]. Uric acid crystals have the capacity to adhere to the surface of renal epithelial cells [141] and induce an acute inflammatory response in such cell lines [142]. In addition to an increased risk of kidney stone formation, such effects have been shown to reduce GFR [140]. Contrary to the role of uric acid crystals in kidney disease, non-crystal effects of uric acid remain contentious because under physiologic concentrations, urate is a powerful antioxidant that can scavenge O2-, .OH, and singlet oxygen [143]. Nevertheless, recent data may implicate mild hyperuricemia in kidney disease onset and progression. Experimentally induced hyperuricemia in rats leads to reduced urinary nitrite levels and systemic and glomerular hypertension [144, 145]. The latter two can be prevented with supplementation of L-arginine, suggesting that uric acid may cause endothelial dysfunction. This conclusion, although controversial, is supported by in vitro experimental studies showing that uric acid decreases nitric oxide production and also may lead to nitric oxide depletion [146]. In addition to a potential role in endothelial dysfunction, experimental hyperuricemia has been reported to cause an afferent renal arteriolopathy and tubulointerstitial fibrosis in the kidney by activating the RAAS [147]. Uric acid also has been shown to activate the cytoplasmic phospholipase A and inflammatory transcription factor nuclear factor-κB (NF-κB), leading to the inhibition of proximal tubular cellular proliferation in vitro [148], the increase of tumor necrosis factor α (TNF-α) [149], and the local expression of chemokines. Consistent with such experimental data, further animal studies suggest that decreasing uric acid levels may slow CKD progression. Sanchez-Lozada LG et al. demonstrated that decreasing uric acid levels, cause a reduction in tubulointerstitial fibrosis in 5/6 nephrectomy animal model [150], also Kosugi T et al. reported similar results in diabetic nephropathy model [151]. However, more interventional studies in humans are required to establish a clear position about the beneficial effects of acid-lowering therapy.

3. Therapies

Treatment of hypertension in CKD is directed at two goals: prevention or slowing of progression of CKD and prevention of cardiovascular (CV) morbidity and mortality, by controlling the BP. The National Kidney Foundation (NKF), American Diabetes Association (ADA), and the Joint National Committee's seventh report (JNC7) have established the target BP as <130/80 mm Hg for individuals with CKD [25]. Recent data from the African American Study of Kidney Disease (AASK) clearly demonstrate that <130/80 mmHg may not be the most appropriate goal to slow nephropathy progression unless proteinuria is >300mg/day. Moreover, there was no difference in outcomes between the group with a mean systolic BP of 140 mm Hg versus that with a mean of 128 mm Hg [68]. The best available data suggest that individuals with CKD and no proteinuria do just as well at <140/90 mm Hg as they do at <130/80 mm Hg, so there is no need to drive BP lower. Individuals with CKD and proteinuria (>300-500 mg/day) appear to benefit from more intensive BP reduction and should have a target of <130/80 mm Hg along with a focus of proteinuria reduction to at least 30% to 40% from pretreatment baseline. Proteinuria reduction, using antihypertensive agents that modify the RAAS, should be a primary goal of therapy [25]. Routine care of individuals with hypertension and CKD should include agents that reduce proteinuria, maintenance of euvolemia, monitoring for CV symptoms and diseases. We will explain each therapy in relation with the factors that may cause hypertension in the CKD.

3.1. Blood Volume and Sodium Homeostasis

3.1.1. Diuretics

Extracellular volume expansion due to water and sodium retention is a strong contributing factor to hypertension seen in CKD. Diuretics are therefore a useful tool to manage volume overload and to achieve strict BP control in these patients [65, 152]. On the other side these diuretics enhance the effect of ACE inhibitors (ACEIs) and angiotensin receptor blockers (ARBs), and reduce CV risks in CKD [153].

Tiazidic and Loop Diuretics

The choice on the right diuretic will depend on the level in renal function:

- If GFR is >30 ml/min/1,73 m^2 (CKD stage 1.3), a tiazidic diuretic should be used 1 once a day
- If GFR is <30 ml/min/1,73 m^2 (CKD stage 4-5), a loop diuretic should be used 1-2 times a day.

Thiazide diuretics, especially chlorthalidone, have a longer antihypertensive effect than the loop diuretics. Loop diuretics are less effective in patients with normal renal function, unless they are given in multiple daily doses. However, as thiazide diuretics are less effective at low levels of GFR, a loop diuretic is preferred in patients with more advanced CKD (<30 ml/min/1,73 m^2), as well as in acute renal failure [13]. Several studies have shown the substantial role of diuretics in CKD. Abe et al. [65] administered a low dose of hydrochlorothiazide to those patients in whom BP is not controlled well by intensive RAS inhibition therapy using the maximum recommended doses of ARBs and ACEIs. In this study hydrochlorothiazide was shown to have a renoprotective effect in hypertensive patients with stage 3–4 CKD, as it significantly decreased BP and urinary protein/creatinine ratio. The use of diuretics as monotherapy is controversial. European [154] and US [155] guidelines on hypertension recommend the use of thiazide diuretics as first-line therapy, [156] but some researchers have a different opinion [157]. This is based on the fact that diuretics induce RAS stimulation, as well as metabolic alterations in glucose and lipids, that may have negative impact on CV outcomes. In numerous large intervention trials, we found that long-term therapy with diuretics, especially when diuretics are combined with b-blockers, reduce glucose tolerance and increases new-onset diabetes risk [158, 159]. Thereby supporting the concept of the negative impact.

Although the majority of the studies so far have limited duration and middle to long-term efficacy in renal protection has not been sufficiently assessed. Control of volume retention remains the most important key to hypertension treatment in patients with CKD.

3.1.2. Aldosterone Receptor Blockers

In CKD patients we found elevated levels of aldosterone. This molecule in and by itself is an important mediator of renal injury [25], inducing inflammation and fibrosis in the kidney by stimulating PAI-1 expression [160], generating reactive oxygen species and transforming growth factor-b expression [161]. ACEIs and ARBs that suppress RAS, generate an action that is not enough to control plasma aldosterone levels, owing to aldosterone escape during long-term blockade of the RAAS [162]. Thus, the ARBs therapy could enhance antihypertensive treatment [163]. There are two types of aldosterone antagonists, these are classified in the non-selective, like spironolactone, and in the newer selective antagonists, like eplerenone. Both substances have been proved to reduce albuminuria in patients with diabetic nephropathy. Rossing et al. [164] have shown that 25 mg of spironolactone, when added to maximum doses of ACEI or ARB treatment, resulted in 33% reduction of albuminuria ($P<0.001$) in patients with type 2 diabetes and nephropathy. An important side effect of aldosterone antagonist therapy is the hyperkalemia, this can be aggravated by concurrent renal insufficiency, diabetes mellitus, severe heart failure, old age and other potassium-sparing drugs. These type of drugs are not recommended when serum creatinine is >2.5 mg/dl or creatinine clearance is <30 ml/min or serum potassium is >5mmol/l [157, 165]. There are not yet studies comparing non-selective to selective aldosterone antagonists, neither studies evaluating the long-term effects of aldosterone antagonists combined to other RAS inhibitors, in terms of kidney function. Therefore, aldosterone antagonists cannot be yet recommended as a routine additional therapy in patients with CKD. It is important to remember that, when diuretics are used, we must monitor the depletion of extracellular volume, renal function, serum potassium, and sodium, and that potassium-sparing diuretics (aldosterone antagonists) should be used prudently in CKD.

3.2. The Renin-Angiotensin-Aldosterone System

It has long been recognized that in patients with CKD the RAAS is "inappropriately" activated in relation to the fluid status [166]. This contributes to the hypertension, and explains why hypertension may persist even after correction of the fluid overload.

3.2.1. Inhibitors of the RAAS

ACE Inhibitors and Angiotensin Receptor Blockers (ARBs)

Control of blood pressure and proteinuria is the cornerstone of preservation of renal function and prevention of complications associated with renal dysfunction in patients with CKD. Proteinuria is a marker of kidney damage, and a risk factor for accelerated progression of kidney disease. It is increasingly recognized as an independent risk factor for all-cause and CV mortality [13, 167, 168]. The K/DOQI guidelines recommend that patients with non-diabetic kidney disease and a random (spot) urine total protein-to-creatinine ratio greater than 200 mg per g, and those with diabetic kidney disease, should be treated with an ACEIs or ARBs, regardless of the presence of hypertension [13]. These two type of drugs are the most effective pharmacological strategy for this purpose, being the first-line therapy for renoprotection in non-diabetic and diabetic patients with CKD, as recommended by current guidelines [153, 169]. ACEIs and ARBs have similar ability to reduce proteinuria, but not enough to prevent the progression of CKD. Combination therapy with an ACEI or plus an ARB causes more complete inhibition of the RAAS compared with monotherapy. Meta-analyses of short-term studies show greater reductions in BP and albuminuria in patients receiving dual-agent RAAS blocking therapy than in those receiving either single agent [170, 171]. Of note, these enhanced therapeutic effects occurred at the expense of an increased incidence of drug-related adverse effects: acute renal impairment (decline in GFR) and hyperkalemia [13, 171, 172]. The majority of current evidence recommends against the combined use of ACEIs and ARBs.

Direct Renin Inhibitors

They are the most recent agents of RAAS inhibitors. The blockade of renin is a very attractive idea, as the interaction of renin with its physiological substrate angiotensinogen is the rate-limiting step in the RAAS cascade. Aliskiren is the first commercially available orally active renin inhibitor [173]. It acts by binding to the active site of renin, thereby inhibiting catalytic activity, and reduces Ang II levels and plasma renin activity without stimulating compensatory increases in plasma renin activity, Ang I and Ang II, as seen with ACEIs and ARBs. Also, it is well tolerated and effective in lowering BP in both the general population of hypertensive patients and specific patient groups, such as obese people [174]. Siddiqi L. et al. [175] were the first in showing that aliskiren reduces sympathetic hyperactivity, quantified by MSNA, in hypertensive patients. This reduction occurs despite the fact that BP was reduced. Moreover, the Evaluation of Proteinuria in Diabetes (AVOID) trial, has shown a reduction of proteinuria in patients using aliskiren. In this study they compared the combination of aliskiren/losartan with losartan as monotherapy in 599 hypertensive patients with type 2 diabetes and nephropathy for a period of 6 months. According to the results, proteinuria in the combined therapy group was reduced by 20% more than in the control group, while adverse events were similar in both treatment groups [176]. Several animal models have shown that aliskiren also has renoprotective, cardioprotective and antiatherosclerotic properties, which are independent of BP reduction [177]. However, we also found risky side effects in patients taking aliskiren in combination with an ACEI or an ARB after 18–24 months. These patients developed renal complications, hyperkalemia, an increased risk for non-fatal stroke and hypotension, causing the early closure of ALTITUDE trial [178].

Further studies to evaluate the renoprotective effect of aliskiren are needed before its safe use in the treatment of hypertension in CKD patients.

3.3. Sympathetic Nervous System

The renal SNS has been identified as a major contributor to the complex pathophysiology of hypertension, states of volume overload (such as heart failure), and progressive renal disease, both in animal models and in humans [179–181]. Sympathetic hyperactivity in CKD can be reduced by several types of antihypertensive medications [182]. During the last few decades, some antihypertensive agents, such as inhibitors of the RAAS, including ACEIs, ARBs, and direct renin inhibitors, have proven to reduce sympathetic activity [183, 184]. These studies are reported in the following section.

3.3.1. Inhibitors of the RAAS

Ang II acts on the kidneys and produces vasoconstriction of efferent arteriole in the glomerulus, which increases glomerular capillary pressure and filtration fraction [185]. Also, Ang II enhances ultrafiltration of proteins and is associated with podocyte injury, resulting in proteinuria [186]. Chronic activation of RAAS perpetuates a cascade of proinflammatory, prothrombotic and atherogenic effects associated with end-organ damage [187].

3.3.2. ACE Inhibitors and ARBs

These agents are effective and safe in CKD patients. Both the ACEI, enalapril and the AT-1 receptor blocker, losartan exerted a profound and comparable antihypertensive effect without altering the 24-h BP profile and without effect on heart rate, baroreceptor sensitivity, or kidney function [188, 189], by reducing the sympathetic overactivity. However, neither of them normalizes MSNA completely [183]. Studies show that enalapril and losartan in usually applied dosages are equally effective in reducing the increased BP and sympathetic activity in normovolemic hypertensive patients with CKD. Differences in modes of action do not result in different effects on sympathetic activity [183]. Both of them lowered the average of BP to levels that are acceptable according to WHO criteria, but BP was still slightly higher than in the healthy control subjects, and control the sympathetic hyperactivity only partially [183]. The combination of an ACEI and an Ang II receptor blockade induces a stronger inhibition of the RAAS, and therefore a higher sympatho-inhibitory effect, than either drug alone. Moreover the addition of spironolactone to ACEI, can also produce a similar effect [190, 191]. Presently, many issues need to be resolved. More experimental evidence is needed to establish whether all Ang II receptor antagonists are equally effective in reducing sympathetic activity at the central and peripheral level [192], and the long-term renal outcomes compared to other treatments.

3.3.3. Adrenergic Blockade

SNS acts on the kidney through its β-1, β-2 and α-1 receptors and affects the vasomotor tone of renal arterioles, in order to maintain a constant glomerular filtration. β-1 receptors cause renin release and increase in cardiac output, β-2 receptors induce vasodilation and increase glycogenolysis, whereas α-1 receptors induce vasoconstriction [177].

3.3.4. B-Adrenergic Receptor Blockade

There are several studies showing renal protection by β - adrenergic receptor blockade in 5/6 nephrectomy [175, 193, 194]. This protection has also been observed in NOS inhibition animal models [195, 196]. Propranolol, carvedilol and labetalol belong to non-selective β–blockers, as they exert blocking action both on β-1 and β-2 receptors. Cardio-selective β–blockers (β-1 selective) include metoprolol, atenolol and nebivolol. Carvedilol and labetalol mediate vasodilation through additional blockade of α-1 receptors [197]. Nebivolol also exerts vasodilation via stimulation of NO [198]. In addition, carvedilol and nebivolol have antioxidant effect [199-202] and a safer metabolic profile [203, 204]. However, β-blockers are underused, in large part due to the tolerability of these agents [205].

When it comes to comparing β-blockers with other antihypertensive drugs, in terms of renal protection, unfortunately, a few studies on long-term renal outcomes are available In the study by Brooks et al. [175] very similar protection was found for carvedilol and captopril. Moreover, they are substantial differences between different β–blocking drugs. Third-generation β–blockers, such as carvedilol and nebivolol, seem to have more protective effects than traditional β-blockers [69], possibly via stimulation of NO release [198]. In fact, carvedilol is even protective in acute renal failure after gentamicin [206]. Third-generation β–blockers (carvedilol and nebivolol) are now rapidly becoming the drug of choice in heart failure in the general population [207]. However, their use in patients with advanced renal failure who experience myocardial infarction is grossly neglected [208].

3.3.5. A-Adrenergic Receptor Blockade

Renal protection by α–adrenergic receptor blockade has also been observed in the 5/6 nephrectomy model [193], and in NOS inhibition [196]. Alpha1-adrenergic blockers (doxazosin, terazosin and prazosin) inhibit vasoconstriction that is induced by SNS and cause vasodilation, reduction of peripheral resistances and BP decrease. To date, studies have not found a special benefit of these drugs in cardiovascular and renal protection. Reddi et al. [209] have shown that combining α–adrenergic blockade (doxazosin) with ACE inhibition only provided slightly better protection than single-drug treatment in spontaneous type 2 diabetes. The ALLHAT study showed that cardiovascular and renal outcomes were not significantly reduced in α-blocker group (doxazosin) comparing with diuretic group in patients with metabolic syndrome, including those without diabetes mellitus (RR=1.18) [210]. α-Blockers used as monotherapy, lack of a potent antihypertensive effect, but they are usually given in combination with other antihypertensive drugs in CKD patients that have resistant hypertension. A combination of α-blockade and β–blockade aimed at preventing both α–adrenergic-mediated ATP release and β–adrenergic-mediated renin release was more effective in reducing renal damage in the subtotal nephrectomy model than α-blockade only [193].

3.4. Centrally Acting Antihypertensives

Centrally acting antihypertensives include drugs like clonidine, α-methyldopa, guanfacine and the newer moxonidine. These drugs cross the blood–brain barrier and act centrally by activating α2-adrenergic receptors in the vasomotor center in the brain stem and hypothalamus, causing a reduction of peripheral sympathetic tone, hence vasodilation and a fall in BP, heart rate and cardiac output [26]. Studies have shown numerous side effects for these drugs, such as dry mouth, fatigue, drowsiness and sedation. But they do not mention any adverse metabolic effects.

3.4.1. Moxonidine

Vonend et al. [211] showed in a prospective, randomized, double-blind study that administration of the centrally acting sympatho-inhibitory drug, moxonidine in patients with CKD or ESRD is safe and effective in reducing creatinine clearance and the occurrence of adverse events, even independent of the BP-lowering effect. Thus, antihypertensive effects with this sympatholytic agent may have renoprotective effects, but this needs to be confirmed in larger trials. Moxonidine has been shown at a regular dose of 0.4 mg/day to reduce sympathetic overactivity [32]. It´s addition to the chronic treatment with an Ang II receptor antagonist normalizes BP and MSNA [212].

3.5. Dialysis

Preliminary data have shown that daily short dialysis or nocturnal long dialysis reduce MSNA when compared with thrice weekly conventional hemodialysis, possibly due to a lowering of ADMA levels. Hemodialysis filtration may be more effective than conventional hemodialysis in removing ADMA, but prospective data are needed [213, 214]. In a retrospective analysis in hemodialysis patients ACEI use, independently of its effect on BP, seems to be associated with a dramatic reduction in mortality [215]. In CKD patients not on dialysis, ACEI therapy also improved survival rates independently of its effect on BP [216].

3.6. Statins

Statins have been shown to reduce sympathetic activity in patients with CKD [217], but to date it is unknown whether these effects have a clinical benefit.

3.7. Renal Denervation

The incomplete normalization of sympathetic activation in pharmacologic treatment and its associated risks, asks for new treatment options [77]. Catheter-based denervation of the renal sympathetic nerves (RD) has been shown to reduce BP and to decrease renal and MSNA in patients with resistant hypertension and offers an attractive option to treat these disease states [218]. The concept of RD is not new, having been explored in animal disease models. The Symplicity HTN-1 trial, published in 2009, was the first multicenter proof of concept and safety study in patients with resistant hypertension [219]. After 4 weeks, a significant reduction in systolic and diastolic office BP by 14 and 10 mmHg was reported, with a further reduction to 27 and 17 mmHg after 12 months. Randomized, multicenter, prospective study Symplicity HTN-2 trial included 106 patients with resistant hypertension, randomized 1:1 to a control group (continuation of drug treatment) and a treatment group (renal denervation plus continued drug treatment) [220]. Six months after RD, mean BP in the treatment group decreased significantly by 32/12 mmHg, without changes in the control group. RD did not adversely affect renal function as measured by cystatin C and GFR, or induce renal artery stenoses or aneurysms as assessed by duplex ultrasound [219]. During renal ischemia, adenosine is released evoking an increase on the traffic in renal afferent nerve, as it can be shown during the infusion of adenosine into the renal uninephrectomized artery of dogs. In rats, induction of renal artery stenosis [47], partial renal ablation by arterial ligation [48] or intrarenal phenol injection [49] causes excitation of the renal afferent nerves, this result in neurogenic hypertension. In these animal models, RD results in a reduction or total prevention of hypertension. Regarding the inhibition of NO in animals, the sympathoexcitatory effect of NO inhibition has been clearly demonstrated during systemic administration of NO synthesis inhibitors and is greatly attenuated by sympathectomy or by RD [58].

3.8. Physiology of the BP-Lowering Effect of Renal Denervation

The hypotensive effect in RD increases over time. The effects of RD occur by functional changes and structural changes such as reversal of vascular hypertrophy. It can be said that the antihypertensive effect is due to a balance on water/sodium altered by the kidneys and by a decrease in peripheral vascular resistance. After RD, the effect of Ang II to increase water and chloride reabsorption was decreased by ≈75% [77]. RD also significantly increased basal renal blood flow, improved dynamic autoregulation of renal blood flow, and increased renal blood flow variability in rats with congestive heart failure and rats with spontaneous hypertension, compared with controls [66].

3.9. Renoprotective Effect of Renal Denervation

Animal studies suggest that RD has a renoprotective effect independent of lowering BP. Experiments in hypertensive rats sensitive to salt, RD produced a sympathetic inhibition without a lowering effect in BP. In addition, there are studies suggesting that RD protects renal function through an antiinflammatory effect [221]. RD offers new opportunities, not only in the treatment of patients, but also in the effort to better understand the pathophysiology in various disease conditions characterized by sympathetic overactivity.

3.10. Oxidative Stress

In physiological conditions, ROS play an important role in cardiovascular and renal biology through highly regulated redox-sensitive signaling pathways. The excessive ROS production and/or not enogh removing, results in OE inducing cardiac and renal injury together with activation of the SNS and arterial hypertension [91]. Based on experimental evidence NADPH oxidase subunits are potential therapeutic targets for CV disease and hypertension. Though the mechanisms of action are still unclear, any compound could act as a competitive inhibitor of the substrate because of its resemblance to NADPH. Some benefits in the use of classical antihypertensive agents such as β-adrenergic blockers, ACE inhibitors, AT1 receptor antagonists may be mediated, in part, by decreasing vascular OE [91]. These effects have been attributed to direct inhibition of NADPH oxidase activity and to intrinsic antioxidant properties of the drugs. However, some studies failed to show changes in OE despite significant BP lowering by classical antihypertensive drugs [91].

On the other hand, recent clinical studies have shown to improve vascular function and lower BP in patients with CKD and pulmonary hypertension.

3.11. Chronic Vitamin C Treatment

In one of the studies it was demonstrated that chronic vitamin C treatment of 2K-1C rats reduced arterial pressure and rSNA, and improved cardiac and renal baroreflex responses. Moreover, vitamin C treatment down regulated ATR1 gene expression in the clipped kidneys only in hypertensive rats and enhanced GPx expression in both clipped and non-clipped kidneys of 2K-1C rats. It can be said that chronic treatment with vitamin C improves significantly any CV function and the sympathetic activity in hypertension, reducing the OE in the kidney.

The renovascular model of arterial hypertension is characterized by increased circulating Ang II levels. The Ang II activates NADPH oxidases (through its interaction with AT1R), increasing ROS production and causing a redox state [103]. Nishi et al. [26] administered Vitamin C (150mg/kg/day) for seven consecutive days, by the sixth week after clipping. The

Vitamin C-mediated reduction in the blood pressure of 2K-1C rats may be related to its antioxidant properties, which have been demonstrated to reduce BP in other hypertensive animal models associated with OE, such as salt-sensitive [222], and deoxycorticosterone acetate–salt hypertensive rats [223], as well as in patients with essential hypertension [224]. Consistent with the previous reports, 2K-1C animals after vitamin C treatment, basal rSNA was reduced only in 2K-1C rats. These effects might be mediated by the interaction of vitamin C with O2-, enhancing central NO bioavailability, which exerts a tonic and chronic inhibition on the central SNS [57, 81]. Although vitamin C reduced BP and SNA only in 2K-1C rats, the BP remained elevated, whereas the SNA normalized after the treatment. This suggests an independently relationship between BP changes and a sympathetic impulse, also a possible role of Ang II in the maintenance of BP in Group 2K - 1 c [225].

3.12. Endothelin-1 Receptor Antagonists

Endothelin-1 (ET-1) is an important vasoconstrictor peptide and activation of ET-B receptor results in vasodilation. On the contrary ET-1 receptors activation causes vasoconstriction and inflammatory reactions. A double-blind randomized multicenter study [226] showed that the substance darusentan, a selective ET-A receptor antagonist, offered additional reduction of BP. In addition, other experimental study with diabetic nephropathy patients, macroalbuminuria and hypertension for twelve weeks, and showed a significant decline in albuminuria in the group where the substance avosentan a non-selective antagonist, was added in the already given treatment with ACEIs or ARBs. In both studies, the main side effect was fluid retention [227]. Although endothelin receptor antagonists have already been approved for the treatment of pulmonary hypertension, the available studies on arterial hypertension and CDK are still insufficient.

Conclusion and Perspectives

The etiology of hypertension in CKD is multifactorial. Therefore, combination of two or three antihypertensive drugs is usually necessary for optimal control of BP. Based on the pathophysiologic mechanisms, this treatment should include an ACEI or ARB, combined with diuretics to maintain normovolemia. In addition, new substances possibly contributing to optimal BP control, such as renin inhibitors, the newest RAAS blockers, and inhibitors of endothelin-1, have been reported. These pharmacological agents have positive effects when combined with ACEIs. There is convincing evidence that kidney injury can cause sympathetic overactivity, which contributes to the development of CV organ damage and possibly also kidney failure progression. Accordingly, RD offers new alternatives, not only in the treatment of patients, but also in the effort for a better understanding of the pathophysiology in various disease conditions characterized by sympathetic overactivity. Experimental and clinical studies have shown beneficial effects of both α- and β-adrenergic blockade. There is a strong interaction with Ang II, which increases central sympathetic tone and peripheral sympathetic action, and with NO, which by its suppressed availability increases the damaging action of sympathetic tone. Furthermore, experimental and clinical investigations have shown that the oxidative damage, caused by the overproduction of ROS, is also important indication of the high incidence of CV complications in patients with CKD. Presently, many issues need to be resolved. It is not known which class or combination of classes is most effective in reducing sympathetic hyperactivity and has the greatest effect on prognosis. Evidence suggests that not all Ang II receptor antagonists are equally effective in reducing sympathetic activity at the central and peripheral level. It is known that production/degradation alterations of ROS can produce OE causing renal and CV damage, and inducing also an increase on BP by activating the SNS. Additionally to these problem, new molecules like urotensin II and uric acid have emerged as potential contributors to the pathophysiology of hypertension in CKD. However, it is not yet clear their specific influence in the disease.

In conclusion, hypertension therapy of CKD patients should be individualized for each case, depending on comorbidities, tolerance and side effects present. Future research should outline, more accurately, the behavior of complex balance of pro-oxidant/antioxidant throughout the evolution on patients with kidney damage, which would allow the design of specific and safe strategies for interventions with antioxidant molecules that guarantee the restoration of the redox balance. In relation of the new molecules more studies are required to define their dominant mechanism, and potential role as therapeutic targets.

References

[1] Mahmoodi BK, Matsushita K, Woodward M, Blankestijn PJ, Cirillo M, Ohkubo T, Rossing P, Sarnak MJ, Stengel B, Yamagishi K, Yamashita K, Zhang L, Coresh J, de Jong PE, Astor BC, Chronic Kidney Disease Prognosis Consortium. Associations of kidney disease measures with mortality and end-stage renal disease in individuals with and without hypertension: a meta-analysis. *Lancet* 2012; 380:1649–1661.

[2] Ravera M, Re M, Deferrari L, Vettoretti S, Deferrari G. Importance of blood pressure control in chronic kidney disease. *J. Am. Soc. Nephrol.* 2006;17:S98–S103.

[3] Herget-Rosenthal S, Dehnen D, Kribben A, Quellmann T. Progressive chronic kidney disease in primary care: Modifiable risk factors and predictive model. *Prev. Med.* 2013; 57:357-362.

[4] Kim MJ, Lim NK, Park HY. Relationship between prehypertension and chronic kidney disease in middle-aged people in Korea: the Korean genome and epidemiology study. *BMC Public Health* 2012; 12:960.

[5] Collins AJ, Foley RN, Chavers B, Gilbertson D, Herzog C, Johansen K, Kasiske B, Kutner N, Liu J, St Peter W, Guo H, Gustafson S, Heubner B, Lamb K, Li S, Li S, Peng Y, Qiu Y, Roberts T, Skeans M, Snyder J, Solid C, Thompson B, Wang C, Weinhandl E, Zaun D, Arko C, Chen SC, Daniels F, Ebben J, Frazier E,Hanzlik C, Johnson R, Sheets D, Wang X, Forrest B, Constantini E, Everson S, Eggers P, Agodoa L.. United States Renal Data System 2011 Annual Data Report: Atlas of chronic kidney disease & end-stage renal disease in the United States. *Am. J. Kidney* Dis 2012; 59: e1-e420.

[6] Coresh J, Selvin E, Stevens LA, Manzi J, Kusek JW, Eggers P, Van Lente F, Levey AS. Prevalence of chronic kidney disease in the United States. *JAMA*. 2007; 298:2038–2047.

[7] Roderick P, Roth M, Mindell J. Prevalence of Chronic kidney disease in England: Findings from the 2009 Health survey for England. *J. Epidemiol. Community Health* 2011; 65:A1–A40.

[8] Singh AK, Farag YM, Mittal BV, Subramanian KK, Reddy SR, Acharya VN, Almeida AF, Channakeshavamurthy A, Ballal HS, P G, Issacs R, Jasuja S, Kirpalani AL, Kher V, Modi GK, Nainan G, Prakash J, Rana DS, Sreedhara R, Sinha DK, V SB, Sunder S, Sharma RK, Seetharam S, Raju TR, Rajapurkar MM. Epidemiology and risk factors of chronic kidney disease in India - results from the SEEK (Screening and early evaluation of kidney disease) study. *BMC nephrology* 2013; 14:114.

[9] Smith DH, Gullion CM, Nichols G, Keith DS, Brown JB. Cost of Medical Care for Chronic Kidney Disease and Comorbidity among Enrollees in a Large HMO Population. *J. Am. Soc. Nephrol.* 2004; 15:1300–1306.

[10] Khan S, Amedia CA. Economic burden of chronic kidney disease. *J. Eval. Clin. Pract.* 2008; 14:422–434.

[11] Ewen S, Ukena C, Linz D, Schmieder RE, Böhm M, Mahfoud F. The Sympathetic Nervous System in Chronic Kidney Disease. *CurrHypertens Rep.* 2013; 15:370-376.

[12] Rao M, Qiu Y, Wang C, Bakris G. Hypertension and CKD: Kidney Early Evaluation Program (KEEP) and National Health and Nutrition Examination Survey (NHANES), 1999-2004. *Am. J. Kidney Dis.* 2008; 51:S30–S37.

[13] K/DOQI. K/DOQI clinical practice guidelines for chronic kidney disease: Evaluation, classification, and stratification. *Am. J. Kidney Dis.* 2002; 39:S1–S266.

[14] Levey AS, Eckardt KU, Tsukamoto Y, Levin A, Coresh J, Rossert J, De Zeeuw D, Hostetter TH, Lameire N, Eknoyan G. Definition and classification of chronic kidney disease: A position statement from Kidney Disease: *Improving Global Outcomes* (KDIGO). Kidney int 2005; 67:2089–2100.

[15] Borrelli S, De Nicola L, Stanzione G, Conte G, Minutolo R. Resistant hypertension in nondialysis chronic kidney disease. *Int. J. Hypertens.* 2013; 2013:929183.

[16] Desai N, Madhavankutty Saraswathy V, Hunter K, McFadden C. Prevalence of true therapeutic inertia in blood pressure control in an academic chronic kidney disease clinic. *Journal of clinical hypertension* (Greenwich, Conn.) 2013; 15:375–379.

[17] Sarafidis PA, Li S, Chen SC, Collins AJ, Brown WW, Klag MJ, Bakris GL. Hypertension awareness, treatment, and control in chronic kidney disease. *Am. J. Med.* 2008; 121:332–40.

[18] De Nicola L, Gabbai FB, Agarwal R, Chiodini P, Borrelli S, Bellizzi V, Nappi F, Conte G, Minutolo R. Prevalence and prognostic role of resistant hypertension in chronic kidney disease patients. *J. Am. Coll. Cardiol.* 2013; 61:2461–2467.

[19] NIH/NHLBI. The Seventh Report of the Joint National Committee (JNC-7) on Prevention, Detection, Evaluation, and Treatment of High Blood Pressure. *National High Blood Pressure Education Program* 2004: 25–33.

[20] Sobotka P, Mahfoud F, Schlaich MP, Hoppe UC, Böhm M, Krum H. Sympatho-renal axis in chronic disease. *Clin. Res. Cardiol.* 2011; 100:1049–1057

[21] Di Daniele N, De Francesco M, Violo L, Spinelli A, Simonetti G. Renal sympathetic nerve ablation for the treatment of difficult-to-control or refractory hypertension in a haemodialysis patient. *Nephrol. Dial. Transplant.* 2012; 27:1689–1690.

[22] Appel LJ, Wright JT Jr, Greene T, Agodoa LY, Astor BC, Bakris GL, Cleveland WH, Charleston J, Contreras G, Faulkner ML, Gabbai FB, Gassman JJ, Hebert LA,

Jamerson KA, Kopple JD, Kusek JW, Lash JP, Lea JP, Lewis JB, Lipkowitz MS, Massry SG, Miller ER, Norris K, Phillips RA, Pogue VA, Randall OS, Rostand SG, Smogorzewski MJ, Toto RD, Wang X; AASK Collaborative Research Group. Intensive blood-pressure control in hypertensive chronic kidney disease. *N. Engl. J. Med.* 2010; 363:918-929.

[23] Kim KE, Onesti G, Schwartz AB, Chinitz JL, Swartz C. Hemodynamics of hypertension in chronic end-stage renal disease. *Circulation* 1972; 46:456-464.

[24] Morgado E, Leão P. Hypertension and Chronic Kidney Disease: Cause and Consequence – Therapeutic Considerations. In: Antihypertensive Drugs, Prof. HosseinBabaei (Ed). *InTech*, Portugal, 2012, 45-66.

[25] Udani S, Lazich I, Bakris G. L. Epidemiology of hypertensive kidney disease. *Nat. Rev. Nephrol.* 2011; 7: 11-21.

[26] Nishi EE, Oliveira-Sales EB, Bergamaschi CT, Oliveira TG, Boim MA, Campos RR. Chronic antioxidant treatment improves arterial renovascular hypertension and oxidativ e stress markers in the kidney in Wistar rats. *Am. J. Hypertens.* 2010; 23:473-480.

[27] Tedla FM, Brar A, Browne R, Brown C. Hypertension in chronic kidney disease: navigating the evidence. *Int. J. Hypertens.* 2011; 2011:132405.

[28] Guyton AC, Coleman TG, Young DB, Lohmeier TE, DeClue JW. Salt balance and long-term blood pressure control. *Annu. Rev. Med.* 1980; 31:15-27.

[29] Ardaillou R, Dussaule JC. Role of atrial natriuretic peptide in the control of sodium balance in chronic renal failure. *Nephron* 1994; 66: 249-257.

[30] Dietz JR. Mechanisms of atrial natriuretic peptide secretion from the atrium. *Cardiovasc. Res.* 2005; 68: 8-17.

[31] Penney MD. Sodium, water and potassium. Clinical Biochemistry: Metabolic and Clinical Aspects. 2008. 1:28-66.

[32] Kotanko P. Cause and consequences of sympathetic hyperactivity in chronic kidney disease. *Blood Purif.* 2006; 24: 95-99.

[33] Ishii M, Ikeda T, Takagi M, Sugimoto T, Atarashi K, Igari T, Uehara Y, Matsuoka H, Hirata Y, Kimura K, Takeda T, Murao S. Elevated plasma catecholamines in hypertensives with primary glomerular diseases. *Hypertension* 1983; 5:545–551.

[34] Converse RL Jr, Jacobsen TN, Toto RD, Jost CM, Cosentino F, Fouad-Tarazi F, Victor RG. Sympathetic overactivity in patients with chronic renal failure. *N. Engl. J. Med.* 1992; 327:1912–1918.

[35] Hausberg M, Kosch M, Harmelink P, Barenbrock M, Hohage H, Kisters K, Dietl KH, Rahn KH. Sympathetic nerve activity in end-stage renal disease. *Circulation* 2002; 106:1974–1979.

[36] Grassi G, Quarti-Trevano F, Seravalle G, Arenare F, Volpe M, Furiani S, Dell'Oro R, Mancia G. Early sympathetic activation in the initial clinical stages of chronic renal failure. *Hypertension* 2011; 57:846–851.

[37] Penne EL, Neumann J, Klein IH, Oey PL, Bots ML, Blankestijn PJ. Sympathetic hyperactivity and clinical outcome in chronic kidney disease patients during standard treatment. *J. Nephrol.* 2009; 22:208–215.

[38] Koomans HA, Blankestijn PJ, Joles JA. Sympathetic hyperactivity in chronic renal failure: a wake-up call. J Am Soc Nephrol 2004; 15:524-537.

[39] Augustyniak RA, Tuncel M, Zhang W, Toto RD, Victor RG. Sympathetic overactivity as a cause of hypertension in chronic renal failure. *J. Hypertens.* 2002; 20: 3–9.

[40] Campese VM, Ye S, Zhong H. Downregulation of neuronal nitric oxide synthase and interleukin-1beta mediates angiotensin II-dependent stimulation of sympathetic nerve activity; *Hypertension.* 2002; 39:519-524.

[41] Klein IH, Ligtenberg G, Oey PL, Koomans HA, Blankestijn PJ. Sympathetic activity is increased in polycystic kidney disease and is associated with hypertension. *J. Am. Soc. Nephrol.* 2001; 12:2427-2433.

[42] [Campese VM, Ye S, Truong RH, Gamburd M. Losartan reduces sympathetic nerve outflow from the brain of rats with chronic renal failure. *J. Renin. Angiotensin. Aldosterone Syst.* 2000; 1:202-208.

[43] Ye S, Zhong H, Duong VN, Campese VM; Losartan reduces central and peripheral sympathetic nerve activity in a rat model of neurogenic hypertension. Hypertension 2002; 39:1101-1106.

[44] Campese VM, Ye S, Zhong H, Yanamadala V, Ye Z, Chiu J. Reactive oxygen species stimulate central and peripheral sympathetic nervous system activity. *Am. J. Physiol. Heart Circ. Physiol.* 2004; 287:H695-H703.

[45] Oliveira-Sales EB, Nishi EE, Carillo BA, Boim MA, Dolnikoff MS, Bergamaschi CT, Campos RR. Oxidative stress in the sympathetic premotor neurons contributes to sympathetic activation in renovascular hypertension. *Am. J. Hypertens.* 2009; 22:484–492.

[46] Campese VM, Ku E, Park J. Sympathetic renal innervation and resistant hypertension. *Int. J Hypertens.* 2011; 20:814354.

[47] Faber JE, Brody MJ. Afferent renal nerve-dependent hypertension following acute renal artery stenosis in the conscious rat. Circ Res 1985; 57:676-688.

[48] Campese VM, Kogosov E, Koss M. Renal afferent denervation prevents the progression of renal disease in the renal ablation model of chronic renal failure in the rat. *Am. J. Kidney Dis.* 1995; 26:861-865.

[49] Ye S, Ozgur B, Campese VM. Renal afferent impulses, the posterior hypothalamus, and hypertension in rats with chronic renal failure. *Kidney Int.* 1997; 51:722-727.

[50] Ye S, Zhong H, Yanamadala V, Campese VM. Renal injury caused by intrarenal injection of phenol increases afferent and efferent renal sympathetic nerve activity. *Am. J. Hypertens.* 2002; 15:717–724.

[51] Campese VM. Neurogenic factors and hypertension in renal disease. *Kidney Int. Suppl.* 2000; 75:S2-S6.

[52] Schlaich MP, Socratous F, Hennebry S, Eikelis N, Lambert EA, Straznicky N, Esler MD, Lambert GW. Sympathetic activation in chronic renal failure. *J. Am. Soc. Nephrol.;* 2009; 20:933–939.

[53] Ditting T, Freisinger W, Siegel K, Fiedler C, Small L, Neuhuber W, Heinlein S, Reeh PW, Schmieder RE, Veelken R. Tonic postganglionic sympathetic inhibition induced by afferent renal nerves? Hypertension 2012; 59:467–476.

[54] Katholi RE, Whitlow PL, Hageman GR, Woods WT. Intrarenal adenosine produces hypertension by activating the sympathetic nervous system via the renal nerves in the dog. *J. Hypertens.* 1984; 2:349-359.

[55] Reid IA. Interactions between ANG II, sympathetic nervous system, and baroreceptor reflexes in regulation of blood pressure. *Am. J. Physiol.* 1992; 262:E763–E778.

[56] Carlson SH, Wyss JM. Neurohormonal regulation of the sympathetic nervous system: new insights into central mechanisms of action. *Curr. Hypertens. Rep.* 2008; 10:233–240.

[57] Ye S, Nosrati S, Campese VM. Nitric oxide (NO) modulates the neurogenic control of blood pressure in rats with chronic renal failure (CRF). *J. Clin. Invest.* 1997; 99:540–548.

[58] Sander M, Hansen PG, Victor RG. Sympathetically mediated hypertension caused by chronic inhibition of nitric oxide; *Hypertension* 1995; 26:691-695.

[59] Chowdhary S, Townend JN. Role of nitric oxide in the regulation of cardiovascular autonomic control. *Clin. Sci.* (Lond) 1999; 97:5-17.

[60] Mallamaci F, Tripepi G, Maas R, Malatino L, Boger R, Zoccali C. Analysis of the relationship between norepinephrine and asymmetric dimethyl arginine levels among patients with end-stage renal disease. *J. Am. Soc. Nephrol.* 2004; 15:435–441.

[61] Grassi G, Seravalle G, Ghiadoni L, Tripepi G, Bruno RM, Mancia G, Zoccali C. Sympathetic nerve traffic and asymmetric dimethylarginine in chronic kidney disease. *Clin. J. Am. Soc. Nephrol.* 2011; 6:2620–2627.

[62] Kielstein JT, Zoccali C. Asymmetric dimethylarginine: a novel marker of risk and a potential target for therapy in chronic kidney disease. *Curr. Opin. Nephrol. Hypertens.* 2008; 17:609–615.

[63] Zoccali C, Mallamaci F, Maas R, Benedetto FA, Tripepi G, Malatino LS, Cataliotti A, Bellanuova I, Böger R, CREED Investigators. Left ventricular hypertrophy, cardiac remodeling and asymmetric dimethylarginine (ADMA) in hemodialysis patients. *Kidney Int.* 2002; 62:339–345.

[64] Shi B, Ni Z, Zhou W, Yu Z, Gu L, Mou S, Fang W, Wang Q, Cao L, Yan Y, Qian J. Circulating levels of asymmetric dimethylarginine are an independent risk factor for left ventricular hypertrophy and predict cardiovascular events in pre-dialysis patients with chronic kidney disease. *Eur. J. Intern. Med.* 2010; 21:444–448.

[65] Abe M, Okada K, Maruyama T, Matsumoto K. Renoprotect and blood pressure lowering effect of low-dose hydrochlorothiazide added to intensive renin-angiotensin inhibition in hypertensive patients with chronic kidney disease. *Int. J. Clin. Pharmacol. Ther.* 2009; 47:525-532.

[66] DiBona GF. Physiology in perspective: The wisdom of the body. Neural control of the kidney. *Am. J. Physiol. Regul. Integr. Comp. Physiol.* 2005; 289:R633–R641.

[67] Vonend O, Okonek A, Stegbauer J, Habbel S, Quack I, Rump LC. Renovascular effects of sympathetic cotransmitters ATP and NPY are age-dependent in spontaneously hypertensive rats. *Cardiovasc. Res.* 2005; 66:345–352.

[68] Singh M, Mensah GA, Bakris G. Pathogenesis and clinical physiology of hypertension. *Cardial. Clin.* 2010; 28:545-558.

[69] Joles JA, Koomans HA. Causes and consequences of increased sympathetic activity in renal disease. *Hypertension* 2004; 43:1803-1817.

[70] Taal MW, Brenner BM. Renoprotective benefits of RAS inhibition: from ACEI to angiotensin II antagonists. *Kidney Int.* 2000; 57:1803-1817.

[71] Tesauro M, Mascali A, Franzese O, Cipriani S, Cardillo C, Di Daniele N. Chronic Kidney Disease, Obesity, and Hypertension: The Role of Leptin and Adiponectin. *Int. J. Hypertens.* 2012; 2012:943605.

[72] Pestana M. Renal Dopaminergic mechanisms in renal parenchymal diseases and hypertension. *Nephrol. Dial. Transplant.* 2001; 16: 53- 59.

[73] Sarafidis PA, Khosla N, Bakris GL. Antihypertensive therapy in the presence of proteinuria. *Am. J. Kidney Dis.* 2007; 49:12-26.

[74] Thethi T, Kamiyama M, Kobori H. The link between the renin-angiotensin-aldosterone system and renal injury in obesity and the metabolic syndrome. *Curr. Hypertens. Rep.* 2012; 14:160–169.

[75] Zemin C, Cooper ME. Role of angiotensive II in tubulointerstitial injury. *Semin. Nephrol.* 2001; 21: 554-562.

[76] Torres C. Insuficiencia renal crónica. *Rev. Méd. Hered.* 2003; 14: 1-4.

[77] Vink EE, Blankestijn PJ. Evidence and consequences of the central role of the kidneys in the pathophysiology of sympathetic hyperactivity. *Front Physiol.* 2012; 20;3:29.

[78] Färbom P, Wahlstrand B, Almgren P, Skrtic S, Lanke J, Weiss L, Kjeldsen S, Hedner T, Melander O. Interaction between renal function and microalbuminuria for cardiovascular risk in hypertension: the Nordic diltiazem study. *Hypertension* 2008; 52:115-122.

[79] Morena M, Delosc S, Dupuy AM, Canaud B, Cristol JP. Overproduction of reactive oxygen species in end-stage renal disease patients: a potential component of hemodialysis-associated inflammation. *Hemodial Int.* 2005; 9:37-46.

[80] Heredia D, Fernández D, Alfonso J, Ballesteros M. El estrés oxidativo en la insuficiencia renal asociada con hipertensión. *Rev. Cubana Invest. Bioméd.* 2012; 31: 16-25.

[81] Oliveira-Sales EB, Dugaich AP, Carillo BA, Abreu NP, Boim MA, Martins PJ, D'Almeida V, Dolnikoff MS, Bergamaschi CT, Campos RR. Oxidative stress contributes to renovascular hypertension. *Am. J. Hypertens.* 2008; 21: 98–104.

[82] Campese VM, Shaohua Y, Huiquin Z. Oxidative stress mediates angiotensin II-dependent stimulation of sympathetic nerve activity. *Hypertension* 2005; 46:533–539.

[83] Lerman LO, Nath KA, Rodriguez-Porcel M, Krier JD, Schwartz RS, Napoli C, Romero JC. Increased oxidative stress in experimental renovascular hypertension. *Hypertension* 2001; 37:541–546.

[84] Welch WJ, Mendonca M, Aslam S, Wilcox CS. Roles of oxidative stress and AT1 receptors in renal hemodynamics and oxygenation in the postclipped 2K,1C kidney. *Hypertension* 2003; 41:692–696.

[85] Bosse HM, Bachmann S. Immunohistochemically detected protein nitration indicates sites of renal nitric oxide release in Goldblatt hypertension. *Hypertension* 1997; 30:948–952.

[86] Schiffrin EL, Lipman ML, Mann JF. Chronic kidney disease: effects on the cardiovascular system. *Circulation* 2007; 116:85–97.

[87] Guérin AP, Pannier B, Marchais SJ, London GM. Cardiovascular disease in the dialysis population: prognostic significance of arterial disorders. *Curr. Opin. Nephrol. Hypertens.* 2006; 15:105-110.

[88] González I, Casanova C, Escobar C, Garcia A, Peraira J, Prieto E, Tejero C. Enfermedad cardiovascular y función renal. Mecanismos patogénicos. *Rev. Esp. Cardiol.* 2008; 8:10-21.

[89] Wilcox CS. Reactive oxygen species: Roles in blood pressure and kidney function. *Curr. Hypertens. Rep.* 2002; 4:160-166.

[90] Stas S, Whaley-Connell A, Habibi J, Appesh L, Hayden MR, Karuparthi PR, Qazi M, Morris EM, Cooper SA, Link CD, Stump C, Hay M, Ferrario C, Sowers JR. Mineralocorticoid receptor blockade attenuates chronic overexpression of the renin-angiotensin-aldosterone system stimulation of reduced nicotinamide adenine dinucleotide phosphate oxidase and cardiac remodeling. *Endocrinology* 2007; 148:3773–3780.

[91] Montezano AC, Touyz RM. Oxidative stress, Noxs, and hypertension: experimental evidence and clinical controversies. *Ann. Med.* 2012; 44:S2-16.

[92] Zimmerman MC, Lazartigues E, Sharma RV, Davisson RL. Hypertension caused by angiotensin II infusion involves increased superoxide production in the central nervous system. *Circ. Res.* 2004; 95:210 –216.

[93] Hirooka Y. Role of reactive oxygen species in brainstem in neural mechanisms of hypertension. *Auton. Neurosci.* 2008; 142:20 – 24.

[94] Wilcox CS. Oxidative stress and nitric oxide deficiency in the kidney: a critical link to hypertension? *Am. J. Physiol. Regul. Integr. Comp. Physiol.* 2005; 289:R913 – R935.

[95] González I, Casanova C, Escobar C, Garcia A, Peraira JR, Prieto E, Tejero C. Enfermedad cardiovascular y función renal. Mecanismos patogénicos. *Rev. Esp. Cardiol. Supl.* 2008; 8:10E-21E.

[96] Hayden MR, Whaley-Connell A, Sowers JR. Renal redox stress and remodeling in metabolic syndrome, type 2 diabetes mellitus, and diabetic nephropathy: paying homage to the podocyte. *Am. J. Nephrol.* 2005; 25:553 – 569.

[97] Manning RD Jr, Tian N, Meng S. Oxidative stress and anti-oxidant treatment in hypertension and the associated renal damage. *Am. J. Nephrol.* 2005; 25:311 –317.

[98] Hisaki R, Fujita H, Saito F, Kushiro T. Tempol attenuates the development of hypertensive renal injury in Dahl saltsensitive rats. *Am. J. Hypertens.* 2005;18:707 – 713.

[99] Ferretti G, Bacchetti T, Masciangelo S, Pallotta G. Lipid peroxidation in hemodialysis patients: effect of vitamin C supplementation. *Clin. Biochem.* 2008; 41:381-386.

[100] Blendea MC, Jacobs D, Stump CS, McFarlane SI, Ogrin C, Bahtyiar G, Stas S, Kumar P, Sha Q, Ferrario CM, Sowers JR. Abrogation of oxidative stress improves insulin sensitivity in the Ren-2 rat model of tissue angiotensin II overexpression. *Am. J. Physiol. Endocrinol. Metab.* 2005; 288:E353–E359.

[101] Ponnuchamy B, Khalil RA. Cellular mediators of renal vascular dysfunction in hypertension. *Am. J. Physiol. Regul. Integr. Comp. Physiol.* 2009; 296:R1001-R1018.

[102] Nuyt AM. Mechanisms underlying developmental programming of elevated blood pressure and vascular dysfunction: evidence from human studies and experimental animal models. *Clin. Sci.* (Lond) 2008; 114:1 –17.

[103] Briones AM, Touyz RM. Oxidative stress and hypertension: current concepts. *Curr.Hypertens. Rep.* 2010; 12:135-142.

[104] Ye S, Zhong H, Yanamadala S, Campese VM. Oxidative stress mediates the stimulation of sympathetic nerve activity in the phenol renal injury model of hypertension. *Hypertension* 2006; 48:309-315.

[105] [Kishi T, Hirooka Y, Kimura Y, Ito K, Shimokawa H, Takeshita A. Increased reactive oxygen species in rostral ventrolateral medulla contribute to neural mechanisms of hypertension in stroke-prone spontaneously hypertensive rats. *Circulation* 2004; 109:2357-2362.

[106] Fujita M, Ando K, Nagae A, Fujita T. Sympathoexcitation by oxidative stress in the brain mediates arterial pressure elevation in salt-sensitive hypertension. *Hypertension* 2007; 50:360-367.

[107] Nagae A, Fujita M, Kawarazaki H, Matsui H, Ando K, Fujita T. Sympathoexcitation by oxidative stress in the brain mediates arterial pressure elevation in obesity-induced hypertension. *Circulation* 2009; 119:978-986.

[108] Hursitoglu M, Tukek T, Cikrikcioglu MA, Kara O, Kazancioglu R, Ozkan O, Cakirca M, Akdogan F, Gundogan E, Aydin S, Beycan I, Gursu M, Dogan S, Erek A. Urotensin II levels in patients with chronic kidney disease and kidney transplants. *Ups. J. Med. Sci.* 2012; 117:22-27.

[109] Pearson D, Shively JE, Clark BR, Geschwind II, Barkley M, Nishioka RS, Bern HA. Urotensin II: a somatostatin-like peptide in the caudal neurosecretory system of fishes. *Proc. Natl. Acad. Sci. USA* 1980; 77:5021-5024.

[110] Douglas SA, Dhanak D, Johns DG. From 'gills to pills': urotensin-II as a regulator of mammalian cardiorenal function. *Trends Pharmacol. Sci.* 2004; 25:76-85.

[111] Giachini FR, Callera GE, Carneiro FS, Tostes RC, Webb RC. Therapeutic targets in hypertension: is there a place for antagonists of the most potent vasoconstrictors? *Expert Opin. Ther. Targets* 2008; 12:327-339.

[112] McDonald J, Batuwangala M, Lambert DG. Role of urotensin II and its receptor in health and disease. *J. Anesth.* 2007; 21:378-389.

[113] Zhu YC, Zhu YZ, Moore PK. The role of urotensin II in cardiovascular and renal physiology and diseases. *Br. J. Pharmacol.* 2006; 148:884-901.

[114] Ng LL, Loke I, O'Brien RJ, Squire IB, Davies JE. Plasma urotensin in human systolic heart failure. *Circulation* 2002; 106:2877-80.

[115] Tian L, Li C, Qi J, Fu P, Yu X, Li X, Cai L. Diabetes-induced upregulation of urotensin II and its receptor plays an important role in TGF-beta1-mediated renal fibrosis and dysfunction. *Am. J. Physiol. Endocrinol. Metab.* 2008; 295:E1234-E1242.

[116] Shenouda A, Douglas SA, Ohlstein EH, Giaid A. Localization of urotensin-II immunoreactivity in normal human kidneys and renal carcinoma. *J. Histochem. Cytochem.* 2002; 50:885-889.

[117] Totsune K, Takahashi K, Arihara Z, Sone M, Satoh F, Ito S, Kimura Y, Sasano H, Murakami O. Role of urotensin II in patients on dialysis. *Lancet* 2001; 358:810-811.

[118] Abdel-Razik AE, Forty EJ, Balment RJ, Ashton N. Renal haemodynamic and tubular actions of urotensin II in the rat. *J. Endocrinol.* 2008; 198:617–624.

[119] Abdel-Razik AE, Balment RJ, Ashton N. Enhanced renal sensitivity of the spontaneously hypertensive rat to urotensin II. *Am. J. Physiol. Ren. Physiol.* 2008; 295: F1239–F1247.

[120] Shi Y, Cao YX, Lu N, Yao T, Zhu YC. Hemodynamic-independent anti-natriuretic effect of urotensin II in spontaneously hypertensive rats. Peptides 2008; 29:783-794.

[121] Song W, Abdel Razik AE, Lu W, Ao Z, Johns DG, Douglas SA, Balment RJ, Ashton N. Urotensin II and renal function in the rat. *Kidney Int.* 2006; 69:1360-1368.

[122] Gruson D, Rousseau MF, Ahn SA, van Linden F, Ketelslegers JM. Circulating urotensin II levels in moderate to severe congestive heart failure: its relations with myocardial functionand well established neurohormonal markers. *Peptides* 2006; 27:1527-1531.

[123] Richards AM, Nicholls MG, Lainchbury JG, Fisher S, Yandle TG. Plasma urotensin II in heart failure. *Lancet* 2002; 360:545-546.

[124] Cheung BM, Leung R, Man YB, Wong LY. Plasma concentration of urotensin II is raised in hypertension. *J. Hypertens.* 2004; 22:1341-1344.

[125] Totsune K, Takahashi K, Arihara Z, Sone M, Ito S, Murakami O. Increased plasma urotensin II levels in patients with diabetes mellitus. *Clin. Sc*i (Lond) 2003; 104:1-5.

[126] Totsune K, Takahashi K, Arihara Z, Sone M, Murakami O, Ito S, Kikuya M, Ohkubo T, Hashimoto J, Imai Y. Elevated plasma levels of immunoreactive urotensin II and its increased urinary excretion in patients with Type 2 diabetes mellitus: association with progress of diabetic nephropathy. *Peptides* 2004; 25:1809-1814.

[127] Matsushita M, Shichiri M, Imai T, Iwashina M, Tanaka H, Takasu N, Hirata Y. Co-expression of urotensin II and its receptor (GPR14) in human cardiovascular and renal tissues. *J. Hypertens.* 2001; 19:2185-2190.

[128] Mosenkis A, Kallem RR, Danoff TM, Aiyar N, Bazeley J, Townsend RR. Renal impairment, hypertension and plasma urotensin II. *Nephrol. Dial. Transplant.* 2011; 26:609-614.

[129] Thompson JP, Watt P, Sanghavi S, Strupish JW, Lambert DG. A comparison of cerebrospinal fluid and plasma urotensin II concentrations in normotensive and hypertensive patients undergoing urological surgery during spinal anesthesia: a pilot study. *Anesth. Analg.* 2003; 97:1501-1503.

[130] Ames RS, Sarau HM, Chambers JK, Willette RN, Aiyar NV, Romanic AM, Louden CS, Foley JJ, Sauermelch CF, Coatney RW, Ao Z, Disa J, Holmes SD, Stadel JM, Martin JD, Liu WS, Glover GI, Wilson S, McNulty DE, Ellis CE, Elshourbagy NA, Shabon U, Trill JJ, Hay DW, Ohlstein EH, Bergsma DJ, Douglas SA. Human urotensin-II is a potent vasoconstrictor and agonist for the orphan receptor GPR14. *Nature* 1999; 401:282-286.

[131] Wang YX, Ding YJ, Zhu YZ, Shi Y, Yao T, Zhu YC. Role of PKC in the novel synergistic action of urotensin II and angiotensin II and in urotensin II-induced vasoconstriction. *Am. J. Physiol. Heart. Circ. Physiol.* 2007; 292:H348-359.

[132] Tölle M, van der Giet M. Cardiorenovascular effects of urotensin II and the relevance of the UT receptor. *Peptides* 2008; 29:743-763.

[133] Böhm F, Pernow J. Urotensin II evokes potent vasoconstriction in humans in vivo. Br J Pharmacol 2002; 135:25-27.

[134] Lim M, Honisett S, Sparkes CD, Komesaroff P, Kompa A, Krum H. Differential effect of urotensin II on vascular tone in normal subjects and patients with chronic heart failure. *Circulation* 2004; 109:1212-1214.

[135] Rossi M, Magagna A, Di Maria C, Franzoni F, Taddei S, Santoro G. Skin vasodilator effect of exogenous urotensin-II in hypertensives not exposed to antihypertensive medication. *Blood Press* 2008; 17:18-25.

[136] Affolter JT, Newby DE, Wilkinson IB, Winter MJ, Balment RJ, Webb DJ. No effect on central or peripheral blood pressure of systemic urotensin II infusion in humans. *Br. J. Clin. Pharmacol.* 2002; 54:617-621.

[137] Jalal DI, Chonchol M, Chen W, Targher G. Uric acid as a target of therapy in CKD. *Am. J. Kidney Dis.* 2013; 61:134-146.

[138] Wright AF, Rudan I, Hastie ND, Campbell H. A 'complexity' of urate transporters. Kidney Int 2010; 78:446-452.
[139] Edwards NL. The role of hyperuricemia and gout in kidney and cardiovascular disease. *Cleve Clin. J. Med.* 2008; 75:S13-S16.
[140] Spencer HW, Yarger WE, Robinson RR. Alterations of renal function during dietary-induced hyperuricemia in the rat. *Kidney Int.* 1976; 9:489-500.
[141] Koka RM, Huang E, Lieske JC. Adhesion of uric acid crystals to the surface of renal epithelial cells. *Am. J. Physiol. Renal. Physiol.* 2000; 278:F989-F998.
[142] Umekawa T, Chegini N, Khan SR. Increased expression of monocyte chemoattractant protein-1 (MCP-1) by renal epithelial cells in culture on exposure to calcium oxalate, phosphate and uric acid crystals. *Nephrol. Dial Transplant.* 2003. 18:664-669.
[143] Ames BN, Cathcart R, Schwiers E, Hochstein P. Uric acid provides an a ntioxidant defense in humans against oxidant- and radical-caused aging and cancer: a hypothesis. *Proc. Natl. Acad. Sci. USA* 1981; 78:6858-6862.
[144] Mazzali M, Hughes J, Kim YG, Jefferson JA, Kang DH, Gordon KL, Lan HY, Kivlighn S, Johnson RJ. Elevated uric acid increases blood pressure in the rat by a novel crystal-independent mechanism. *Hypertension* 2001; 38:1101-1106.
[145] Sánchez-Lozada LG, Tapia E, López-Molina R, Nepomuceno T, Soto V, Avila-Casado C, Nakagawa T, Johnson RJ, Herrera-Acosta J, Franco M. Effects of acute and chronic L-arginine treatment in experimental hyperuricemia. *Am. J. Physiol. Renal. Physiol.* 2007; 292:F1238-F1244.
[146] Gersch C, Palii SP, Kim KM, Angerhofer A, Johnson RJ, Henderson GN. Inactivation of nitric oxide by uric acid. *Nucleosides Nucleotides Nucleic Acids* 2008; 27:967-978.
[147] Mazzali M, Kanellis J, Han L, Feng L, Xia YY, Chen Q, Kang DH, Gordon KL, Watanabe S, Nakagawa T, Lan HY, Johnson RJ. Hyperuricemia induces a primary renal arteriolopathy in rats by a blood pressure-independent mechanism. *Am. J. Physiol. Renal. Physiol.* 2002; 282:F991-F997.
[148] Han HJ, Lim MJ, Lee YJ, Lee JH, Yang IS, Taub M. Uric acid inhibits renal proximal tubule cell proliferation via at least two signaling pathways involving PKC, MAPK, cPLA2, and NF-kappaB. *Am. J. Physiol. Renal. Physiol.* 2007; 292:F373-F381.
[149] Netea MG, Kullberg BJ, Blok WL, Netea RT, van der Meer JW. The role of hyperuricemia in the increased cytokine production after lipopolysaccharide challenge in neutropenicmice. *Blood* 1997; 89:577-582.
[150] Sánchez-Lozada LG, Tapia E, Soto V, Avila-Casado C, Franco M, Wessale JL, Zhao L, Johnson RJ. Effect of febuxostat on the progression of renal disease in 5/6 nephrectomy rats with and without hyperuricemia. *Nephron. Physiol.* 2008; 108:69-78.
[151] Kosugi T, Nakayama T, Heinig M, Zhang L, Yuzawa Y, Sanchez-Lozada LG, Roncal C, Johnson RJ, Nakagawa T. Effect of lowering uric acid on renal disease in the type 2 diabetic db/db mice. *Am. J. Physiol. Renal. Physiol.* 2009; 297:F481-F488.
[152] Segura J, Ruilope LM. Should diuretics always be included as initial antihypertensive management in early-stage CKD? *Curr. Opin. Nephrol. Hypertens.* 2009; 18:392-396
[153] K/DOQI. K/DOQI clinical practice guidelines on hypertension and antihypertensive agents in chronic kidney disease. *Am. J. Kidney Dis.* 2004; 43: S1-S290.
[154] Mancia G, De Backer G, Dominiczak A, Cifkova R, Fagard R, Germano G, Grassi G, Heagerty AM, Kjeldsen SE, Laurent S, Narkiewicz K, Ruilope L, Rynkiewicz A,Schmieder RE, Boudier HA, Zanchetti A, Vahanian A, Camm J, De Caterina R,

Dean V, Dickstein K, Filippatos G, Funck-Brentano C, Hellemans I, Kristensen SD, McGregor K, Sechtem U, Silber S, Tendera M, Widimsky P, Zamorano JL, Erdine S, Kiowski W, Agabiti-Rosei E, Ambrosioni E, Lindholm LH, Viigimaa M, Adamopoulos S, Bertomeu V, Clement D, Farsang C, Gaita D, Lip G, Mallion JM, Manolis AJ, Nilsson PM, O'Brien E, Ponikowski P, Redon J, Ruschitzka F, Tamargo J, van Zwieten PA, Waeber B, Williams B. 2007 Guidelines for the Management of Arterial Hypertension: The Task Force for the Management of Arterial Hypertension of the European Society of Hypertension (ESH) and of the European Society of Cardiology (ESC). *J. Hypertens.* 2007; 25: 1105–1187.

[155] Chobanian AV, Bakris GL, Black HR, Cushman WC, Green LA, Izzo Jr JL, Jones DW, Materson BJ, Oparil S, Wright Jr JT, Roccella EJ. The Seventh Report of the Joint National Committee on Prevention, Detection, Evaluation, and Treatment of High Blood Pressure: the JNC 7 report. *JAMA* 2003; 289:2560–2572.

[156] Wright JM, Musini VM. First-line drugs for hypertension. *Cochrane Database Syst. Rev.* 2009; 8: CD001841.

[157] Messerli FH, Nussberger J, Phung S. Thiazide diuretic monotherapy for hypertension: diuretic's dark side just got darker. *Kidney Int.* 2008; 74:825.

[158] Brown MJ, Palmer CR, Castaigne A, de Leeuw PW, Mancia G, Rosenthal T, Ruilope LM. Morbidity and mortality in patients randomised to double-blind treatment with a long-acting calcium-channel blocker or diuretic in the International Nifedipine GITS study: Intervention as a Goal in Hypertension Treatment (INSIGHT). *Lancet* 2000; 356: 366–372.

[159] Lindholm LH, Persson M, Alaupovic P, Carlberg B, Svensson A, Samuelsson O. Metabolic outcome during 1 year in newly detected hypertensives: results of the Antihypertensive Treatment and Lipid Profile in a North of Sweden Efficacy Evaluation (ALPINE study). *J. Hypertens.* 2003; 21: 1563–1574.

[160] Brown NJ, Nakamura S, Ma L, Nakamura I, Donnert E, Freeman M, Vaughan DE, Fogo AB. Aldosterone modulates plasminogen activator inhibitor-1 and glomerulosclerosis in vivo. *Kidney Int.* 2000; 58: 1219–1227.

[161] Juknevicius I, Segal Y, Kren S, Lee R, Hostetter TH. Effect of aldosterone on renal transforming growth factor-beta. *Am. J. Physiol. Renal. Physiol.* 2004; 286:F1059–F1062.

[162] Schjoedt KJ, Andersen S, Rossing P, Tarnow L, Parving HH. Aldosterone escape during blockade of the renin-angiotensin-aldosterone system in diabetic nephropathy is associated with enhanced decline in glomerular filtration rate. *Diabetologia* 2004; 47: 1936–1939.

[163] Epstein M. Aldosterone blockade: an emerging strategy for abrogating progressive renal disease. *Am. J. Med.* 2006; 119: 912–919.

[164] Rossing K, Schjoedt KJ, Smidt UM, Boomsma F, Parving HH. Beneficial effects of adding spironolactone to recommended antihypertensive treatment in diabetic nephropathy: a randomized, double-masked, cross-over study. *Diabetes Care* 2005; 28: 2106–2112.

[165] Lindenfeld J, Albert NM, Boehmer JP, Collins SP, Ezekowitz JA, Givertz MM, Katz SD, Klapholz M, Moser DK, Rogers JG, Starling RC, Stevenson WG, Walsh MN. HFSA 2010 Comprehensive Heart Failure Practice Guideline. *J. Card. Fail.* 2010; 16: e1–e194.

[166] Schalekamp MA, Beevers DG, Briggs JD, Brown JJ, Davies DL, Fraser R, Lever AF, Medina A, Morton JJ, Robertson JI, Tree M: Hypertension in chronic renal failure. *Am. J. Med.* 1973; 55: 379–390.

[167] Hemmelgarn BR, Manns BJ, Lloyd A, James MT, Klarenbach S, Quinn RR, Wiebe N, Tonelli M. Alberta Kidney Disease Network; Relation between kidney function, proteinuria, and adverse outcomes. *JAMA* 2010; 303:423-429.

[168] Chronic Kidney Disease Prognosis Consortium, Matsushita K, van der Velde M, Astor BC, Woodward M, Levey AS, de Jong PE, Coresh J, Gansevoort RT. Association of estimated glomerular filtration rate and albuminuria with all-cause and cardiovascular mortality in general population cohorts: a collaborative meta-analysis. *Lancet* 2010; 375:2073-2081.

[169] American Diabetes Association. Standards of medical care in diabetes--2012. *Diabetes Care* 2012; 35: S11–S63.

[170] Kunz R, Friedrich C, Wolbers M, Mann, JF. Meta-analysis: effect of monotherapy and combination therapy with inhibitors of the renin angiotensin system on proteinuria in renal disease. *Ann. Intern. Med.* 2008; 148: 30–48.

[171] Jennings DL, Kalus JS, Coleman CI, Manierski C, Yee J. Combination therapy with an ACE inhibitor and an angiotensin receptor blocker for diabetic nephropathy: a metaanalysis. *Diabet Med.* 2007; 24:486–493.

[172] MacKinnon M, Shurraw S, Akbari A, Knoll GA, Jaffey J, Clark HD. Combination therapy with an angiotensin receptor blocker and an ACE inhibitor in proteinuric renal disease: a systematic review of the efficacy and safety data. *Am. J. Kidney Dis.* 2006; 48:8–20.

[173] Van den Meiracker AH, Jan Danser AH. Aliskiren: the first direct renin inhibitor for hypertension. *Curr. Cardiol. Rep.* 2007; 9:470–476.

[174] Pimenta E, Oparil S. Role of aliskiren in cardio-renal protection and use in hypertensives with multiple risk factors. *Vasc. Health Risk Manag.* 2009; 5:453–463.

[175] Brooks DP, Short BG, Cyronak MJ, Contino LC, DiCristo M, Wang YX, Ruffolo RR, Jr. Comparison between carvedilol and captopril in rats with partial ablation-induced chronic renal failure. *Br. J. Pharmacol.* 1993; 109: 581–586.

[176] Parving HH, Persson F, Lewis JB, Lewis EJ, Hollenberg NK. Aliskiren combined with losartan in type 2 diabetes and nephropathy. *N. Engl. J.Med 2008*; 358:2433–2446.

[177] Ptinopoulou AG, Pikilidou MI, Lasaridis AN. The effect of antihypertensive drugs on chronic kidney disease: a comprehensive review. *Hypertens. Res.* 2013; 36:91-101.

[178] Parving HH, Brenner BM, McMurray JJ, de ZD, Haffner SM, Solomon SD, Chaturvedi N, Ghadanfar M, Weissbach N, Xiang Z, Armbrecht J, Pfeffer MA. Aliskiren Trial in Type 2 Diabetes Using Cardio-Renal Endpoints (ALTITUDE): rationale and study design. *Nephrol. Dial. Transplant.* 2009; 24: 1663–1671.

[179] DiBona GF. The sympathetic nervous system and hypertension: recent developments. *Hypertension* 2004; 43:147–150.

[180] Alexander BT, Hendon AE, Ferril G, Dwyer TM. Renal denervation abolishes hypertension in low-birth-weight offspring from pregnant rats with reduced uterine perfusion. *Hypertension* 2005; 45:754 –758.

[181] Schlaich MP, Markus P., Paul A. Sobotka, Henry Krum, Robert Whitbourn, Anthony Walton, and Murray D. Esler. Renal Denervation as a Therapeutic Approach for

Hypertension Novel Implications for an Old Concept. *Hypertension* 2009; 54: 1195-1201.

[182] Neumann J, Ligtenberg G, Oey L, Koomans HA, Blankestijn PJ. Moxonidine normalizes sympathetic hyperactivity in patients with eprosartan-treated chronic renal failure. *J. Am. Soc. Nephrol.* 2004; 15: 2902–2907.

[183] Klein IH, Ligtenberg G, Oey PL, Koomans HA, Blankestijn PJ. Enalapril and losartan reduce sympathetic hyperactivity in patients with chronic renal failure. *J. Am. Soc. Nephrol.* 2003; 14:425–430.

[184] Siddiqi L, Oey PL, Blankestijn PJ. Aliskiren reduces sympathetic nerve activity and blood pressure in chronic kidney disease patients. *Nephrol. Dial. Transplant.* 2011; 26:2930–2934.

[185] Kobori H, Nangaku M, Navar LG, Nishiyama A. The intrarenal renin-angiotensin system: from physiology to the pathobiology of hypertension and kidney disease. *Pharmacol. Rev.* 2007; 59:251-287.

[186] Wolf G, Ziyadeh FN. Cellular and molecular mechanisms of proteinuria in diabetic nephropathy. *Nephron. Physiol.* 2007; 106:26–31.

[187] Dielis AW, Smid M, Spronk HM, Hamulyak K, Kroon AA, ten CH, de Leeuw PW. The prothrombotic paradox of hypertension: role of the renin-angiotensin and kallikreinkinin systems. *Hypertension* 2005; 46: 1236–1242.

[188] Toto R, Shultz P, Raij L, Mitchell H, Shaw W, Ramjit D, Toh J, Shahinfar S. Efficacy and tolerability of losartan in hypertensive patients with renal impairment. *Hypertension* 1998; 31: 684–691.

[189] Schulz E, Bech JN, Pedersen EB, Mûller GA. A randomized, double-blind, parallel study on the safety and antihypertensive efficacy of losartan compared to captopril in patients with mild to moderate hypertension and impaired renal function. *Nephrol. Dial. Transplant.* 1999; 14: 27–28.

[190] Sakata K, Yoshida H, Obayashi K, Ishikawa J, Tamekiyo H, Nawada R, Doi O. Effects of losartan and its combination with quinapril on the cardiac sympathetic nervous system and neurohormonal status in essential hypertension; *J. Hypertens.* 2002; 20:103-110.

[191] Kasama S, Toyama T, Kumakura H, Takayama Y, Ichikawa S, Suzuki T, Kurabayashi M. Effect of spironolactone on cardiac sympathetic nerve activity and left ventricular remodeling in patients with dilated cardiomyopathy. *J. Am. Coll. Cardiol.* 2003; 41:574-581.

[192] Esler M. Differentiation in the effects of angiotensin II receptor blocker class. *J. Hypertens.* 2002; 20:S13–S19.

[193] Amann K, Koch A, Hofstetter J, Gross ML, Haas C, Orth SR, Ehmke H, Rump LC, Ritz E. Glomerulosclerosis and progression: effect of subantihypertensive doses of alpha and beta blockers. *Kidney Int.* 2001; 60:1309–1323.

[194] Takamitsu Y, Nakanishi T, Nishihara F, Hasuike Y, Izumi M, Inoue T, Hiraoka K, Itahana R, Miyagawa K. A nitric oxide-generating beta-blocking agent prevents renal injury in the rat remnant kidney model. Comparative study of two beta-blocking drugs, nipradilol and propranolol. *Nephron. Physiol.* 2003; 93:42-50.

[195] Inada H, Ono H, Minami J, Ishimitsu T, Matsuoka H. Nipradilol prevents L-NAME-exacerbated nephrosclerosis with decreasing of caspase-3 expression in SHR. *Hypertens. Res.* 2002; 25:433–440.

[196] Wangensteen R, O' Valle F, Del Moral R, Vargas F, Osuna A. Chronic alpha1-adrenergic blockade improves hypertension and renal injury in L-NAME and low-renin L-NAME-DOCA hypertensive rats. *Med. Sci. Monit.* 2002; 8:BR378–BR384.

[197] Cleophas TC, Van Der Meulen, J. Beta-blockers: ancillary properties important after all? 2013. *Eastern. J.* Med 2013; 4:1-5.

[198] Kalinowski L, Dobrucki LW, Szczepanska-Konkel M, Jankowski M, Martyniec L, Angielski S, Malinski T. Third-generation beta-blockers stimulate nitric oxide release from endothelial cells through ATP efflux: a novel mechanism for antihypertensive action. *Circulation* 2003; 107: 2747–2752.

[199] Gomes A, Costa D, Lima JL, Fernandes E. Antioxidant activity of beta-blockers: an effect mediated by scavenging reactive oxygen and nitrogen species? *Bioorg. Med. Chem.* 2006; 14: 4568–4577.

[200] Mason RP, Kubant R, Jacob RF, Walter MF, Boychuk B, Malinski T. Effect of nebivolol on endothelial nitric oxide and peroxynitrite release in hypertensive animals: Role of antioxidant activity. *J. Cardiovasc. Pharmacol.* 2006; 48: 862–869.

[201] Bakris GL, Fonseca V, Katholi RE, McGill JB, Messerli F, Phillips RA, Raskin P, Wright Jr JT, Waterhouse B, Lukas MA, Anderson KM, Bell DS. Differential effects of betablockers on albuminuria in patients with type 2 diabetes. *Hypertension* 2005; 46: 1309–1315.

[202] Giner V, Tormos C, Chaves FJ, Saez G, Redon J. Microalbuminuria and oxidative stress in essential hypertension. *J. Intern. Med.* 2004; 255:588–594.

[203] Bakris GL, Fonseca V, Katholi RE, McGill JB, Messerli FH, Phillips RA, Raskin P, Wright Jr JT, Oakes R, Lukas MA, Anderson KM, Bell DS. Metabolic effects of carvedilol vs metoprolol in patients with type 2 diabetes mellitus and hypertension: a randomized controlled trial. *JAMA* 2004; 292: 2227–2236.

[204] Bakris GL. Role for beta-blockers in the management of diabetic kidney disease. *Am. J. Hypertens. 2003*; 16: 7S–12S.

[205] Bakris GL, Hart P, Ritz E. Beta blockers in the management of chronic kidney disease. *Kidney Int.* 2006; 70:1905-1913.

[206] Kumar KV, Shifow AA, Naidu MU, Ratnakar KS. Carvedilol: a beta blocker with antioxidant property protects against gentamicin-induced nephrotoxicity in rats. *Life Sci.* 2000; 66:2603–2611.

[207] Packer M, Fowler MB, Roecker EB, Coats AJ, Katus HA, Krum H, Mohacsi P, Rouleau JL, Tendera M, Staiger C, Holcslaw TL, Amann-Zalan I, DeMets DL. Effect of carvedilol on the morbidity of patients with severe chronic heart failure: results of the carvedilol prospective randomized cumulative survival (COPERNICUS) study. *Circulation* 2002; 106:2194 –2199.

[208] Shlipak MG, Heidenreich PA, Noguchi H, Chertow GM, Browner WS, McClellan MB. Association of renal insufficiency with treatment and outcomes after myocardial infarction in elderly patients. *Ann. Intern. Med.* 2002; 137:555–562.

[209] Reddi AS, Nimmagadda VR, Lefkowitz A, Kuo HR, Bollineni JS. Effect of antihypertensive therapy on renal injury in type 2 diabetic rats with hypertension. *Hypertension* 2000; 36:233–238.

[210] Wright Jr JT, Probstfield JL, Cushman WC, Pressel SL, Cutler JA, Davis BR, Einhorn PT, Rahman M, Whelton PK, Ford CE, Haywood LJ, Margolis KL, Oparil S, Black

HR, Alderman MH. ALLHAT findings revisited in the context of subsequent analyses, other trials, and meta-analyses. *Arch. Intern. Med.* 2009; 169: 832–842.

[211] Vonend O, Marsalek P, Russ H, Wulkow R, Oberhauser V, Rump LC. Moxonidine treatment of hypertensive patients with advanced renal failure. *J. Hypertens.* 2003; 21:1709–1717.

[212] Neumann J, Ligtenberg G, Oey L, Koomans HA, Blankestijn PJ. Moxonidine normalizes sympathetic hyperactivity in patients with eprosartan-treated chronic renal failure. *J. Am. Soc. Nephrol.* 2004; 15: 2902–2907.

[213] Zilch O, Vos PF, Oey LP, Cramer MM, Koomans HA, Blankestijn PJ. Daily dialysis reduces peripheral vascular resistance and sympathetic activity (abstract*). J. Am. Soc. Nephrol. 2001*; 12.

[214] Schroder M, Riedel E, Beck W, Deppisch RM, Pommer W. Increased reduction of dimethylarginines and lowered interdialytic blood pressure by the use of biocompatible membranes. *Kidney Int. Suppl.* 2001; 78:S19–S24.

[215] Efrati S, Zaidenstein R, Dishy V, Beberashvili I, Sharist M, Averbukh Z, Golik A, Weissgarten J; ACE inhibitors and survival of hemodialysis patients. *Am. J. Kidney Dis.* 2002; 40:1023–1029.

[216] Mann JF, Gerstein HC, Pogue J, Bosch J, Yusuf S. Renal insufficiency as a predictor of cardiovascular outcomes and the impact of ramipril: The HOPE randomized trial. *Ann. Intern. Med.* 2001; 134:629–636.

[217] Siddiqi L, Joles JA, Oey PL, Blankestijn PJ. Atorvastatin reduces sympathetic activity in patients with chronic kidney disease. *J. Hypertens*. 2011; 29:2176–80.

[218] Mahfoud F. [Renal denervation in hypertension - pro]; Dtsch Med Wochenschr 2012; 137:720.

[219] Krum H, Schlaich M, Whitbourn R, Sobotka PA, Sadowski J, Bartus K, Kapelak B, Walton A, Sievert H, Thambar S, Abraham WT, Esler M. Catheter-based renal sympathetic denervation for resistant hypertension: a multicentre safety and proof-of-principle cohort study. *Lancet* 2009; 373:1275–1281.

[220] Esler MD, Krum H, Sobotka PA, Schlaich MP, Schmieder RE, Böhm M. Renal sympathetic denervation in patients with treatment-resistant hypertension (The Symplicity HTN-2 Trial): a randomised controlled trial. *Lancet* 2010; 376:1903–1909.

[221] Veelken R, Vogel EM, Hilgers K, Amann K, Hartner A, Sass G, Neuhuber W, Tiegs G. Autonomic renal denervation ameliorates experimental glomerulonephritis. *JAmSoc. Nephrol.* 2008; 19:1371–1378.

[222] Tian N, Thrasher KD, Gundy PD, Hughson MD, Manning RD Jr. Antioxidant treatment prevents renal damage and dysfunction and reduces arterial pressure in salt-sensitive hypertension. *Hypertension* 2005; 45:934-939.

[223] Elhaïmeur F, Courderot-Masuyer C, Nicod L, Guyon C, Richert L, Berthelot A. Dietary vitamin C supplementation decreases blood pressure in DOCA-salt hypertensive male Sprague-Dawley rats and this is associated with increased liver oxidative stress. *Mol. Cell Biochem.* 2002; 237:77-83.

[224] Rodrigo R, Prat H, Passalacqua W, Araya J, Bächler JP; Decrease in oxidative stress through supplementation of vitamins C and E is associated with a reduction in blood pressure in patients with essential hypertension; *Clin. Sci.* (Lond) 2008; 114:625-634.

[225] Vaziri ND. Roles of oxidative stress and antioxidant therapy in chronic kidney disease and hypertension. *Curr. Opin. Nephrol. Hypertens.* 2004; 13:93-99.

[226] Weber MA, Black H, Bakris G, Krum H, Linas S, Weiss R, Linseman JV, Wiens BL, Warren MS, Lindholm LH. A selective endothelin-receptor antagonist to reduce blood pressure in patients with treatment-resistant hypertension: a randomised, doubleblind, placebo-controlled trial. *Lancet* 2009; 374: 1423–1431.

[227] Wenzel RR, Littke T, Kuranoff S, Jurgens C, Bruck H, Ritz E, Philipp T, Mitchell A. Avosentan reduces albumin excretion in diabetics with macroalbuminuria. *J. Am. Soc. Nephrol.* 2009; 20: 655–664.

Index

B

C

D

E

F

G

H

I

N

O

P

T

U

V